Every Decker book is accompanied by a CD-ROM.

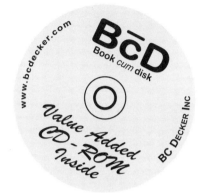

The CD ROM for *Tooth-Colored Restoratives: Principles and Techniques, 9/e* appears in the front of each copy, in its own sealed jacket. Affixed to the front of the book will be a distinctive BcD sticker **"Book *cum* disk."**

The CD ROM contains the complete text and illustrations of *Tooth-Colored Restoratives: Principles and Techniques, 9/e*, in fully searchable PDF files. The book and disk are sold *only* as a package; neither is available independently, and no prices are available for the items individually.

BC Decker Inc is committed to providing high-quality electronic publications that complement traditional information and learning methods. We trust you will find the book/CD package invaluable and invite your comments and suggestions.

Brian C. Decker
CEO and Publisher

TOOTH-COLORED RESTORATIVES

PRINCIPLES AND TECHNIQUES

Ninth Edition

Harry F. Albers, DDS

2002
BC Decker Inc
Hamilton • London

BC Decker Inc
20 Hughson Street South
P.O. Box 620, L.C.D. 1
Hamilton, Ontario L8N 3K7
Tel: 905-522-7017; 1-800-568-7281
Fax: 905-522-7839; 1-888-311-4987
e-mail: info@bcdecker.com
website: www.bcdecker.com

© 2002 Harry F. Albers, DDS

All rights reserved. No part of this publication may be reproduced, stored in a retrieval system, or transmitted, in any form or by any means, electronic, mechanical, photocopying, recording, or otherwise, without prior written permission from the publisher.

02 03 04 /UTP/ 9 8 7 6 5 4 3 2 1

ISBN 1-55009-155-7

Printed in Canada

Sales and Distribution

United States
BC Decker Inc
P.O. Box 785
Lewiston, NY 14092-0785
Tel: 905-522-7017; 1-800-568-7281
Fax: 905-522-7839; 1-888-311-4987
e-mail: info@bcdecker.com
website: www.bcdecker.com

Canada
BC Decker Inc
20 Hughson Street South
P.O. Box 620, L.C.D. 1
Hamilton, Ontario L8N 3K7
Tel: 905-522-7017; 1-800-568-7281
Fax: 905-522-7839; 1-888-311-4987
e-mail: info@bcdecker.com
website: www.bcdecker.com

Japan
Igaku-Shoin Ltd.
Foreign Publications Department
3-24-17 Hongo, Bunkyo-ku
Tokyo 113-8719, Japan
Tel: 81 3 3817 5680
Fax: 81 3 3815 6776
e-mail: fd@igaku-shoin.co.jp

U.K., Europe, Scandinavia, Middle East
Elsevier Science
Customer Service Department
Foots Cray High Street
Sidcup, Kent   DA14 5HP, UK
Tel: 44 (0) 208 308 5760
Fax: 44 (0) 181 308 5702
e-mail: cservice@harcourt_brace.com

Singapore, Malaysia, Thailand, Philippines, Indonesia, Vietnam, Pacific Rim, Korea
Elsevier Science Asia
583 Orchard Road
#09/01, Forum
Singapore 238884
Tel: 65-737-3593
Fax: 65-753-2145

Australia, New Zealand
Elsevier Science Australia
Customer Service Department
STM Division
Locked Bag 16
St. Peters, New South Wales, 2044
Australia
Tel: 61 02 9517-8999
Fax: 61 02 9517-2249
e-mail: stmp@harcourt.com.au
website: www.harcourt.com.au

Foreign Rights
John Scott & Company
International Publishers' Agency
P.O. Box 878
Kimberton, PA 19442
Tel: 610-827-1640
Fax: 610-827-1671
e-mail: jsco@voicenet.com

Notice: The authors and publisher have made every effort to ensure that the patient care recommended herein, including choice of drugs and drug dosages, is in accord with the accepted standard and practice at the time of publication. However, since research and regulation constantly change clinical standards, the reader is urged to check the product information sheet included in the package of each drug, which includes recommended doses, warnings, and contraindications. This is particularly important with new or infrequently used drugs.

Contents

Preface v
Introduction vii

1. Materials Science 1
2. Diagnosis 19
3. Glass Ionomers 43
4. Resin Ionomers 57
5. Uses of Ionomers 69
6. Resin Polymerization 81
7. Resins 111
8. Resin Bonding 127
9. Placement and Finishing 157
10. Anterior Restorations 183
11. Direct Posterior Composites 203
12. Esthetics 237

Appendix A: Nomenclature For Curing Composite Resins 271
Appendix B: Universal Restorative Tray 275
Appendix C: Magnification 283
Appendix D: Air Abrasion 289
Index 293

Preface

I began teaching continuing education courses in restorative dentistry in 1978, at the genesis of resin bonding. My students' questions motivated me to produce handouts on materials science and the usage of composites. The handouts quickly grew in length and number, and became a book. The first edition of *Tooth-Colored Restoratives* (whose title was inspired by Dr. Ralph Phillips' then annual lecture, at the University of California, San Francisco) was published in 1980 for sale at the University of the Pacific bookstore. Eight editions later, *Tooth-Colored Restoratives* is available around the world and in numerous languages. I am still teaching in San Francisco and producing handouts, in preparation for two additional texts: *Indirect Bonded Restorations* and *Concepts in Cosmetic Dentistry*.

Over the past 20 years, I have observed that dentists are accustomed to working with materials they do not understand. The most common question I am asked in class or at a cocktail party is "What branded product should I use?" for a given restoration. Rarely am I asked how to use a product or about the nature of its makeup. I believe this question exemplifies dentists' tendency to become enamored of a material and assume that a good material secures a good result, rather than recognize that its full value depends on the clinician's skill and knowledge. How a material is used is always considerably more important than which material is used. The belief that a product can itself provide an answer leads many dentists astray. The practitioner with this perspective is likely to switch product brands—perhaps a number of times—without improving the quality of his or her dental care, and without questioning his or her method. Yet it is choice of material and command of technique, not brand, that determines restoration outcome.

What disappoints me most about dental education today is that a dentist must go to extra lengths to gain knowledge of materials. The common practice of rote technique in the absence of understanding produces inconsistent treatment outcomes and failures that otherwise could be avoided. No dentist would expect an orange to behave like an apple, even if marketed as a "Washington Orange Delicious." But a continual influx of new materials, and marketing schemes that interweave science and speculation, has confused dentists into thinking products can cross the bounds of nature. Plastic is plastic and porcelain is porcelain; the dentist who believes one can be made to behave like the other does not adhere to reality. Unfortunately, commercial interests are influencing larger and larger portions of dental education, which promotes allegiance to brands as opposed to recognition of generic classes of materials or the importance of technique. Product packaging often does not indicate whether a product is glass ionomer, resin, or some other class of material, forcing dentists into guesswork. Such obfuscation leads unwary dentists to believe there is, for example, only Bayer® aspirin, when instead, aspirin is a generic class having many equivalent products.

I have avoided using brand names in the clinical sections of this book because products in the same generic class behave similarly. In the materials sections, I have grouped into classes (eg, resins, glass ionomers, etc) many commonly used products to help readers understand which materials are alike, which are different, and how they differ. (Given the rapid rate of product introductions, I also provide up-to-date materials information by product name at the Adept Institute Web site: www.AdeptInstitute.com.)

This text has been under development for over 20 years. My goal is to help clinicians understand the basics of how composite materials work and to show how to apply that knowledge in materials selection and use. The chapters on materials science, diagnosis, and the different classes of materials are supported by published literature. The chapters on application are supported by two decades of personal clinical experience and roughly 700 dentists' involvement in study group evaluations of techniques and results. These data provide sound clinical guidance for excellence in direct restorations.

For encouragement, I am most grateful to all my teachers, especially the late Ralph Phillips, who provided enormous support in my early teaching years. His impact on my development is immeasurable. I hope to return to the profession a portion of what he and other teachers gave me.

I also appreciate the continued support of the hundreds of graduates from my 2-year clinical study group programs. Without the wealth of information provided by these talented professionals this text could not deliver as many insights. I am especially grateful to the dentists who have volunteered as assistant teachers in my study groups. Among them are Dr. Scott Baxter, Dr. Jerry Becker, Dr. Jennifer Buchanan, Dr. Rad Eastman, Dr. Brian Faber, Dr. Darryl Farley, Dr. Tom Fasanaro, Dr. Alfred Funston, Dr. Dewin Harris, Dr. David Layer, Dr. George McCully, Dr. Lee Mlejnek, Dr. Mike Perona, Dr. Steve Pitzer, Dr. Leslie Plack, Dr. Mary Lou Ramsey, Dr. Creed Roman, Dr. Tom Sharp, Dr. Bill Thompson, and Dr. Vaughn Tidwell.

For technical assistance, particularly in the tedious job of editing, I thank Dr. Jerry Aso, who has assisted me for over a decade and reviewed previous editions of this text countless times. His attention pervades every aspect of my work. His encouragement over the years has been an inspiration, especially through the difficult times.

Without the inexhaustible efforts of my significant other, Dorothy Foster, this edition would not have reached your hands. Her training as a professional science writer and editor, and her wisdom as a practicing psychotherapist, have made this work my best to date. Dorothy has the perseverance of purpose and unending optimism to bring out the best in my ability. I am so very lucky to have her in my life and feel confident that with her help my work will continue to flourish.

I am just as excited to talk about tooth-colored restoratives today as I was in 1978. Since that time, composites have leapt into the foreground to become the primary restorative material in the profession, which I expect they will remain for many years to come. Few dental techniques are as versatile and immediate as direct placement of tooth-colored resins. As the gap between the clinical performance of direct and indirect treatments narrows, composite use will expand to all but the most complicated restorative cases. Direct-placement tooth-colored restoratives are the most conservative, most esthetic, most easily placed, and most cost-effective materials available to dentists today. The public has embraced them with open arms, and their future is bright.

Harry F. Albers
December 2001

Introduction

The dental profession is a young one in the field of health care. So young that in many cases the inventors of today's materials and technologies are still alive to witness the profession accept their innovations. Although dental products change at a rapid rate, the basic science governing how dental materials work remains constant. Many of what may seem significant advances in products and techniques are merely modifications that build on the fundamentals.

Dentistry has not always quickly embraced new ideas. A short list of anniversaries can help put in perspective the limited experience we have with tooth-colored restoratives.

- One hundred and twenty-eight years ago, in 1873, Thomas Fletcher introduced the first tooth-colored filling material, silicate cement. Silicate did not become popular until Steenbock introduced an improved version in 1904, but even the improved silicates discolored easily and lasted only a few years.

- Sixty-one years ago, in the early 1940s, German chemists developed the first acrylic resins. The first dental acrylic resin product was introduced in 1948. These acrylics demonstrated better color stability but significant shrinkage, limited stiffness, and poor adhesion.

- Fifty years ago, in 1951, Swiss chemist Oscar Hagger developed the first dimethacrylate molecule, which allowed for a cross-polymerized matrix. The first dental product to use the more durable and color-stable dimethacrylate was produced in 1964, but it was not accepted by clinicians.

- Forty-six years ago, in 1955, Michael Buonocore published a milestone article that described a simple method of increasing the adhesion of acrylic fillings to enamel. His ideas resulted in the development of dental adhesives with the ability to bond to tooth structure. The first tooth-colored restorative using bonding was not introduced until two decades later.

- Thirty-nine years ago, in 1962, Ray Bowen and others developed a large-molecule, hydrophobic dimethacrylate monomer (Bis-GMA), a key advance in resin chemistry. Bis-GMA forms the basis of present-day composite resins because of its limited shrinkage and fracture resistance. It was first used in a composite in 1969.

- Thirty-eight years ago, in 1963, Dennis Smith developed the polyelectrolyte cement that led to the polycarboxylate adhesive cements, the key component for developing glass-ionomer cement.

- Twenty-seven years ago, in 1974, Wilson and Kent, with the assistance of John McLean, developed the first glass-ionomer cement.

- Twenty-one years ago, in 1980, the first edition of *Tooth-Colored Restoratives* was published, the result of my teaching a newly established course at the University of the Pacific, "Composite Fillings."

Most dentists currently entering the profession do not realize how much has changed in so little time. In addition to the advances in materials, several trends, as described below, have contributed to public interest in tooth-colored restoratives. Other trends could be said to conspire against innovations in patient care.

AMALGAM AND MERCURY

For 200 years, amalgam was the mainstay of dentistry. It now has a dim future because of patient concern about mercury toxicity. Research has shown a correlation between blood mercury levels and amalgam restorations. Controversy surrounds the question of whether or not mercury in the blood presents a health hazard. For healthy adult patients, there is little evidence that amalgam is not a safe and effective restorative material. Whereas many published testimonials claim the removal of amalgam cures assorted ailments, few of these claims have been substantiated with sound scientific research.

Amalgam is a forgiving material for both dentist and patient. It has saved more teeth than any other restorative material in the profession—and not just because it is older, but because of its ease of use and toxicity to caries. Tooth-colored restoratives are a safe albeit less forgiving and more technically complicated alternative.

DEMAND FOR ESTHETICS

The dental profession has spent most of its history restoring the effects of dental disease, but currently, the majority of restoration work is replacement or repair of prior treatment. One reason for the change is enormous strides over the past several decades in dental disease prevention. Specifically, fluoridation programs and the increased availability of dental care have reduced the need for traditional caries-related restorative dentistry. At the same time, the average life span has increased in developed countries, which means more restorations live long enough to require repair.

Another factor is the population's burgeoning interest in health and beauty, which is driving increased demand for cosmetic dental procedures. Historically, for many adults, the achievement of a pretty smile has meant submission to extensive invasive procedures and high-cost fixed prosthodontics. Improvements in tooth-colored restoratives and bonding technology have made cosmetic dental procedures more palatable and feasible. In addition, newer technology allows the general practitioner to handle many previously complex esthetic problems more simply, conservatively, and economically.

These factors together mean the average general practitioner is performing elective procedures more frequently. This results in a fundamental shift from a patient pool that visited the dentist as a health-warranted necessity to a patient pool that now often presents for elective cosmetic treatment. In recognition of this trend, there are now more professional organizations devoted to esthetic dentistry than to any other dental specialty; and specialties such as periodontics and surgery, which used to deal only with pathology, are now devoting significant portions of their treatments to esthetics.

DENTAL INSURANCE

Dental insurance was introduced in the early 1960s in southern California. The first plan, Delta Dental, was run by dentists and gave patients an annual $1000 maximum limit for care, which provided adequate funds to treat most situations. Currently, most dental plans, including the original, are run by business firms with a financial motivation. Their annual limits are unrealistically low. For example, Delta Dental still has an annual $1000 maximum on most of its plans. Indeed, the benefits of most dental plans do not cover the cost of one of the most common events in dentistry: a single abscessed molar. To treat this situation within the standard of care requires endodontic therapy, a post and core, and a cast restoration.

Thus, dental insurance plans and their representatives seem to encourage dentists to treat patients down to a price rather than up to a standard. Third-party payers have an obvious conflict of interest in providing coverage for more advanced techniques and technologies, since they are more costly to perform. This shortsighted thinking often has negative results for both dentist and patient. For example, many plans deny coverage of such preventive procedures as sealants and yet cover the cost of amalgam restorations.

Many third parties try to convince patients that treatment based on a lower cost is in their best interest. They recruit and promote "preferred dentists" who accept the insurance-dictated terms of coverage. Unfortunately, most patients are blind to this process that so compromises their treatment. It is vital to educate patients to the realities of good dental care and have them deal directly with their dental plan representatives. This forces the third parties to rationalize their behavior directly to health-plan buyers. A more informed American public can force third parties to make the needed changes to their policies.

This book explains and teaches dental procedures of potentially great value to patients. It is up to the dentist to ensure that the benefits of these sophisticated procedures are fully realized by his or her patients. One good book is not enough. Acquisition of the knowledge and skills to perform these more technically demanding procedures takes a dedicated effort. This text provides a starting point for learning the best practices in tooth-colored restoration, but hands-on learning is essential to attain mastery of the techniques and technologies involved. Keeping step with evolving improvements to ensure patients continue to receive the most conservative, most esthetic, and longest-lasting treatment available requires ongoing academic and hands-on training. This ninth edition assembles current knowledge of tooth-colored restoratives in a comprehensive set of building blocks.

*Dedicated to those who practice
the art and science of dentistry
and aspire to become the best they can be.*

A special thanks to those who inspired me and helped me grow: Hans and Leni Albers, Saundra Albers, Arthur Krol, Mike O'Brien, Jerry Aso, Arthur Hoffman, Dorothy Foster, and most of all, my students, who have taught me more than I have taught them.

*Read not to contradict
nor to take for granted,
but to weigh and consider.*

Francis Bacon
1561–1626

Chapter 1

Materials Science

Our dignity is not what we do, but what we understand.

George Santayana

The ideal tooth-colored restorative (ie, direct restorative) would have the capacity to

- adhere to enamel and dentin,
- maintain a smooth surface,
- maintain desired color,
- resist water (insolubility),
- resist wear,
- resist fracture,
- resemble tooth structure in stiffness,
- react to temperature change like other tooth structures,
- resist leakage,
- maintain marginal integrity,
- not irritate pulpal tissues,
- inhibit caries,
- place easily, and
- repair easily.

No available restorative can meet all of these requirements; however, by matching the characteristics of various materials to the needs of a specific tooth, it is possible to approach this ideal for each restoration undertaken.

Clinicians who understand the chemical nature and physical properties of a material are more likely than those who do not to make good decisions concerning its use and application. This book begins with a review of basic concepts in material and restorative science to provide a foundation for improved understanding of dental materials.

CHEMISTRY OF TOOTH-COLORED RESTORATIVES

A direct restorative transforms in the mouth from a fluid or putty-like material into a tooth-like solid. There are three common mechanisms by which direct tooth-colored restoratives undergo transformation: acid–base reactions, polymerization reactions, and precipitation reactions.[1–3]

Acid–base reactions

Many dental materials undergo an acid–base reaction when they set. The resulting material is chemically referred to as a salt. Examples of this reaction in everyday life are commonplace (eg, concrete). The first tooth-colored restoratives to undergo this type of setting were the silicate cements. All acid–base reactions are similar. Acid molecules (a configuration of atoms) have a shortage of electrons, and base molecules have an excess of electrons. When acids and bases react, they transfer electrons between them, creating a more stable compound. This exchange of electrons results in heat generation during the setting reaction. Since the ions required to initiate a setting reaction exist only in water, all acid–base materials contain water. Once an acid–base reaction is complete, however, the resulting salt typically does not include water.

There are two types of acid–base reactions: those involving inorganic components and those involving organic components. Examples of an inorganic acid–base reaction are zinc phosphate cement and silicate cement. Examples of an organic acid–base reaction are glass-ionomer cement and polycarboxylate cement. Acid–base reactions that contain inorganic components are generally stable outside the mouth in the absence of moisture, whereas those containing organic components are generally not stable. For example, zinc phosphate cement is stable in a dry environment whereas glass-ionomer cement is not.

Polymerization reactions

The most common type of setting reaction for direct tooth-colored restoratives involves the formation of

2 Tooth-Colored Restoratives

resin polymers. A polymer is a molecule or group of molecules made up of repeating single units that are covalently bonded. The individual units of a polymer are referred to as monomers. "Poly" means many, and "mono" means one. Hence, polymethyl methacrylate is a polymer made up of multiple methacrylate monomers. Polymers form from one or more types of monomer. The process of converting monomers into a polymer is called polymerization. If two or more different monomers are polymerized, the resulting material is a copolymer (Figure 1–1). Combining different monomers creates materials with unique properties that reflect the characteristics of the individual monomers.

All monomers have at least one carbon–carbon double bond (C=C) that becomes a single carbon–carbon bond when they join to form a polymer. Monomers with two or more carbon–carbon double bonds can transform to cross-linked polymers (Figure 1–2, A). Cross-linking usually results in improved physical properties in dental materials. Most dental restorative polymers contain cross-linked copolymer components for durability (Figure 1–2, B).

An initiation system starts the transformation of monomers into polymers and copolymers. The initiation reaction creates a molecule with a free radical (an unpaired electron). This unpaired electron makes the radical highly reactive. When a free radical collides with a monomer's double bond, it pairs with one of the electrons of the double bond, leaving the other member of the pair free. Thus, the monomer itself becomes a free radical that can react with another monomer. Ideally, this process continues until all of the monomers become polymerized. The degree to which monomers convert into a polymer is referred to as the degree of conversion. The most common polymers used in the dental field contain methacrylates. Methacrylates with two double bonds are called dimethacrylates. The advantage of a dimethacrylate is that it allows for cross-linking, as illustrated in Figure 1–2. Most resins used in dentistry have a conversion of about 40 to 60% when polymerized in the mouth and over 60% to nearly 100% when cured in a laboratory.

Polymerization shrinkage patterns
All polymerizing resins shrink during curing. Composite resin shrinkage is about 2 to 5% by volume, depending on the filler loading (filler particles do not shrink) and the percentage of conversion. The less the filler loading and the higher the rate of conversion, the greater the shrinkage. In the laboratory, or when cured outside the mouth, chemically cured materials shrink toward their center, because the initiators are mixed throughout the material (Figure 1–3). Light-cured materials, on the other hand, shrink toward the source of initiation, which is the curing light (Figure 1–4).

In clinical use, shrinkage patterns are much more complex. Active bonding agents placed on a tooth usually start the initiation process when the composite contacts them. Some researchers also believe a tooth's inherent heat causes curing to occur along the tooth interface sooner than it does along cooler portions of composite away from tooth structure. Thus, composites generally start to shrink toward cured bonding agents, since the polymerization process has already started there. When a composite is placed against a light-cured bonding agent and then light-cured, the composite is initiated from two sides. However, the rate of polymerization is not equal on the two sides in that the composite facing the light polymerizes more quickly and has larger effect on the direction of composite shrinkage (see Figure 1–4).

Precipitation reactions
Precipitation reactions involve the loss of a solvent. In this case, the liquid materials commonly contain resins diluted in an organic solvent. When exposed

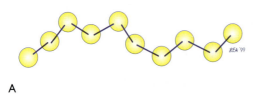

A

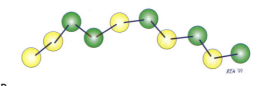

B

Figure 1–1. *A,* A linear polymer is made up of multiple units of one type of monomer. *B,* A copolymer includes more than one type of monomer.

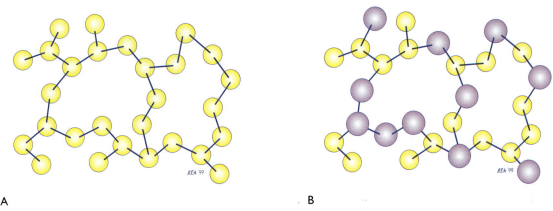

Figure 1–2. *A*, Cross-linking of polymer. Monomers with two carbon–carbon double bonds make cross-linking possible. *B*, Polymers with cross-linked components have better durability.

to air, the solvent evaporates and concentrates the resin into a solid. Examples of these reactions are wall paint, fingernail polish, dental varnish, etc. The setting reaction is referred to as drying. Presently, few dental restoratives set through a precipitation reaction. Precipitation is used, however, in setting bonding agents, cavity varnishes, and some surface coatings. With bonding agents, the solvent enhances the agent's penetration of the tooth. Evaporation of the solvent concentrates the monomer prior to polymerization and improves durability.

Most materials that set by drying contain a large molecule (resin) that is suspended in a volatile solvent (thinner). During drying, the loss of the solvent brings the component of greater molecular weight out of the solution and turns it into a solid (Figure 1–5). Precipitation materials used in the mouth must be insoluble in water (at least the resulting resin) to avoid reversal of this process in the oral fluids. Precipitation reactions result in the least durable restoratives and are recommended only for temporary treatment of tooth structure.

PHYSICAL PROPERTIES AND DESTRUCTIVE FORCES

Knowledge of the physical properties of restorative materials can help predict their susceptibility to breakage under occlusal function.

Compressive strength

Compressive strength is a measure of the amount of force a material can support in a single impact before breaking (Figure 1–6). This physical property is one of the easiest to measure and is often cited in advertisements for dental materials. Compressive strength is such a commonly used physical property that it has acquired a greater respectability in the profession than is appropriate

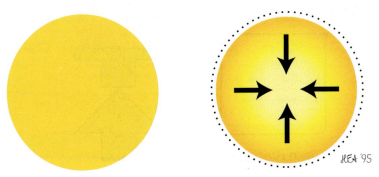

Figure 1–3. Autocured resin, polymerization shrinkage pattern. The left sphere represents the volume of an autocured material prior to polymerization. The right sphere represents the volume and shrinkage pattern of the material after polymerization.

4 Tooth-Colored Restoratives

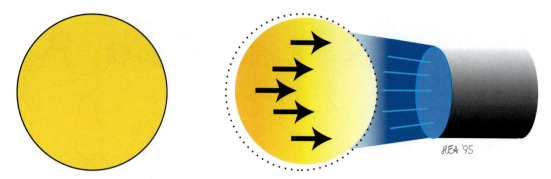

Figure 1–4. The left sphere represents the volume of light-cured composite prior to polymerization. The right sphere represents the volume and shrinkage pattern of the material after polymerization when not attached to any surface. Note how the material moves toward the light of the curing tip at the right.

to its actual clinical relevance. There is no direct correlation between compressive strength and clinical performance. However, compressive strength does measure strength, and it gives an indication of a material's resistance to creep and plasticity. In conjunction with a sound understanding of the clinical purpose of a dental material, measurement of compressive strength is sometimes used as a screening test in the development of new materials.

Tensile strength

Tensile strength is the amount of force that can be used to stretch a material in a single impact prior to breaking (Figure 1–7). This physical property is more difficult to measure than compressive strength. The tolerance of the measuring device is critical. Materials must be pulled at an exact 180-degree angle from each other to eliminate the influence of shear forces. The clinical relevance of tensile strength is limited.

Diametrical tensile strength

This is a theoretical tensile strength measurement that is calculated by measuring the compressive strength of a disc of material (Figure 1–8). This test is easier to perform and is more consistent than the normal tensile strength test.

Shear strength

Shear strength is the maximum shear stress that a material can absorb in one impact before failure

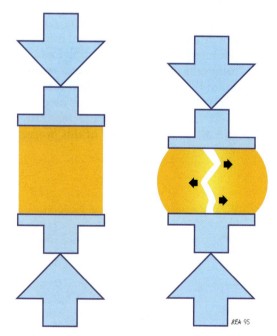

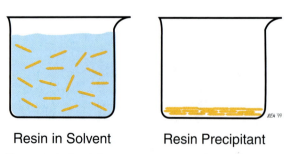

Figure 1–5. Precipitation reaction. A volume of solvent evaporates and leaves a solid behind.

Figure 1–6. Compressive strength. The amount of force a material can support in a single impact.

Materials Science 5

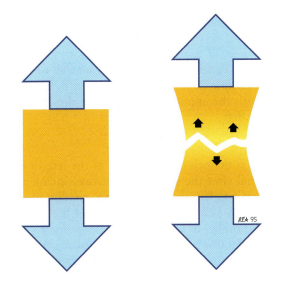

Figure 1–7. Tensile strength. The amount of stretching force a material can withstand.

(Figure 1–9). The punch test is a common method of measuring shear strength. In this test, shear strength is calculated from the compressive force applied, the diameter of the punch, and the thickness of the material tested. Shear strength has been used to measure the bond strength between different materials. In this test, a disc of material is bonded to a surface, a chisel instrument is placed above the disc, or a loop of wire is attached. The force required to shear the disc from the bonded surface is the bond strength of the tested adhesive (Figure 1–10). This test is easier to perform than a tensile test on two bonded materials.

Unfortunately, the punch test has no direct correlation to the clinical performance of a material. Further, there is little agreement in the research community on how to conduct this test, although standards are being developed. Shear strength data from different testing laboratories show extremely large variations are possible even when testing the same materials with the same instruments.

Stiffness

Stiffness is also called the modulus of elasticity, elastic modulus, or Young's modulus. Stiffness determines resistance to flexure and deformation, or the amount of bending when loaded (Figure 1–11). The measure of stiffness has been related to predicting the potential results of cyclic loading outside the oral environment. Stiffness can be measured by placing a force on a material and measuring the deformation. It can be calculated in a nondestructive way by measuring the harmonics of a material when vibrated.

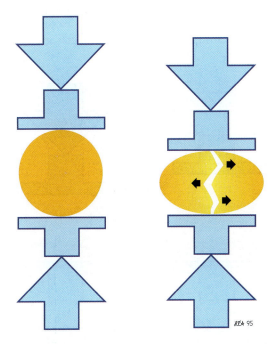

Figure 1–8. The diametrical tensile strength test is used to calculate tensile strength.

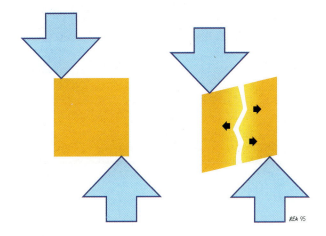

Figure 1–9. Shear strength. The maximum shear stress a material can absorb in one impact.

6 Tooth-Colored Restoratives

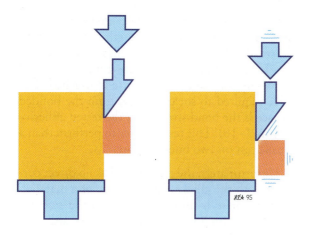

Figure 1–10. Bond strength. The force required to shear a disc of material from the surface to which it is bonded.

Stress and strain are related in that the elastic modulus is the ratio of stress over strain. Elastic modulus is expressed in the same units as stress. Most dental composites have an elastic modulus between 5 and 15 GPa (gigapascals). The elastic modulus indicates the amount of stress that needs to be applied to achieve a certain strain, or, if the strain is known, what level of stress is in effect.

Stress

Stress is defined as force per unit area, expressed in newtons per square millimeter (N/mm²) or pounds per square inch (psi). The unit N/mm² is properly known as the pascal and abbreviated Pa. The pascal is a small unit; for dental applications, stress forces are usually expressed as megapascals or MPa. For example, adhesive bonds to dentin typically fail with the application of stress in the 20 to 30 MPa range.

Strain

Strain is defined as the change in the length of a material after the application of stress divided by its original length—a unit with no dimensions (Figure 1–12). A material capable of high strain, such as rubber or latex, can tolerate strain values of 0.5 to 50.0% before failure. For most solid materials, strain is expressed as microstrain in parts per million (ppm) or 10^{-6} strain.

Fatigue

Fatigue occurs in all rigid materials undergoing continual stress and strain. Fatigue occurs in a tooth when a functional cusp can no longer support occlusal forces. It is also a common cause of conventional restoration failure. Over time, fatigue results in cohesive microcracks and external chipping in a restoration. It occurs in direct placement composites under heavy function. The intraoral degradation of restorative materials is a complex process that has not been mimicked to any great extent by simple laboratory tests. Each group of

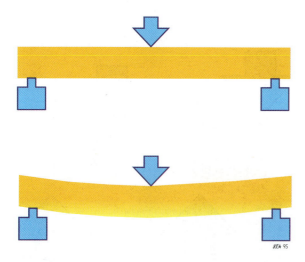

Figure 1–11. Stiffness. The resistance of a material to flexure and deformation when loaded.

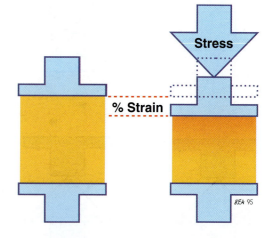

Figure 1–12. Stress and strain. Strain is measured as the percentage of change in length when a stress is applied in a single application.

Materials Science 7

materials—metals, polymers, and cements—seems to fail by mechanisms specific to that group, making generalization difficult. The phenomenon is called fatigue because, under certain loading conditions, a component appears to tire, losing strength over a period of time in service. Two types of loading conditions can cause these symptoms: (1) cyclic loading and (2) steady loading. Both are more severe in the presence of a chemically active agent. The progressive loss of strength that accompanies cyclic loading is attributable to the gradual spread of cracks. Cyclic loading is illustrated in Figure 1–13.

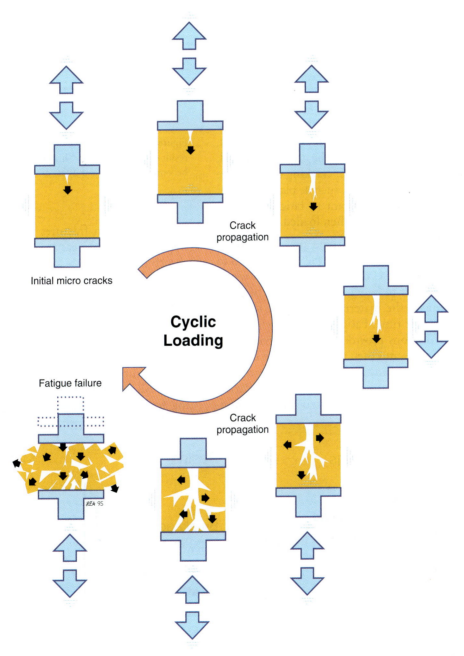

Figure 1–13. The progressive and cumulative damage that occurs during cyclic loading. The restoration eventually fails.

8 Tooth-Colored Restoratives

The mouth is unique in that it combines cyclic loading with a chemically active environment. The most common chemically active agent in dentistry is saliva, which contains varying amounts of water and other components. Saliva varies from patient to patient, and individual differences can explain some of the atypical results seen in some mouths. A patient's diet may also contain substances that are chemically reactive to teeth and restorations.

Cyclic loading might appear less harmful to restorative materials than steady loading, because the average deflection (over the cyclic period) is less than the steady deflection. In practice, it is the cyclically loaded materials that break first from occlusal forces; statically loaded materials, such as those maintaining, for example, resting contact points, last considerably longer. Since the growth of a crack requires plastic deformation, cracking occurs more rapidly in ductile materials, such as plastics. Stiffer restoratives are more resistant to fatigue, because they are under less strain when loaded.

The clinical effects of fatigue are important in all dental restoratives, because the force needed to cause failure decreases over time. The rate of weakening is thought to be related to the rate of crack propagation in the material in response to stress absorption over time. Fatigue explains why many dental restorations provide excellent service for a number of years and then suddenly break under a relatively minor load. Figure 1–14 illustrates the relation between stress and time in restoration breakage, demonstrating the fatigue phenomenon.

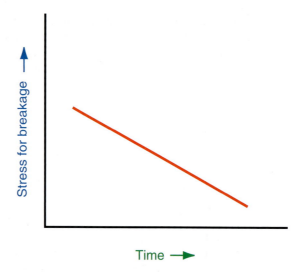

Figure 1–14. The weakening of a material over time as a result of cyclic loading. Clinically, this means that materials become more brittle and less durable over time.

Most restoration fractures occur in the marginal ridge areas. These areas are the least supported and absorb the most static and cyclic stress and strain; thus, they are the most inclined to fracture.

Fracture toughness

Fracture toughness is an important measure of a material's susceptibility to fatigue. Stress is the amount of force placed on an object, and strain is the amount of deformation that occurs under that stress. All materials undergo strain (such as a bending force) when stressed. Figure 1–15 illustrates

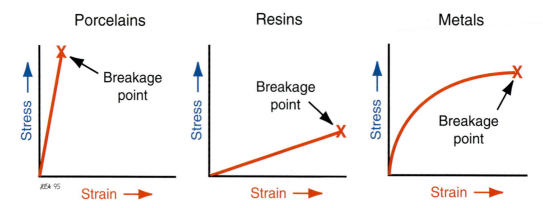

Figure 1–15. The stress–strain curves of a material show the amount of flexure it produces under a given stress. At a critical stress, the material fractures, because its maximum amount of deformation (elastic limit) has been exceeded.

how different materials react to stress up to their breaking point. As shown, porcelain bends little, even when placed under considerable stress. Resins (plastics) are different in that they bend a lot even under low stress. Metals can tolerate considerable stress and bending.

Fracture toughness is defined as the area under the curve when viewing a plot of the stress and strain relation of a restorative material. It is a measure of the total amount of stress a material can take before failing (Figure 1–16). It is related to the energy needed for flexure to a breaking point, which is called flexural strength. Flexural strength, bending strength, and fracture resistance are terms used interchangeably. Owing to its ease of measurement, flexural strength is the physical property most commonly used to indicate the fracture toughness of a material. However, many researchers believe that fracture toughness is the best physical property to measure to predict the wear and fracture resistance of a restorative.

The graphs in Figure 1–16 indicate the differences in fracture toughness among porcelains, resins, and metals. The clinical performance of metal restorations bears out their fracture resistance. Porcelain and resins used alone have a long history of breakage under stress; to extend their longevity, they are often supported with metal. The way in which these materials are used together can profoundly affect the physical properties of the resulting restoration.

Surface hardness

Surface hardness is the resistance of a material to deformation from compressive contact with a predetermined object (Figure 1–17). There are many ways to measure hardness, depending on the shape of the object used to deform the surface of the material being tested.

Brinell hardness, one of the oldest hardness test methods used in dentistry, measures resistance to penetration by a small steel ball, 1.6 mm (1/16 inch) in diameter, when subjected to a force of 27.7 pounds. The resulting number, known as the Brinell hardness number (BHN), is calculated by a formula that uses load, area, and indentation as variables.

Knoop hardness uses a specially made diamond indenting tool. The Knoop hardness number (KHN) is also calculated using the variables of load, area, and indentation. The units of Knoop hardness are measured in kilograms per square millimeter (Kg/mm^2).

Vickers hardness uses a 136-degree diamond pyramid; it is used in applied loads. It is commonly used in dentistry and is about 2.45 N for enamel.

Rockwell hardness is a rapid testing method in which an instrument applies a load to a material and a dial quickly calculates a hardness number. This method is commonly used with plastics, since the device can be kept on the material for varying amounts of time to measure percent of recovery.

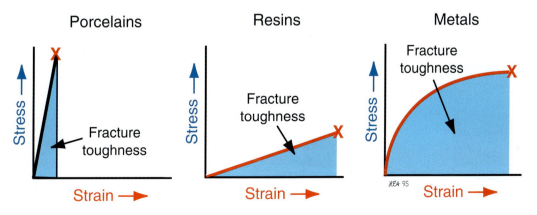

Figure 1–16. Fracture toughness is related to the area under the stress–strain curve. Note that metals are far superior to porcelains and resins.

10 Tooth-Colored Restoratives

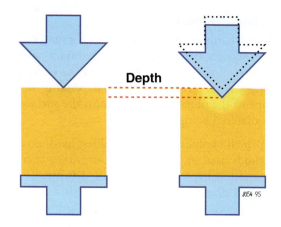

Figure 1–17. Surface hardness. The resistance of a material to deformation during compression.

Abrasion

Abrasion, or wear, is the progressive loss of material from the surface because of relative motion. Wear is related to a material's coefficient of friction. It explains why metals perform so well in high-stress areas whereas heterogeneous glass-containing plastics and ionomers wear more rapidly.

One result of wear in a heterogeneous material is roughness at the microscopic level. Because of roughness, contact between the surfaces of two objects can result in frictional forces that microscopically fracture off pieces from the surface, resulting in material loss (Figure 1–18).

There are four types of wear: adhesive wear, loss of material owing to contact between filler shearing points; abrasive wear, deformation of a softer material by a harder one; fatigue wear, breaking away of material as a result of cyclic loading; and corrosive wear, removal or chemical softening of a surface.

Erosion

Erosion is the loss of substance from a material by chemical means. In dentistry, acid from foods and gastric fluids (eg, bulimia) are the most common sources of erosion (Figure 1–19).

Roughness or smoothness

Roughness refers to the surface texture of a material. There are two types: the smoothness resulting from a finishing process, referred to as applied or acquired smoothness, and the smoothness of an unpolished material, referred to as inherent smoothness. Inherent smoothness depends on the filler particle size of the material. A finished material will always return to its inherent smoothness. For example, if a material has filler particles of 1 to 10 μm, it will always return to a smoothness of 10 μm; therefore, if it is polished to 5 μm, its roughness will double over time (Figure 1–20). The clinical significance of roughness is discussed in greater detail in Chapter 9. Smoothness or roughness is measured in microns or in grit. A smoothness of less than 1 μm or a grit greater than 600 is considered as smooth as enamel.

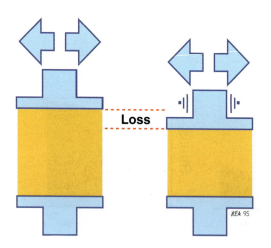

Figure 1–18. Wear and abrasion. The progressive loss of material from its surface as a result of relative motion.

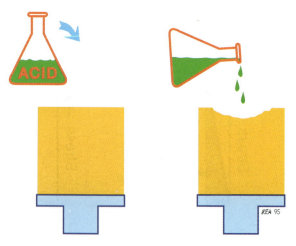

Figure 1–19. Erosion. The loss of substance from a material by chemical means.

Materials Science

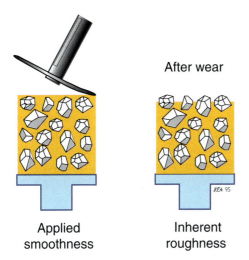

Figure 1–20. Roughness or smoothness is measured in grit and microns. Many materials can be polished to a high luster, referred to as applied polish or smoothness. After a period, each material reverts to an inherent polish based on the size of its heterogeneous components.

Cutting instruments are commonly measured in grit whereas polishing instruments are frequently measured in microns.

As a general rule for dental uses, a roughness of less than 300 grit is coarse, 300 to 600 grit is intermediate, and 600 to 1200 grit is smooth enough for a final finish equal to or better than enamel.

Coefficient of thermal expansion

The coefficient of thermal expansion refers to the amount of expansion and contraction a material undergoes in relation to temperature (Figure 1–21). A tooth expands and contracts with thermal changes. A high coefficient of thermal expansion indicates a relatively high degree of dimensional change in reaction to temperature (also referred to as a high coefficient). Studies show that there is a direct relation between marginal leakage and thermal changes. The greater the difference in the thermal coefficient between the tooth structure and the restorative, the greater the leakage.

Water sorption

Water sorption is a critical physical property for direct restoratives because increased absorption of water increases the volume of a restorative (Figure 1–22). This property has great clinical significance when polymers are used for buildups since, through water sorption, a polymer can enlarge in the lapse time between impression-taking and cementation appointments. More important, water is a softener of plastics and increases the deterioration of the resin matrix. In addition, water sorption usually decreases color stability since water-soluble stains can penetrate the restoration.

Fluoride release

Fluoride release is an important feature of a dental restorative. Fluoride release should not be confused with fluoride content. Many materials contain fluoride but do not release it. The minimum amount of fluoride release necessary to effectively inhibit recurrent decay is unknown, but it is probably over 20 ppm per day.

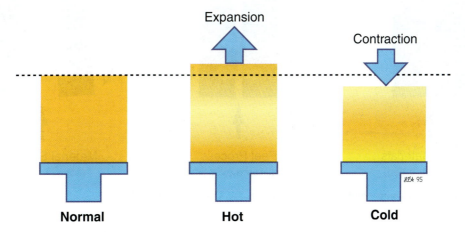

Figure 1–21. Coefficient of thermal expansion. The amount of expansion and contraction a material demonstrates in relation to temperature.

12 Tooth-Colored Restoratives

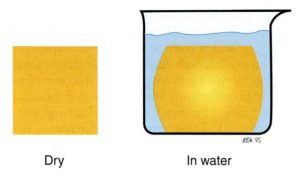

Figure 1–22. Water sorption. The volume of water a material can absorb.

The amount and duration of fluoride release varies greatly among dental materials. Most fluoride-releasing materials that have demonstrated clinical effectiveness share common features: (1) the materials contain water, which is necessary to transport the fluoride ions out of the material; (2) the fluoride is retained in the material in an inorganic state as a soluble salt; and (3) the materials produce some acid–base reactions that initiate the release of the inorganic fluoride in an ionic state. Alternatively, in some cases, a rare earth, such as ytterbium trifluoride (YbF_3), is added to a composite resin as filler, resulting in short-term, low-level fluoride release. The caries-inhibiting effectiveness of this type of composite material is not as great as that of aqueous ion-containing systems.

Peel strength

In the peel strength test, all of the forces are placed at the end of the bonded specimen rather than in the middle, such that the force is exerted on one area at a time. By contrast, when testing compressive strength, the forces are equally spread over every molecule used for attachment. Over time, peel stress separates substances with a relatively small amount of force (10% or less of the required

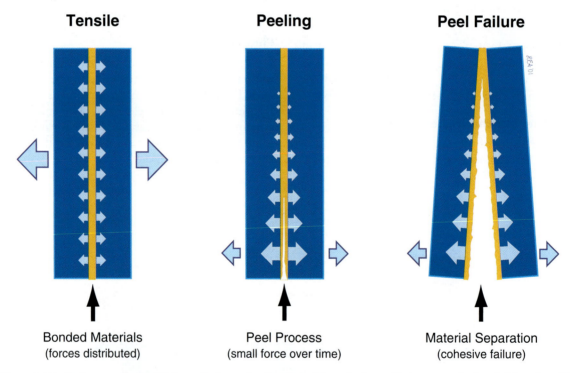

Figure 1–23. Peel versus tensile. With tensile force, the direction of force is always 90 degrees to the bonded interface. This distributes the stress over the entire adhesive surface. With peel force, the force is placed on one small area, which results in a more rapid failure of a portion of the bond. Once the bond is broken, the force moves along the surface and breaks another small portion of the bond, and so on, until the entire system fails.

tensile force with adhesives), especially in the presence of cyclic loading (Figure 1–23). Peel strength failure can be greatly reduced or eliminated by the use of resistance form in a restoration, which prevents stress on the interface. Clinically, peel strength has a much more significant effect than tensile strength.

Peel energy: Boeing test

Peel energy, otherwise known as the energy of adherence, the wedge test, or the Boeing test (because of its use in testing aircraft structures) is the force required to sustain a peel motion (Figure 1–24). This physical property is often used to measure the failure rate of air foils in aircraft designs. Although not commonly used in dentistry, this physical property could provide meaningful information about an adhesive interface, because it contributes to cyclic fatigue.

Contact angle

Contact angle is the measure of how well a fluid wets a solid. A smaller contact angle indicates that a liquid has good ability to penetrate the micromechanical porosities of a surface. The angle between an adhesive and a bondable substance is of enormous significance in determining micromechanical retention and the potential for chemical adhesion. The measurement of contact angle and a demonstration of its applied effects are shown in Figure 1–25.

COHESIVE FORCES

The bonding forces that hold materials together are called cohesive forces. Generally, the atoms in these materials have positive or negative charges and are referred to as ions. A positive ion is short one or more electrons, and a negative ion has one or more extra electrons. Bonds are formed when atoms combine to reduce these charges.

Primary bonds

Primary bonds are chemical in nature and are formed through the attraction of positive and negative ions. There are three types of primary bonds:

1. Ionic bonds occur when atoms transfer electrons (eg, sodium chloride, Na$^+$Cl$^-$). Materials that result from acid–base reactions are called salts (Figure 1–26).

2. Covalent bonds occur when two atoms share electrons (eg, polymers). These bonds often form between the carbon and hydrogen atoms found in most organic materials (Figure 1–27).

3. Metallic bonds occur when many atoms share available electrons. These primary bonds are responsible for the strength, elasticity, and fracture toughness of the crystalline solids called metals (Figure 1–28).

Secondary bonds

Secondary bonds involve complex physical interactions between various kinds of molecules. Common secondary bonds are van der Waals forces and dipole forces. These forces hold liquids and nonrigid solids (plastics) together and include attractions between polar molecules (fluctuating dipoles), hydrogen bonds (permanent dipoles), and other secondary molecular attractions. The

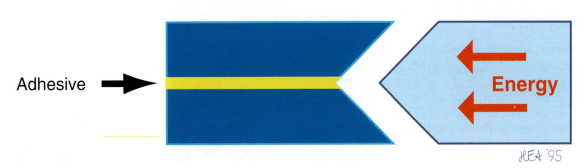

Figure 1–24. Peel energy. The energy of adherence (also called the wedge test and Boeing test) is the peel energy required to sustain a peel reaction over time.

14 Tooth-Colored Restoratives

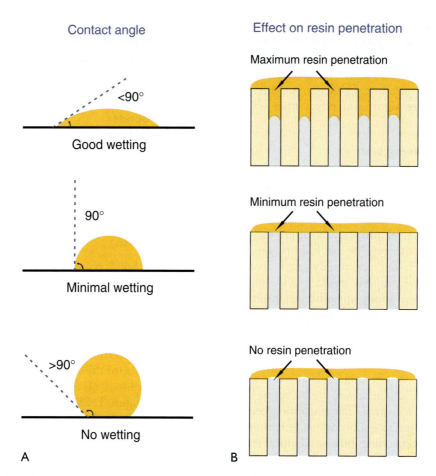

Figure 1–25. Effect of wetting on surface adhesion. *A*, The relation between the contact angle and the wetting of a substance. *B*, Improved adhesive penetration on a porous dentin surface as the contact angle of the adhesive decreases.

most common example of this bonding is water. Secondary bonds are responsible for viscosity and resistance to deformation (Figure 1–29).

WHY MEASURE PHYSICAL PROPERTIES?

Physical properties are measures of a material. These properties have great significance in dental research because they provide the information needed to assess the characteristics of and improvements in materials under development. The physical properties of a tooth set the standard for materials attached to a tooth. Theory suggests that if a restorative can be made to hold properties similar to those of natural tooth structure, it should perform as well as an original tooth. In the field of civil engineering, certainly, new designs are built and tested under conditions that exactly match or well approximate those under which they are to perform. Unfortunately, in dentistry, this type of testing is seldom done. Few of today's newer materials have undergone long-term clinical testing prior to marketing. This makes the dental practitioner who purchases a new material,

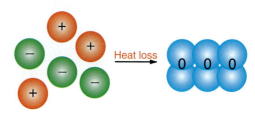

Figure 1–26. Tight packing of molecules in acid–base reactions that form ionic bonds.

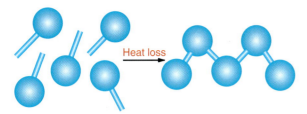

Figure 1–27. The carbon–carbon bonding links formed in polymer reactions create covalent bonds.

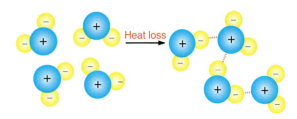

Figure 1–29. Strong attraction between molecules of negative and positive charge creates the secondary bonds that hold together liquids including water.

and the patients who have the material placed in their mouths, the actual test site.

To the dentist, success is measured not by physical properties but by clinical performance. A material that displays some good physical properties during development is not necessarily a material that will perform well in the mouth. The individual properties that scientists measure usually are not the cause of restoration failure in the mouth. Thus, the only real assurance a dentist has of a material's safety and reliability is the test of time. Generally, if a dental material has been on the market unchanged for over 5 years, it has proven itself reasonably safe and reliable. In the absence of manufacturer-funded clinical testing, therefore, 5-year clinical reports from the field are a good way of assessing which materials are proving their value.

Although commonly measured physical properties are a poor predictor of clinical success, these properties are useful in comparing materials to one another. Success in clinical dentistry is based on a chain of events, from the material and its placement to the host response. Physical properties allow a dentist to measure a single link in this complex chain. The measures of physical properties are useful only if they measure characteristics that are significant to the success of a single restoration in a single tooth in an individual. These variables are enormous, but useful trends do exist.

UNITS AND CONVERSIONS

Below is a partial listing of the units of measure used to determine the physical properties, state, temperature, and size of dental systems. Each description includes a small amount of history on the unit and its most common conversions.[4]

Weight units

Weight units are the gravitational forces applied by an object irrespective of the area of the object.

Grain. A unit of weight based on the weight of a grain of wheat taken as an average of the weight of grains from the middle of the ear and equal to 0.0648 grams.

Carat. A unit of weight based on the weight of four grains. In the United States before 1913, one carat was equal to 205.3 milligrams (mg). After 1913, the international standard for the carat was adopted, which was then standardized at 200 mg. This unit is mainly used to measure the weight of precious stones and pearls.

Pound (lb). A unit of weight equal to 12 troy ounces (historically 1 pound = 5760 grains = 0.3732 kilograms). Presently, English-speaking people use the avoirdupois pound, which is now the most commonly used: 1 pound equals 7000 grains or 0.4536 kilograms.

Ounce (oz). A unit of weight that represents 1/16 of the present-day pound (technically referred to as the avoirdupois pound).

Gram (g). A unit of weight based on the weight of 1 cubic centimeter (cm^3) of water at its maximum

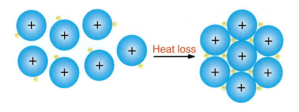

Figure 1–28. The compacting and sharing of electron charges that form in metals.

density. This unit is the standard for the metric system of weights.

Conversions
One kilogram (kg) equals 1000 grams; 1 milligram (mg) equals one thousandth of a gram; 1 nanogram (ng) equals one billionth of a gram.

Force units
Newton (N). A force scale named after British mathematician Sir Issac Newton in 1727. It is the unit of force required to give a free mass of 1 kilogram an acceleration of 1 meter per second per second (second^2). On a larger scale, 1 meganewton (MN) is 1 million (10^6) newtons. On a smaller scale, 1 newton equals 1 million (10^6) dynes.

The normal biting force generated on the first molars in a human mouth ranges from 400 to 800 newtons, or 90 to 200 pounds (mean, 550 N or 125 lb).

Dyne. The unit of force required to give a free mass of 1 gram an acceleration of 1 centimeter per second per second (second^2).

Conversions
One newton equals 0.225 pounds and 1 pound equals 4.44 newtons; 1 newton equals 1 million dynes.

Length units
Foot (ft). A unit of length based on the length of a British king's foot. One foot is equal to 0.3048 meters, or 3.28 feet = 1 meter.

Inch (in). A unit of length equal to 1/12 of a foot. One inch is equal to 2.54 centimeters.

Meter (m). A unit of length equal to the distance between two lines on a platinum-iridium bar kept at the International Bureau of Weights and Measures near Paris. One meter is equal to 39.37 inches and is equal to 1,650,763.73 wavelengths of the orange-red light of the excited krypton of mass number 86. Use of this constant allows this unit of length to be reproduced anywhere.

Conversions
One centimeter (cm) equals 1/100 of a meter; one millimeter (mm) equals 1/1000 of a meter; one micrometer (μm) equals one millionth of a meter; one nanometer (nm) equals one billionth of a meter.

Stress units
Stress is the unit force applied per unit area. Stress units are commonly used to measure bond strengths associated with dental materials. Currently, the preferred unit in dental science is the megapascal.

Megapascal (MPa). A force scale named after French scientist Blaise Pascal in 1662. It is a measure of force over area. The megapascal is equal to 1 meganewton (MN) per meter per meter (m^2), which is equivalent to 1 N/mm^2.

Conversions
One MPa equals 10.196 kg/cm^2; 1 psi equals 0.07032 kg/cm^2; 1 kg/cm^2 equals 14.22 psi; 1 MPa equals 145 psi; 1 psi equals 0.00689 MPa; 1 kg/cm^2 equals 0.098077 MPa.

Thermometric units
Fahrenheit (°F). A thermometric scale named after German physicist Gabriel D. Fahrenheit in 1736. In this thermometric scale, the boiling point of water is 212°F, whereas the freezing point of water is 32°F, under standard atmospheric pressure. The zero point of the Fahrenheit scale approximates the temperature produced by mixing equal quantities by weight of snow and common salt.

Centigrade or Celsius (°C). A thermometric scale on which the interval between two standard points, the freezing and the boiling point of water, is divided into 100 degrees, 0° representing the freezing point and 100° the boiling point.

Conversions
x°C equals x°F − 32 × 5/9.

Kelvin (°K). A thermometric scale named after British physicist William Lord Kelvin in 1907. In this thermometric scale, centigrade degrees are related to absolute zero (defined as 0°K). 1° Kelvin is the equivalent of −276.16°C.

The Kelvin thermometric scale is used in photography to measure the temperature of light sources used to illuminate objects. Color-corrected lighting, which is equivalent to average daylight, is 5400°K.

Conversions
x°K equals x°C + 276.16 and x°C equals x°F − 32 × 5/9.

REFERENCES

1. Phillips RW. Skinners' science of dental materials. 9th ed. Philadelphia: WB Saunders, 1991.

2. Craig RG. Restorative dental materials. 8th ed. St. Louis: CV Mosby, 1989.

3. O'Brien WJ. Dental materials: properties and selection. Chicago: Quintessence, 1989.

4. Gove PB (after Webster N [1758–1843]). Webster's third new international dictionary of the English language (unabridged). Springfield, MA: G&C Merriam, 1902 to present.

Chapter 2

Diagnosis

It is more important to know what kind of patient one has than what kind of disease the patient has.

Harold Shyrock, MD

As noted by McLean, "The diagnosis and treatment of early dental caries remains an area of controversy and arouses great emotion among clinicians and academicians. Phrases such as 'overprescribing' and 'supervised neglect' are good examples of the divergence of opinion."[1] This chapter reviews the physiology of dental caries, the various procedures for caries detection, and the diagnosis of several related clinical conditions (dentin sensitivity, cervical lesions, and anorexia and bulimia).

PHYSIOLOGY OF DENTAL CARIES

A considerable amount of information has been acquired over the past several decades about the caries process. Knowledge of the process aids in caries detection. The process of decay has a relatively large reversibility component—up to the point of destruction of the protein matrix.

Caries in enamel

Dental caries is a dynamic process of alternating demineralization and remineralization (Figure 2–1). According to researcher Kidd, "Sound enamel may become carious in time if plaque bacteria are given the sugary substrate they need to produce acid. However, saliva is an excellent remineralization fluid particularly if it contains the fluoride ion. If the disease can be diagnosed in its earliest stages, the balance can be tipped in favor of repair by the use of fluoride, modifying diet and attempting to remove plaque."[2]

Caries in dentin

Caries in dentin has two basic differentiated layers.[3-5] Distinguishing between the two is of key importance to the clinician.[6] The first layer, *infected carious dentin*, has been demineralized, and a large number of bacteria reside in the dentinal tubules.[7]

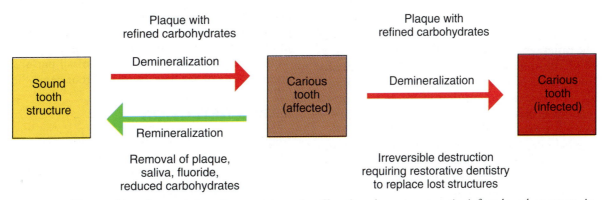

Figure 2–1. The transitions from sound tooth structure to caries-affected tooth structure to caries-infected tooth structure. As long as the protein matrix that supports the enamel or dentin is intact, as is true in sound and caries-affected tooth structure, the potential for remineralization of the matrix exists. However, once the protein matrix has been denatured, the caries process is irreversible.

This layer is infected beyond the point of remineralization and must be removed during tooth preparation. The second layer, *affected carious dentin*, has been demineralized by the acidic byproducts of the caries process but contains far fewer, if any, bacteria.[8,9] This layer, which still has an intact organic matrix, is reversibly diseased and any remaining bacteria will arrest after restoration placement.[10,11] Clinically, this portion of the dentin should not be removed, since the demineralized area will remineralize in oral fluids.[12] Each of these layers is chemically distinct such that it stains differently when various dyes are applied.[13,14]

Caries incidence

Pit and fissure caries

The decline in smooth surface decay with the introduction of systemic fluoride has resulted in increased treatment of pit and fissure caries. Surveys by the National Institute of Dental Research (NIDR) indicate that pit and fissure caries now constitutes a higher proportion of the total caries incidence among teens and children than in the past.[4,5] First-time caries is now being detected many years later in young adults.[15,16] Carious lesions now progress more slowly and are commonly arrested in high-fluoride groups.[17] In addition, the rate of carious lesion growth slows with increasing patient age. Fluoride greatly reduces caries in enamel but has less impact on dentin. Clinicians have observed that about 60 to 80% of asymptomatic stained pits and fissures with no radiographic or tactile evidence of caries have caries in the dentin and may even have near-pulpal exposures.[3]

Traditionally, although occlusal surfaces constituted only 12% of the permanent dentition surface area, they have been the site of more than 50% of the caries reported among school-aged children.[7-9] With the initiation of municipal water fluoridation and the use of fluoride supplements in nonfluoridated areas, the proportion of pit and fissure to smooth surface decay has changed dramatically.[10,11] A study by the NIDR of more than 30,000 school-aged children found that from 1980 to 1987, the incidence of pit and fissure caries was reduced by 31%, whereas caries in other surfaces dropped by 51 to 59%, a dramatic decline.[11]

Occlusal caries

With the fluoridation of community drinking water, the overall rate of occlusal caries has declined about 12%, which is down a third since the 1980s.[18-20] The combination of high fluoride exposure and an older population is expected to continue to decrease the future incidence of occlusal carious lesions.

Proximal caries

The rate of proximal caries has changed considerably over the past decade. Proximal caries, even with systemic or topical fluoride, can be rampant in children. Caries development and advancement is generally a much slower process in adults over 35 years of age. In many adults, a proximal carious lesion may take up to 4 years to progress through the enamel.[21-27] Despite this general trend in well-kept mouths, factors such as medical problems, medications that cause xerostomia, poor oral hygiene, high intake of simple carbohydrates, and even frequent use of "sugar-free" breath mints, can significantly increase rates of lesion development and progress.

Root caries

The incidence of root caries is increasing in our aging population.[28] Periodontal treatment has resulted in higher tooth retention with more exposed root surfaces for the average patient and, therefore, a growing incidence of root caries. Root caries is now present in about a quarter of the retired population.[29-31] Root caries is most often associated with the use of sugar in coffee and tea and is less common among patients who brush often and visit a dentist regularly.[32] Mints, chewing gum, or other sugar-containing foods that remain in the mouth for long periods of time can prompt root caries development in relatively short periods of time. Clinical studies show that 57 to 67% of all persons between 50 and 65 years of age have had one or more incidents of root decay.[33,34] These data also indicate that 37% of all persons over 50 years of age have untreated root decay.[33]

CARIES DETECTION

Magnification, caries detection devices, and improved access to enlarged radiographic images help take the guesswork out of caries diagnosis. As is true in pulp testing, no one test is perfect, but clinicians who use a combination of diagnostic measures and sound clinical judgment can routinely achieve more accurate assessments of disease.

Diagnosis of smooth-surface caries

The easiest type of caries to detect is a smooth-surface caries that is not on a proximal surface. Typically, a clinician places a sharp explorer into a suspected carious lesion (usually because the area is discolored) and, if the explorer sinks in or sticks, makes a diagnosis of caries. This method is useful in detecting gross carious involvement, but it is less useful in detecting precarious decalcification (affected tooth structure), which might be treatable by topical fluoride application. Caries indicators, which are discussed later this chapter, can assist in determining the nature and extent of these lesions. They can also assist in determining the appropriate method of treatment.

Diagnosis of pit and fissure caries

Owing to variations in tooth morphology, pit and fissure caries is more difficult to accurately diagnose than smooth-surface caries. Errors are made when a sharp explorer sticks into normal anatomy and gives a clinician the feel of caries when none exist (Figure 2–2). Hence, the profession is reevaluating the methods of detecting pit and fissure lesions and questioning the adequacy of the explorer to probe for caries.[1,2,12–14,17] Fluoridation makes it difficult to distinguish a surface stain in enamel from a darker organic plug that can promote caries within a pit or fissure. In addition, fluoride-containing enamel is stronger and less likely to fracture and collapse than is nonfluoridated enamel, even when undermined by carious dentin.[12] The appearance of strength makes detecting diseased dentin more difficult. A very thin, very sharp explorer (eg, a sharp Suter No. 2) may stick in these grooves. Clinicians also look for color shifts through the enamel. If the color is darker than the surrounding enamel, caries should be suspected.[33] Studies question the effectiveness of radiographs in diagnosing pit and fissure caries, because the decay is hidden by the sound enamel, and the current emphasis on reducing exposure to radiation has resulted in less film contrast.[12,28] To improve detection, clinicians should dry radiographs well and view them under high magnification. Mounting films and projecting them onto a large screen helps detect early-stage dentin lesions. Digital radiographs are easily magnified, and specialized software can enhance image reading.

Caries in fissures begins with the formation of a white spot lesion bilaterally on the walls; such a lesion is not easy to see.[35] As the lesion advances to the dentin–enamel junction, it forms a triangle with the junction as its base. Unfortunately, a fissure that looks caries-free may histologically show signs of early lesion formation, and a so-called sticky fissure may be caries-free even though a sharp explorer can enter and bind on the walls, producing the tactile sensation of carious dentin. For these reasons, diagnosis of early fissure caries should depend more on visual examination than on tactile exploration.

The following list outlines procedures for achieving an accurate diagnosis of caries in fissures (modified from Wilson and McLean).[1]

1. Use magnifying loupes or intraoral camera magnification.

2. Use excellent lighting (operatory head lamp or fiber optic).

3. Clean and dry the teeth (ideally with an air abrasion cleaning device or a water abrasion device such as Prophy Jet [Dentsply/Caulk, Milford, Delaware, USA] or Prophy Flex [KaVo, Biberach, Germany]).

4. Use caries indicators and caries detection devices.

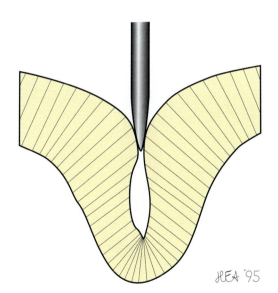

Figure 2–2. A healthy occlusal fissure can clinically result in an explorer sticking in the fissure even though the enamel within the fissure is caries-free.

5. Transilluminate teeth, especially along the dentin–enamel junction.

6. Use accurate bitewing radiographs and view them with magnification.

7. To avoid binding in the grooves, use only light pressure with an explorer. An explorer is best used as a diagnostic device to determine only the width and depth of a fissure orifice.

If a pit or fissure of a tooth has inaccessible areas where plaque removal is impossible, sealing the area as soon as the tooth erupts into the mouth greatly reduces the likelihood of future caries (Figure 2–3). Sealing limits the potential for caries development along the enamel walls of the internal parts of the fissure.

Clinicians are becoming increasingly aware of the danger of missing occlusal caries. The reports of belated discovery of significant caries can no longer be regarded as anecdotal; they reveal a definite pattern of change in the disease. It is generally easy to detect caries in teeth with low fluoride content (Figure 2–4), since the enamel breaks down in conjunction with increased dentin involvement (Figure 2–5). Fluoride-enriched enamel is hard and firm, but bacteria still gain access through cracks and open fissures. These lesions are harder to detect visually (Figure 2–6).

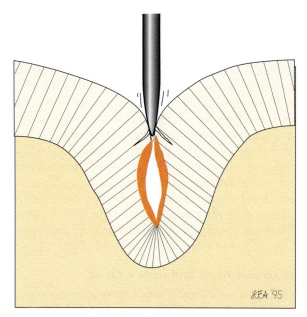

Figure 2–4. Small caries is easier to detect in a tooth with low fluoride content than in a tooth with high fluoride content. Because caries begins in the outer enamel, an explorer can break through the enamel and stick in the affected pits and fissures.

Undetected lesions can develop into a large "mushroom" of caries, even though the opening in the enamel seems benign (Figure 2–7). Opening the occlusal surface of the tooth then reveals extensive caries. Reports of strange patterns of caries under

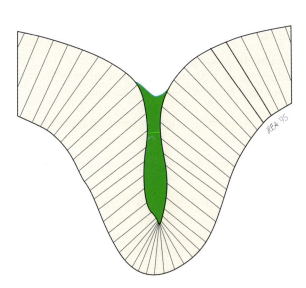

Figure 2–3. Sealing a pit or fissure greatly reduces the likelihood of future caries.

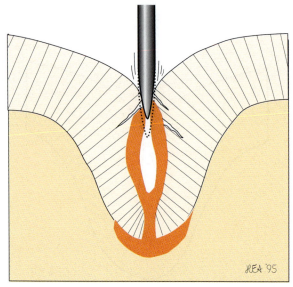

Figure 2–5. Large caries in a tooth with limited exposure to fluoride is easy to detect because the superficial enamel is broken and the lesion generally is discolored.

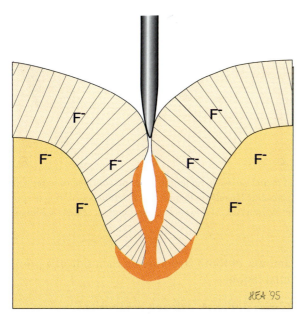

Figure 2–6. Small caries in fluoridated teeth is difficult to detect because the enamel is largely unaffected and it is difficult to access the underlying carious dentin with an explorer.

occlusal fissures have increased since the fluoridation of water. Clearly, good bitewing radiographs and routine dental examinations are essential in detecting dentin caries.

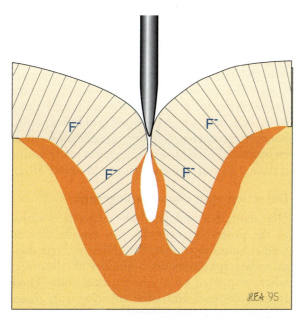

Figure 2–7. Large caries in fluoridated teeth is somewhat less difficult to detect than small caries because it shows on radiographs; however, clinically there is no stick with an explorer and minimal discoloration of the lesion.

Shaw and Murray showed that even with the best of modern aids and techniques, the trained epidemiologist is only 70 to 80% reliable in detecting pit and fissure problems.[36] Examiner variability is at least as important as the type of test used. A "wait-and-see" policy can have devastating effects, because pit and fissure caries is much more rapid and destructive in its progress in dentin than in enamel.

Diagnosis of proximal caries

Visual examination with an explorer is useful in detecting proximal caries of moderate size. Unfortunately, this method does not easily detect decay at or just under the contact area. Radiographic examination and transillumination, discussed later in this chapter, are the primary methods for detecting proximal caries.

Detection with radiographs

Smooth-surface caries

With the exception of the proximal areas, smooth-surface caries is difficult to detect radiographically.

Pit and fissure caries

Radiographs can detect occlusal caries but only when the decay is advanced. Radiographs are more useful in detecting decay under existing amalgam, composite, or sealant restorations, particularly in posterior teeth (see Figures 2–4 to 2–7).

Proximal caries

The most common method of detecting proximal caries is the radiograph. Unfortunately, this method can only detect 40 to 60% of the size of a lesion and requires patient exposure to electromagnetic radiation.

The following list outlines a ranked diagnosis of caries using radiographs (Figure 2–8).

1. No lesion. Enamel is apparently sound, no treatment is required (see Figure 2–8, *A*).

2. Lesion confined to outer half of enamel. Where radiolucency is confined to the enamel, preventive measures, such as fluoride treatments and dietary changes, should be instituted (see Figure 2–8, *B*).

3. Lesion penetrating dentin–enamel junction. Make decisions at this point based on the history of the lesion. In older patients, lesions of this depth that remain unchanged do not require restorative treatment. The lack of cari-

24 Tooth-Colored Restoratives

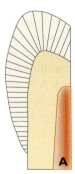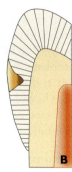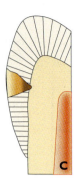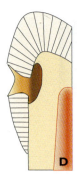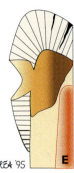

Figure 2–8. Suggested ranking system for radiographic diagnosis of dental caries: *A*, no lesion; *B*, lesion confined to outer half of enamel; *C*, lesion penetrating dentin–enamel junction; *D*, lesion spreading laterally in dentin; and *E*, lesion penetrating deeply in dentin, with the possibility of pulpal involvement. (Modified from Wilson AD, McLean JW. Glass-ionomer cement. Chicago: Quintessence, 1988.)

ous growth indicates the lesion is arrested. In younger patients, however, when preventive measures have not stopped these lesions from progressing to this level, restorative treatment is indicated (see Figure 2–8, *C*).

4. Lesion spreading laterally in dentin. This degree of carious involvement should be treated restoratively (see Figure 2–8, *D*).

5. Lesion penetrating deeply into dentin, with the possibility of pulpal involvement. These teeth should be treated as soon as possible: remove decay and place a sedative temporary (eg, glass ionomer restorative or material containing zinc oxide). Use pulp capping materials on or near small pulpal exposures (see Figure 2–8, *E*). The teeth should be observed for signs of possible irreversible pulp damage.

All smaller proximal carious lesions require monitoring with bitewing radiographs to assess the effectiveness of preventive measures. Once caries has penetrated dentin, monitoring becomes difficult and lesions can spread rapidly. Restorative dentistry is highly recommended.

Monitoring early proximal lesions

Proximal carious lesions are classified based on their progress into the enamel and dentin (see Figure 2–8).[37] Although a bitewing radiograph does not reveal the full extent of a carious lesion, it gives some indication of the progress of the lesion into dentin. Histologically, a carious lesion is always larger than it appears in a radiograph. Typical radiographs show less than 50% of a carious lesion, since they are blocked by the large amount of tooth structure on each side of a proximal lesion.

Caries under an existing composite

It is difficult to detect dental caries under composite by visual inspection. Experienced clinicians who were asked to diagnose caries under a composite were incorrect in 7 to 44% of cases.[28,38] Thus, aids such as radiographs and transillumination are essential.

Radiopaque composites used with radiopaque bases help in caries detection, particularly in posterior teeth. Note, however, that not all radiolucencies under radiopaque composites are carious. One study showed that about one-third are pooled unfilled bonding agent.[39] Diffuse radiolucent patterns that travel up the dentin–enamel junction are likely to be carious. Distinct radiolucencies visible in the corners of preparations or uniformly along inner walls have a high probability of being pooled bonding agent. Hence, follow-up radiographs must be compared with earlier radiographs to determine if there is an enlargement that would signify caries.

Detection with digital radiographs

Digital intraoral radiographs have become available to the profession over the past decade. Several studies have shown that, theoretically, direct digital radiography provides a number of advantages when compared with conventional film. These include contrast and edge enhancement, image enlargement, lower radiation dose, image compression, and automated image analysis. Although there is little clinical evidence as yet to support these claims, properly used digital intraoral radiographic systems seem to be as accurate in caries detection as currently available dental films.

Digital systems are either storage-based or direct sensor-based. In the storage-based systems, a film containing a memory medium (or plate), usually phosphoric, stores the image until it is digitized by a reading device. Sensor-based systems use an electronic sensor, usually a charge coupled device (CCD), and send the image directly to a computer via a wired or wireless device. Digital radiographs, taken by either method, are of minimum value in the detection of initial occlusal or proximal lesions in enamel. However, they are helpful in detecting both types of lesions that have radiolucency in dentin. Dentin lesions are more easily distinguished, with a 5 to 10% occurrence of false-positive results.

A number of issues await further clarification. For example, whereas a reduction in radiation dose is suggested, this has not been clinically shown for either the storage or the sensor systems, and there is no evidence of a reduction in the number of retakes. Further, it is not known how many images are needed with the various CCD-based systems compared with conventional bitewing radiographs, nor how stable these systems are in daily clinical use. Maintenance of proper cross-infection control in relation to scanning the storage phosphoric plates or handling the sensors and cable is still a question. There is only sparse evidence that the enhancement facilities are used when interpreting images, and none that this has changed working practices or treatment decisions.[40]

The most significant advantage of digital radiography is its versatility in clinical practice: images are available immediately and can be enlarged for easy viewing without the use of magnification.

Detection with transillumination

Using transillumination
Transillumination works best with longer wavelengths of light in the yellow and orange range, because they have higher penetration properties. Blue light used for curing is the least effective, owing to decreased penetration and increased scattering. Blue light should be avoided, since it is harmful to the eyes. A major advantage of transillumination is that the patient can easily see the problems that the practitioner is addressing. It can be used as a screening device to determine if a radiograph is necessary.

Transillumination works best when a small light source is used in a dark field. The optimal approach is to turn the operatory light away and use an incandescent yellow-to-white light source about 1-mm wide. The most contrast is achieved when the light source is placed against the side of the tooth that has the most enamel and then viewed from the side of the tooth with the largest mass of restoration (Figure 2–9). In anterior teeth, the light source is usually placed on the facial, and the dentist views from the lingual. Moving the light back and forth improves the likelihood of detecting pathology.

Transillumination devices
There are many devices that can transilluminate a tooth. The standard light for an ear, nose, and throat examination works well. Some composite curing lamps have filtered tips that change the wavelength of light to yellow-orange so the lamp can be used for transillumination. Small light probes used in electronics (that look like tiny flashlights) also work well.

An easy-to-use alternative is the fiber optics built into most delivery systems for lighting handpieces. Fiber optics yield an intense white light with a small spot-size. Simply remove the bur from the handpiece and turn the operatory light away. Then turn on the fiber-optic light and use the handpiece as a light wand. It is best to place the light opposite the tooth under inspection. Rotating the light source in a dark field can reveal carious lesions, cracks, stains, and retained restorations. Headlamps should be turned off, and sometimes turning the room lamps off or low is helpful.

In addition to application for caries detection, transillumination is useful, after a tooth is prepared, to evaluate the integrity of the remaining tooth structure. When cracks remain, the clinician can better decide if a restoration providing cusp coverage is indicated. Transillumination would also reveal any stains that could affect the esthetics of composite placement.

Proximal caries
Transillumination is a good method of detecting proximal decay in anterior teeth. It is less effective in detecting decay in premolars and molars. Transillumination is an excellent adjunct to radiographs. In many cases, it can be more effective in determining the extent of a lesion (see Figure 2–9, *A–C*).

26 Tooth-Colored Restoratives

Caries under existing composite
When a tooth is filled with a radiolucent composite, the best and usually the only method of checking for decay is transillumination. Discoloration along the dentin–enamel junction is usually decay, whereas uniform discoloration around a restoration can be simply discoloration in the resin bonding agent (see Figure 2–9, *D* and *G*).

Digital imaging fiber-optic transillumination
Another option in transillumination, the Digital Imaging Fiber-Optic Transillumination (DIFOTI)

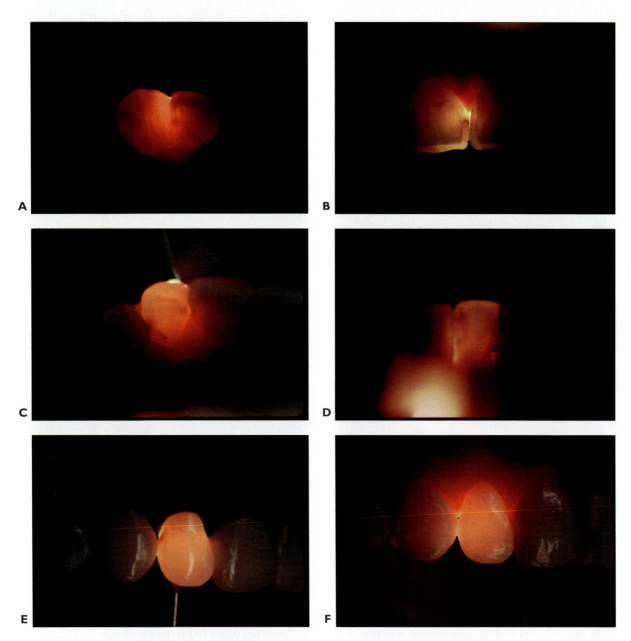

Figure 2–9. Transilluminated view of a small proximal carious lesion in enamel. *A*, Note the diffuse borders along the axial wall of the preparation. This indicates the presence of an active carious lesion. *B*, A medium proximal carious lesion in dentin. *C*, A small mesial and larger distal proximal carious lesion. *D*, Recurrent caries under an existing composite restoration. *E*, Proximal caries prior to treatment. *F*, The same tooth post-treatment. Transillumination enables a dentist to check that all the stain has been removed.

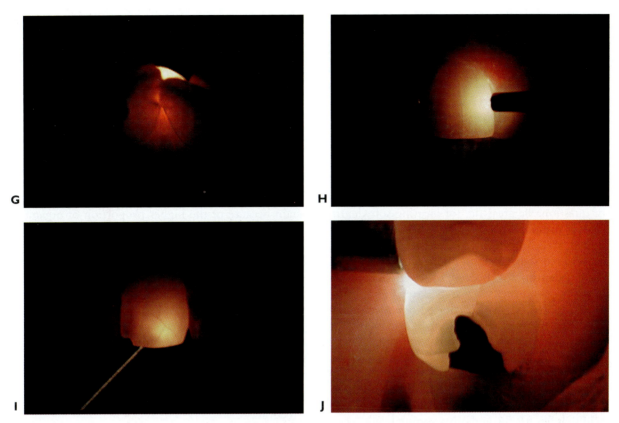

G, Recurrent caries under an existing composite restoration. *H,* A vertical fracture in enamel—little was detected under normal lighting. *I,* A complex fracture from a traumatic injury—nothing was detected under normal lighting. *J,* A fracture in a marginal ridge.

system from Electro-Optical Sciences Inc. (Irvington, New York) uses white light, a CCD camera, and computer-controlled image acquisition and analysis to detect caries (Figure 2–10). The mouthpiece carries a single fiber-optic illuminator. Directed toward a smooth surface of a tooth, the light travels through enamel and dentin and scatters toward the tooth's nonilluminated areas. The CCD camera in the handpiece digitizes the light emerging from the smooth surface oppo-

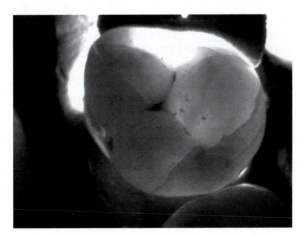
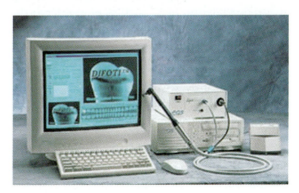

Figure 2–10. The DIFOTI (Electro-Optical Sciences Inc.) uses white light, a CCD camera, and computer-controlled image acquisition and analysis to detect caries.

site the illuminated surface or the occlusal surface for real-time display on a computer monitor. Caries is detected via computer analysis using dedicated algorithms. The DIFOTI device has been tested by imaging teeth in vitro. The results suggest it can sensitively detect proximal, occlusal, and smooth-surface caries.[41,42]

Detection with chemical dyes
Tactile and visual inspection are still the best methods of determining the presence of caries in a cavity.[43] Dyes are a diagnostic aid for detecting caries in questionable areas (ie, for locating soft dentin that is presumably infected).[44] Fusayama introduced a technique in 1972 that used a basic fuchsin red stain to aid in differentiating layers of carious dentin.[7,45,46] Because of potential carcinogenicity, basic fuchsin was replaced by another dye, acid red 52, which showed equal effectiveness.[47] Products based on acid red 52 are marketed by a number of manufacturers (eg, Caries Detector™, Kuraray, Osaka, Japan). A pharmacist can prepare this dye from acid red crystals obtained from most medical or chemical supply dealers. Many clinicians also have had good success with acid reds 50, 51, 54, and other commercially available caries detectors. Some caries detection products contain a red and blue disodium disclosing solution (eg, Cari-D-Tect, Gresco Products, Stafford, Texas). These products stain infected caries dark blue to bluish-green.[48]

Studies show dye stains are about 85% effective in detecting all caries in a tooth. Clinical removal of caries without the aid of a dye is 70% effective.[44,47] Clinical trials involving the use of dyes in cavities prepared by dental students and judged to be caries-free by their clinic instructors revealed dye-stained dentin in 57 to 59% of cavities at the enamel–dentin junction.[49,50] These studies did not correlate dye-stained material with infection but rather with lower levels of mineralization.[50]

How chemical dyes work
Caries-detecting stains differentiate mineralized from demineralized dentin in both vital and nonvital teeth. Outer carious dentin is stainable because the irreversible breakdown of collagen cross-linking loosens the collagen fibers. Inner carious dentin and normal dentin are not stained because their collagen fibers are undisturbed and dense. In other words, dyes do not stain bacteria but instead stain the organic matrix of poorly mineralized dentin.[43,51] Yip and others confirmed the lack of specificity of caries-detector dyes in 1994 by correlating the location of dye-stainable dentin with tooth mineral density.[52] The dyes neither stained bacteria nor delineated the bacterial front but did stain collagen associated with a less mineralized organic matrix. Importantly, use of the dyes on caries-free, freshly extracted human primary and permanent teeth showed that sound circumpulpal dentin and sound dentin at the dentin–enamel junction took up the stain because of the higher proportion of organic matrix normally present in these sites. Clearly, using these dyes without an understanding of their distinct limitations can result in excessive removal of sound tooth structure. Also, quantification of the intensity of staining is critical when assessing for caries. The contrast afforded by dyes helps identify carious dentin when tactile discrimination is insufficient. For example, the same intensity of dye that is found to be indicative of caries may be present in other areas of the tooth where tactile evaluation is inconclusive.

Accuracy
Unfortunately, false positives for infection are common. In one study, not all dye-stainable dentin was infected: 52% of the completed preparations for cavities showed stain in some part of the dentin–enamel junction, but subsequent microbiologic analysis detected only light levels of infection of no clinical significance.[53]

False staining of healthy tooth structure in deeper areas of dentin is also common. The tubules in these areas usually are wide and easily absorb stain by diffusion rather than by reaction with the denatured infected caries. It is important to use each tooth as its own control. Since carious areas absorb more dye, they stain darker than other areas, yielding a sort of quantitative measure of the infected tooth structure. To check for false positives, first remove the area of darker stain. Then, when working in the more lightly stained area, use a spoon excavator to check for firmness: where it is firm, protein matrix remains and tooth structure should not be removed. Hence, all stains lighter than this should be left in place. False negatives have also been demonstrated in that the absence of stain does not ensure elimination of bacteria.[13,14] Most practitioners would not remove nonstained infected dentin that is hard.

Technique
The process of caries detection using chemical dyes is shown in Figure 2–11.

1. The area to be tested is rinsed with water and then blotted dry (excess water dilutes a stain).
2. Dye is applied for 10 seconds.
3. The tooth is rinsed with water and suctioned, then excess water is removed.

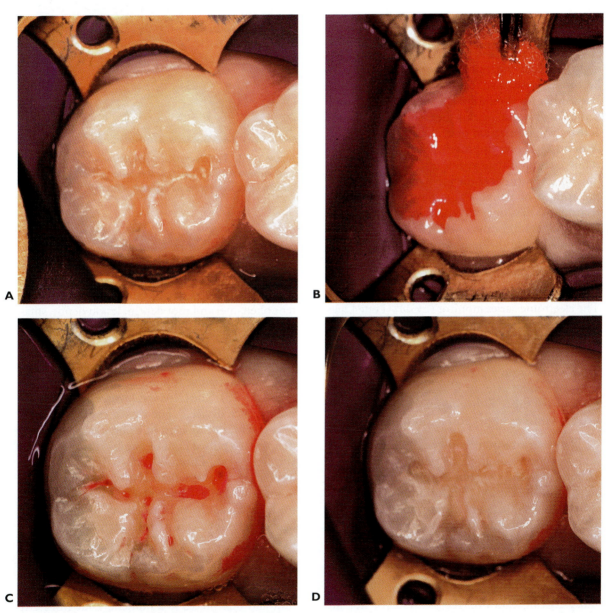

Figure 2–11. *A,* Prepared tooth before adding caries indicator. *B,* The tooth is treated with a 1% acid red 52 solution for 10 seconds. *C,* After rinsing with water for 10 seconds, some tooth structure shows discoloration. The stain indicates decalcified dentin. If the stained tooth structure is soft and appears carious, it should be removed. *D,* After removal of soft, carious tooth structure, some harder, less stained tooth remains, giving a pink appearance to some areas of this tooth. This healthy, stained tooth structure should not be removed.

30 Tooth-Colored Restoratives

4. Stained decay is removed with a spoon excavator and evaluated by tactile sensation.

Care should be taken not to remove any hard, calcified tooth structure. The procedure is repeated until there is no level of staining that was previously determined to indicate caries. It should be noted that a light residual or background stain usually remains, especially in deep areas of the preparation where the tubules are widest. This is usually healthy dentin and should not be removed.

When removing stained caries, it is important to be conservative near the pulp. Any questionable stained dentin should be left in place; remineralization will occur in this area, and the bacterial activity will be arrested once the tooth is restored. A more aggressive approach is appropriate when stained dentin is removed near the dentin–enamel junction. Dentin near the junction, being close to the surface of the tooth, is most susceptible to recurrent caries, since any microleakage associated with a restoration can continue to feed any bacteria remaining in the dentin.

Caries detection with devices

Electronic caries monitor

The electronic caries monitor (ECM) (Lode Diagnostics, Germany), measures a tooth's electric resistance during controlled air drying to determine its mineral content (Figure 2–12). The data are used to screen a patient for differences among teeth of similar size, or for changes in measurements over time. Either result would indicate a need for further inspection to rule out decay.

The electric resistance value of any given area of a tooth depends on the local porosity, the amount of liquid present, the temperature, the mobility of the liquid, and the ion concentration of the liquid. To avoid the influence of surface liquid (saliva), the ECM technique involves drying the tooth surface using a standardized airflow procedure. Interpreting the measurements is relatively complex since there is no standard representing different levels of caries. (The lack of a standard is a problem with most existing caries diagnostic systems, not just ECM.) The ECM protocol encourages a dentist to measure each patient's teeth at regular time intervals, as part of a standard checkup routine, to develop patient-specific baselines for the detection of tooth decay or healing. Results from in vitro

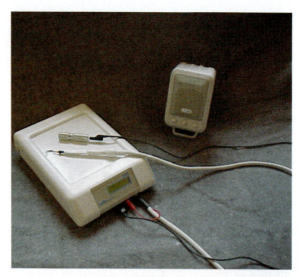

Figure 2–12. The electronic caries monitor (Lode Diagnostics) measures a tooth's electrical resistance during controlled air drying to determine its mineral content.

studies suggest that ECM can be an accurate diagnostic tool for the diagnosis of early, noncavitated occlusal lesions on posterior teeth.[54] Evaluation studies show good correlation with mineral content of enamel and root dentin, lesion depth, small structural changes, and chemical activity.

Laser fluorescence

Laser fluorescence and dye-enhanced laser fluorescence are alternative techniques for caries detection (Figure 2–13). The DIAGNOdent (KaVo) is a laser fluorescence device.[55] The device contains a diode laser (such as those used in computer disc readers) that emits a pulsed light of one specific wavelength (Figure 2–14). Directed onto a tooth, the light wavelength is consistent until it encounters a change in tooth structure. Changes in structure attributable to decay cause the light to refract (break up) and change color (owing to a loss of energy, which results in a longer wavelength). This changes the pulse of fluorescent light reflected back to a sensor. The device translates these changes into a qualitative reading that is subsequently displayed by the control unit and interpreted as a numeric value from 1 to 99. When the unit shows a value of less than 30, the tooth is usually sound.[56] A sound signal can be correlated to the digital readout. The device is easy to use and is calibrated to a standard, which allows comparison of current readings to those of previous

Diagnosis 31

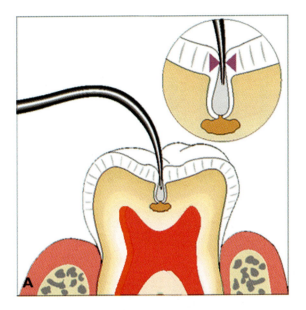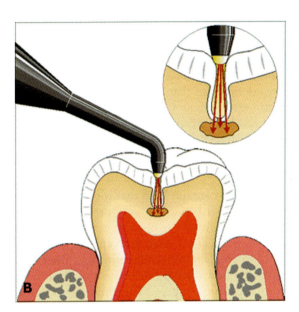

Figure 2–13. *A,* It is difficult to get an explorer to detect decay at the bottom of a fissure. *B,* A laser sensor detects the reduced density of a carious area.

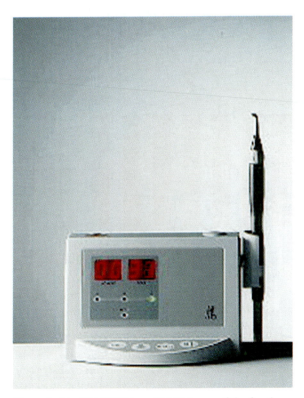

Figure 2–14. DIAGNOdent (KaVo) is one of the first laser fluorescence units for caries detection.

or subsequent patient visits. Readings are taken in a process similar to that for periodontal probing. The qualitative measurements can help track the progress of a carious lesion.

Several studies indicate good occlusal caries diagnostic accuracy. One study showed that the accuracy of DIAGNOdent was significantly better than that of radiography for occlusal lesions.[57] Another showed that the device could diagnose pit and fissure lesions with 92% accuracy and that it was 100% accurate in identifying virgin teeth (a reading of 30 or less).[56] A third investigation reported the DIAGNOdent has higher diagnostic validity than the ECM for occlusal caries and good in vitro reproducibility of findings. This suggests that laser devices could be valuable tools for the longitudinal monitoring of caries and for assessing the outcome of preventive interventions.[58]

DENTIN SENSITIVITY

In 1884, Calvo stated, "There is great need of a medicament, which while lessening the sensitivity of dentin, will not impair the vitality of the pulp."[59] Well over 100 years later, hypersensitivity, despite considerable research, is still difficult to manage.

Tooth-Colored Restoratives

Dentin physiology

Histology

One square millimeter of dentin can contain as many as 30,000 tubules (depending on the depth). The odontoblasts that line the pulpal surface of the dentin extend about 0.5 to 1 mm into each tubule. The ends of the many nerve fibers located at the pulp periphery (called C-fibers) are in synaptic connection with the odontoblasts and often extend into the tubules along the protoplasmic protrusions.[60]

The pulp contains fluid that is much like other tissue fluid with a hydrostatic pressure of about 30 mm Hg toward the outside. Because these tissues are normally covered with enamel or cementum, which are relatively impermeable, there is an extremely slow outward movement of fluid in the normally sealed tubule. The fluids hydrate the dentin and enamel, which enables different stimuli to reach the pulp.[61] However, if the enamel or cementum is removed through tooth preparation or erosion, the rate of outward fluid flow increases sharply and can result in extreme sensitivity.

Normally, exposed tubules become plugged by contents of the dentinal fluid, saliva, or gingival cervicular fluid that have become insoluble.[62] Cutting a tooth produces fine particles that contribute to the development of a smear layer on the surface and can also obstruct the tubules.[63,64] This mechanism generally accounts for sealing over 85% of the tubules.[64] Unfortunately, this layer is highly susceptible to acids. Thus, any excess acid from etching could affect the dentin after cutting. Removal of the tubular seal causes excessive stimulation of the odontoblast within the tubule.

Cause of sensitivity

Considerable research has confirmed that dentin hypersensitivity is mainly caused by the transmission of pain to the pulp through a hydrodynamic mechanism.[65–67] Based on this, it is thought that teeth with cervical sensitivity have at the dentin surface open tubules that connect to the pulp. The most common goal of treatment includes occlusion of the tubules or reduction of their diameter.

Since the nerve fiber is interwoven along the odontoblast, desiccation can trigger a pain response. Excess desiccation can draw the odontoblast into the tubule and result in a chronic inflammatory response of the odontoblastic cells (Figure 2–15).

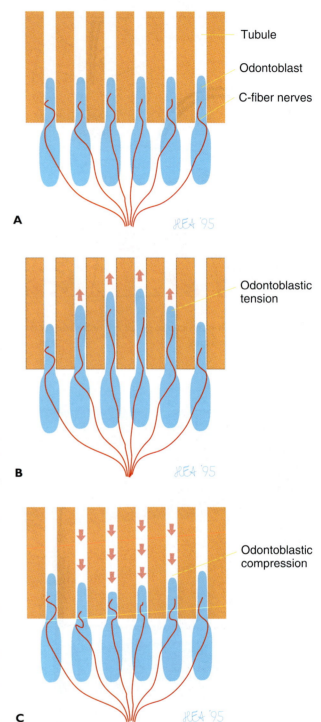

Figure 2–15. *A*, Schematic diagram illustrating normal dentin. *B*, Depiction of the way in which the hydrodynamic theory explains pain resulting from tooth exposure to air drying, cold, and hyperosmotic solutions and, *C*, from exposure to heat and hypo-osmotic solutions.

If the stimuli and sensitivity persist, the pulp either produces a barrier of secondary or sclerotic dentin to protect it, or the pulp tissues become irritated or damaged by the trauma.

C-fibers

C-fibers are nerve fibers that are myelinated, fast-conducting, and have a low threshold. Stimulating these fibers results in sharp localized pain. C-fibers are the fibers that most commonly respond to dentin sensitivity.

A-fibers

A-fibers are fibers that are unmyelinated, slow-conducting, and have a high threshold. Stimulation of A-fibers results in a dull, poorly localized pain. A-fibers are the fibers most likely to respond to chronic pulpitis and heat sensitivity.[67]

Sensitive teeth generally have open dental tubules that are wider and more numerous than the tubules in nonsensitive teeth.[68] The sensitivity is similar to that of stimulating C-fibers.

Incidence of hypersensitivity

The incidence of hypersensitive teeth in the general population is estimated as 9 to 30%.[69–71] Hypersensitivity is most common among patients between 20 and 30 years of age,[69,70] and occurs equally in males and females. Cold is the most common stimulus (74%).[72]

The most commonly sensitive teeth are the canines (25%), followed by first premolars (24%). Sensitivity occurs most commonly on facial surfaces (93%) associated with gingival recession (68%). Generally, sensitive incisors are the most painful, followed by premolars, and then molars. This descending order of sensitivity can be attributed to the thickness of enamel and cementum on these teeth. Older teeth are generally less sensitive than younger teeth. This can be attributed to the progressive deposition of secondary dentin, and the narrowing of the pulp chamber.

Common pain stimuli

Desiccation

If a dry cotton pellet placed on exposed dentin causes pain and a wet cotton pellet does not, this generally indicates that open tubules exist and pain is the result of tubular fluid movement.[73,74]

Air pressure

Short air blasts evaporate fluid and trigger a pain response. Prolonged air blasts evaporate water and condense proteins and other constituents, which produces a precipitate of debris that can close off tubules and reduce pain.[62]

Changes in osmolarity

Changes in osmolarity can alter intertubular flow and trigger pain. Sweet beverages are usually highly hyperosmotic and stimulate outward movement of tubular fluid.

Thermal stimuli

Fluid expands under heat and contracts under cold. A mechanical stimulation results because the thermal expansion of dentinal fluids is over 10 times that of the tubule wall.[75]

Treatment

Many materials have been used to treat dentin sensitivity: strontium, fluoride, formaldehyde, and oxalates are the most common.

Silver nitrate has strong protein-precipitating properties.[76] The risk with its use is that silver ions, if transmitted to the pulp, can cause pulpal inflammation. Hence, this material is generally not recommended.

Potassium oxalate used at a concentration of 3 to 10% creates calcium oxalate crystals on a tooth. These crystals have low solubility and can obstruct dentin tubules and prevent the penetration of fluids and acids.[77,78] Some research shows that the effect of this treatment is equal to or better than that of a cavity varnish, which is minimal.[79–81] Potassium oxalate is found in products such as DDS™ (O.P. Laboratories) and Protect™ (Butler, Chicago, Illinois).

Sodium fluoride promotes the deposition of calcium phosphate in fluorapatite.[82,83] It is also effective against root caries that often accompanies sensitivity.[28] However, sodium fluoride works slowly. Numerous fluoride gels (neutral pH is best) are available (eg, Prevident™ Colgate, Canton, Massachusetts). Fluoride is the treatment of choice for most mild to moderate cases of dentin sensitivity.

Strontium chloride, when combined with the phosphate in the dental tubule, produces strontium phosphate crystals that close off tubules.[76]

These crystals are the active ingredients in Sensodyne® (Block Drug Company, Jersey City, New Jersey) and Thermodent™ (Johnson and Johnson, Jersey City, New Jersey) dentifrices.

Potassium nitrate reduces dentin sensitivity without causing pulpal changes.[84] It is fast-acting and has some anesthetic properties. Potassium nitrate (usually 5%) is the most common active ingredient in over-the-counter products for tooth sensitivity (including Promise™, Sensodyne-F®, and Colgate Sensitive Maximum Strength dentifrices, Colgate Pharmaceuticals, Canton, Massachusetts). Potassium nitrate is also available in pharmacies as potash. Used in liquid form, it can help severely sensitive teeth.

Glutaraldehyde as a 5% solution in water or saline is effective in reducing acute sensitivity. It fixes the fluid in the dentin tubules and forms collagen plugs. These plugs reduce intertubular fluid flow and, therefore, dentin sensitivity. Collagen plugs also form a matrix that can later be mineralized by saliva. Glutaraldehyde is applied to sensitive dentin with a cotton pellet for 5 to 10 seconds and then rinsed off.

Many other materials are entering the market for the treatment of dentin sensitivity, such as chlorhexidine. One such product is Hemaseal (Advantage Dental Products, Lake Orion, Michigan), which is 4% chlorhexidine.

Primers and resins

A number of resin treatments have been proposed for sensitive roots. Many feel these treatments, although basically restorative, are ideal for moderate and severe cases of sensitivity. Some dentin bonding agents contain desensitizing components. For example, Gluma Desensitizer (Heraeus Kulzer, South Bend, Indiana) contains 5% glutaraldehyde.

Brännstrom was one of the first researchers to recommend filling tubules with resin.[66] The steps of the technique are as follows:

1. Treat the surface with EDTA to remove the smear layer.
2. Wash and dry the surface with water.
3. Place a free-flowing resin on the surface.
4. Remove excess water with a cotton pellet.
5. Cure.

Jensen and Doering recommended using a phosphate dentin bonding agent over the smear layer.[85] They reported higher success with this method than with sodium fluoride and strontium chloride. Fusayama used a variation of Brännstrom's method, but he acid etched the dentin for 30 to 60 seconds with a phosphoric etching solution prior to placing a resin.[86] He recommended etching as a necessary step to retain the resin coating. Currently, a number of products (eg, Seal & Protect, Dentsply/Caulk and All-Bond, Bisco, Chicago, Illinois) are available for this purpose.

Resins remain a good alternative treatment when more conservative topical agents, such as potassium nitrate, are ineffective.

CERVICAL LESIONS

There are three common causes of noncarious Class V lesions: mechanical wear, stress corrosion, and chemical erosion (Figure 2–16). It is important to determine lesion etiology prior to treatment to minimize the need for retreatment. Failure to adjust the occlusion in abfractions reduces the life span of these restorations. Failure to remove causes of erosion may result in premature wear or more erosion alongside any restoration.

Mechanical wear

Mechanical wear is the easiest to prevent. Careful home care instruction with regular follow-up dental visits can demonstrate to a patient that small amounts of force are required to remove plaque.

Mechanical wear presents as a uniform loss of tooth structure along a group of teeth (usually on the facial) caused by a wear factor, such as excessive toothbrushing. These losses usually occur on the left side of the mouth in right-handed patients and on the right side in left-handed patients. Loss of structure on a single tooth below the dentin–enamel junction is often from flossing in a sawing motion.

Stress corrosion

Stress corrosion, abfractions, or stress-induced cervical lesions (all three terms are used) are more difficult to treat since they involve both acids from the diet and the control of lateral occlusal forces. These lesions should be restored to prevent oral fluids from corroding excessively stressed portions of the

Diagnosis 35

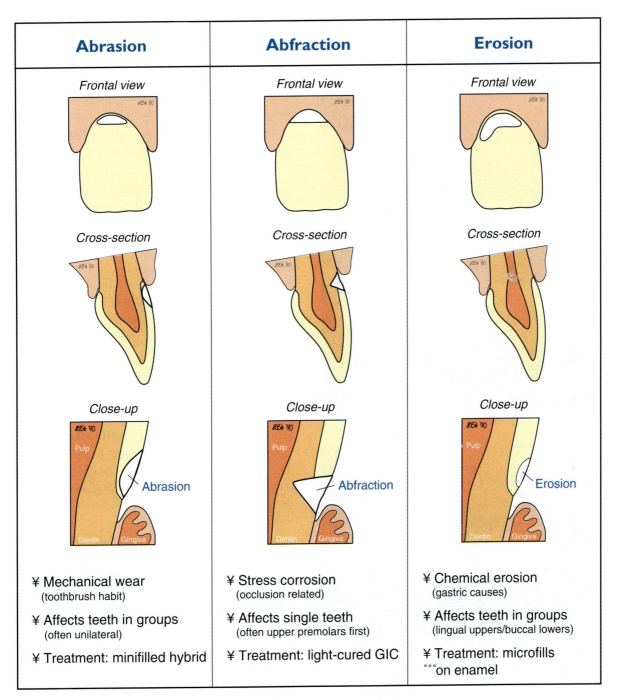

Figure 2–16. Three common types of noncarious Class V lesions.

tooth. Occlusal correction and the removal of fremitus are critical to prevent these lesions from increasing in size. Figure 2–17, *A* and *B*, show the type of lesion most often associated with lateral movement during centric loading. Notice that the premolar with the abfracted lesion has a large centric holding stop on the cusp incline rather than at the cusp tip. These lesions can threaten the

36   Tooth-Colored Restoratives

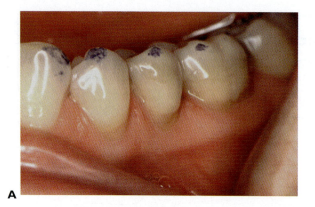

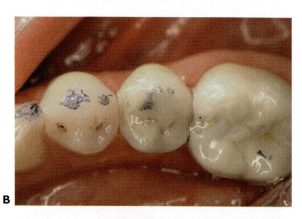

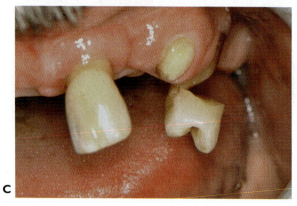

Figure 2-17. *A*, Buccal and, *B*, occlusal views showing articulator markings that indicate the patient's habitual occlusion. This is the typical clinical appearance of the kind of Class V abfraction that can rapidly develop following placement of reinforced ceramic. The occlusion was high and the opposing tooth contacted mainly on the cusp incline. This is the most common clinical finding associated with these lesions. *C*, Unaltered photograph of a Class V abfraction that had no dental intervention during its progress. At this point, the first premolar had fractured off, and the coronal portion of the clinical crown on the second premolar was threatened. (Courtesy of Dr. Roger Lawrence, Beaverton, Oregon.)

integrity of the coronal portions of the clinical crown, as illustrated in Figure 2-17, *C*. There are two types of lesions: active and static.

Active (progressive) lesions are lighter in color, have a dull (not shiny) surface, are nonsclerotic, and often are hypersensitive.

Static (arrested) lesions are darker in color, have a shiny surface, often are sclerotic and are insensitive.

When an abfraction is a progressive lesion it should be restored. Following restoration, the occlusion should be checked. A nightguard should be made if these treatments do not work.

Chemical erosion
Chemical erosion is often associated with dietary habits, such as sucking on citrus fruit. More severe cases are associated with bulimia (Figure 2-18).

Chemically eroded teeth are shiny, smooth edged, and amorphous. Erosion from gastric purging is usually seen on the lingual of the upper maxillary teeth and on the facial of the lower molar teeth. Erosion from citric acid is usually found on the facial of anterior teeth.

ANOREXIA NERVOSA AND BULIMIA
A number of medical and mental health disorders damage teeth. Among the most common disorders affecting teeth are anorexia nervosa and bulimia. Both are mental health disorders that affect eating habits.

Anorexia usually starts in early adolescence, bulimia in later adolescence. Between them, these disorders affect 1 of every 200 people between 12 and 18 years of age. The typical patient is female, white, upper middle class, intelligent, obedient, highly motivated, and popular with her peers. (Only about 10% of cases are male.) Many of these girls feel pressured to be perfect, to achieve, and to obtain parental approval. Many are overprotected by their parents and feel they have little control over their lives. Depression is often an associated symptom.

Anorexia nervosa
Anorexia nervosa is self-induced starvation characterized by an obsession with being thin. The diagnosis is made when there is intentional loss of over 20% of body mass.[87] The term anorexia means loss of appetite. This is a striking symptom

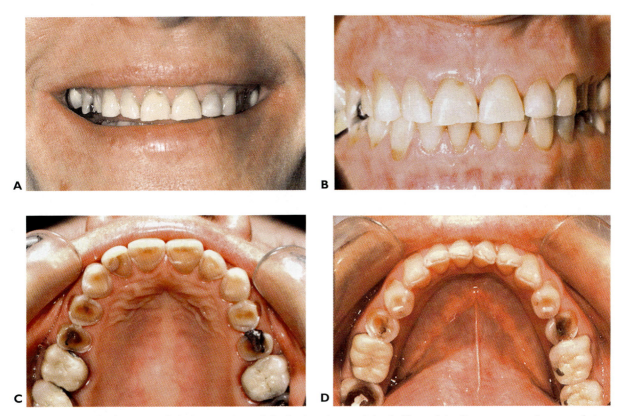

Figure 2–18. The dentition of a bulimic patient. *A*, Smile view shows minimal effects of the disease process; *B*, retracted view shows tooth damage; *C*, maxillary occlusal view shows severe loss of enamel from the maxillary central teeth as a result of the path of purging gastric contents; and *D*, the mandibular view shows less loss of enamel since the tongue usually covers these areas during purging.

of this disease: these girls refuse to eat and have no apparent hunger. Note that a subgroup of anorexics do experience hunger and resolve this with a pattern of binging and purging that often develops into a coexisting diagnosis of bulimia. An anorexic-bulimic creates weight loss through self-induced vomiting, diuretics, and laxatives.

Medical referral

Almost all anorexics deny their illness and refuse therapy; over 24% die of starvation.[88] If a dentist confronts the patient with the disorder, she often discontinues treatment. Referral to psychiatric professionals, although a delicate issue, is highly recommended. To overcome the denial barrier, it is sometimes helpful to suggest that the patient's oral problems may be caused by an ulcer. On this basis, she may accept a referral to a physician. This approach avoids alarming the patient; she does not know that the dentist is aware of her "secret." The best referral is to a physician (or therapist) who specializes in eating disorders. The clinician should be informed of the dentist's findings and concern that anorexia exists, since the patient is unlikely to disclose her disorder. In many cases, referrals are successful. In others, the denial is too strong. In the latter case, family intervention may be necessary to force the anorexic into needed treatment.

Bulimia

Bulimia designates a disorder that has been reported from before Roman times. The word is from the Greek language and means "ox hunger." It is characterized by episodes of binging followed by vomiting or purging with laxatives or diuretics. Unlike anorexia, it does not include self-starvation; in fact, bulimics are typically normal weight.

The psychological component does not have a consciously self-destructive intent.

Bulimia, an epidemic in the United States affecting 19% of women and 5% of men,[89] is commonly found among individuals 15 to 30 years of age. They are typically white, college-educated, self-supporting, and success-oriented individuals with low self-esteem. Like anorexics, they are perfectionists and are obsessed with achievement. Bulimics often lack self-control and are impulsive; they often battle alcoholism and kleptomania (stealing). Bulimics generally hide their disorder by arranging their schedules to allow time to binge and purge privately. Some bulimics binge and purge numerous times during the course of a day.[90]

Oral manifestations

Dental destruction caused by bulimia is generally the most common nonreversible manifestation of these disorders. Hellstrom first described the oral effects of bulimia-associated purging in 1974.[91] He described the loss of enamel and dentin along the lingual surfaces of teeth caused by the chemical and mechanical effects of regurgitating gastric contents; he called the condition "perimylolysis."

Hellstrom noted maxillary teeth were the most severely affected, since the accumulation of hydrochloric acid on the papillae of the tongue increases acid contact there. The extent of perimylolysis varies from a mild polish on the lingual surfaces to extreme erosion of the facial, occlusal, and the lingual aspects of the teeth. In severe cases, pulp exposure can result. The mandibular teeth are protected by the lips, cheeks, and tongue position (see Figure 2–18).

Systemic effects on oral tissues

Related vitamin deficiencies can affect oral tissues. Riboflavin deficiencies have caused glossitis, papillary atrophy, paleness of lips, and cheilosis. Nicotinic acid deficiency causes a burning sensation of the tongue and leads to ulceration of the gingival papillae. Pyridoxine deficiency causes angular cheilosis.

Restorative treatment
Palliative treatment

Patients with perimylolysis should rinse with a solution of sodium bicarbonate to reduce oral acidity after purging and should be told not to brush their teeth immediately after regurgitation, since this may burnish acids into the enamel and increase dental erosion.[87] A daily application of 0.05 to 0.20% neutral fluoride rinse can slow the erosion. Antacid tablets may increase salivary flow and help neutralize acids. Eating cheese counteracts xerostomia, by increasing the pH of the mouth, and provides needed calcium.

Restorative treatment

Treat areas of lingual erosion by bonding a microfilled composite to the exposed enamel and dentin surfaces. Macrofills and glass ionomers are more susceptible to dissolution from gastric contents if the disorder continues after treatment. Bruxism often accompanies the disorder; a nightguard helps protect the teeth.

REFERENCES

1. Wilson AD, McLean JW. Treatment of early carious lesions. In: Glass-ionomer cement. Chicago: Quintessence, 1988:179–95.

2. Kidd EAM. The histopathology of enamel caries in young and old permanent teeth. Br Dent J 1983;155: 196–8.

3. Kuboki Y, Ohgushi K, Fusayama T. Collagen biochemistry of the two layers of carious dentin. J Dent Res 1977;56:1233–4.

4. Bernick S, Warren O, Baker RF. Electron microscopy of carious dentin. J Dent Res 1954;33:20–6.

5. Tukuma S, Kurahashi Y. Electron microscopy of various zones in a carious lesion in human dentin. Arch Oral Biol 1962;7:439–53.

6. Masseler M, Pawiak J. The affected and infected pulp. Oral Surg Oral Med Oral Pathol 1977;43:929–47.

7. Ohgushi K, Fusayama T. Electron microscopic structure of the two layers of carious dentin. J Dent Res 1977;54:1019–26.

8. Eidelman E, Finn SB, Koulourides T. Remineralization of carious dentin treated with calcium hydroxide. J Dent Child 1965;32:218–25.

9. Shovelton D. A study of deep carious dentine. Int Dent J 1968;18:392–405.

10. Miyauchi H, Iwaku M, Fusayama T. Physiological recalcification of carious dentin. Bull Tokyo Med Dent Univ 1978;25:169–79.

11. Kato S, Fusayama T. Recalcification of artificially decalcified dentin in vivo. J Dent Res 1970;49:1060–7.

12. Massler M. Therapy conducive to healing of the human pulp. Oral Surg Oral Med Oral Pathol 1972;34:122–30.

13. Miller W, Masseler M. Permeability and staining of active and arrested lesions in dentin. Br Dent J 1961;112:187–97.

14. Wirthlin M. Acid-reacting stains, softening and bacteria invasion in human carious dentin. J Dent Res 1970;49:42–6.

15. Foreman FJ. Sealant prevalence and indication in a young military population. J Am Dent Assoc 1994;125:182–4, 186.

16. Eriksen HM. Has caries merely been postponed? Acta Odontol Scand 1998;56:173–5.

17. Pitts NB, Rensen CE. Monitoring the behavior of posterior proximal carious lesions by image analysis or serial standardized bitewing radiographs. Br Dent J 1987;162:15–21.

18. Stahl JW, Katz RV. Occlusal dental caries incidence and implications for sealant programs in a US college student population. J Public Health Dent 1993;53:212–8.

19. Ogaard B. [Continued reduction of incidence of caries among children and young adults in USA]. Nor Tannlaegeforen Tid 1989;99:758–62.

20. Brown LJ, Wall TP, Lazar V. Trends in total caries experience: permanent and primary teeth. J Am Dent Assoc 2000;131:223–31.

21. Backer-Dirks O. Longitudinal dental caries study in children 9–15 years of age. Arch Oral Biol 1961;6 (Spec Suppl):94–108.

22. Berman DS, Slack GL. Dental caries in English school children: a longitudinal study. Br Dent J 1973;133:529–38.

23. Berman DS, Slack GL. Caries progression and activity in approximal tooth surfaces: a longitudinal study. Br Dent J 1973;134:51–7.

24. Berman DS, Slack GL. Susceptibility of tooth surfaces to carious attack: a longitudinal study. Br Dent J 1973;134:135–9.

25. Marthaler TM, Wiesner PK. Rapidity of penetration of radiolucent areas through mesial enamel of the first permanent molars. Helv Odontol Acta 1973;17:19–26.

26. Zamir T, Fisher D, Sharrar Y. A longitudinal radiographic study of the rate of spread of human approximal dental caries. Arch Oral Biol 1976;21:523–6.

27. Granath L, Kahlmeter A, Matsson L, Schroder V. Progression of proximal enamel caries in early teens related to caries activity. Acta Odontol Scand 1980;38:247–51.

28. Seichter U. Root surface caries: a critical literature review. J Am Dent Assoc 1987;115:305–10.

29. Lawrence HP, Hunt RJ, Beck JD, Davies GM. Five-year incidence rates and intraoral distribution of root caries among community-dwelling older adults. Caries Res 1996;30:169–79.

30. Louw AJ, Carstens IL, Hartshorne JE, van Wyk Kotze TE. Root caries in a sample of elderly persons. J Dent Assoc S Afr 1993;48:183–7.

31. Joshi A, Douglass CW, Feldman H, et al. Consequences of success: Do more teeth translate into more disease and utilization? J Public Health Dent 1996;56:190–7.

32. Vehkalahti MM, Paunio IK. Occurrence of root caries in relation to dental health behavior. J Dent Res 1988;67:911–4.

33. Locker D, Slade GD, Leake JL. Prevalence of and factors associated with root decay in older adults in Canada. J Dent Res 1989;68:768–72.

34. Beck JD, Hunt RJ, Hand JS, Field HM. Root caries: prevalence of root and coronal caries in a non-institutionalized older population. J Am Dent Assoc 1985;111:964–7.

35. Mortimer KV. Some histological features of fissure caries in enamel. In: Hardwick JL, Dustin J-P, Meld HR, eds. Advances in fluorine research and dental caries prevention. Vol. 2. Proceedings of the 10th Congress of the European Organization for Research on fluorine and dental caries prevention. Oxford, England: ORCA, and New York: Pergamon Press, 1964.

36. Shaw L, Murray JJ. Inter-examiner and intra-examiner reproducibility in clinical and radiographic diagnosis. Int Dent J 1975;25:280–8.

37. Kidd EAM. The diagnosis and management of the "early" carious lesion in permanent teeth. Dent Update 1984;11:69–78.

38. Sewerin IB. Radiographic identification of simulated carious lesions in relation to fillings with Adaptic radiopaque. Scand J Dent Res 1980;88:377–81.

39. Hardison JD, Rafferty-Parker D, Mitchell RJ, Bean LR. Radiolucent halos associated with radiopaque composite resin restorations. J Am Dent Assoc 1989;118:595–7.

40. Wenzel A. Digital radiography and caries diagnosis. Dentomaxillofac Radiol 1998;27:3–11.

41. Keem S, Elbaum M. Wavelet representations for monitoring changes in teeth imaged with digital imaging fiber-optic transillumination. IEEE Trans Med Imaging 1997;16:653–63.

42. Schneiderman A, Elbaum M, Shultz T, et al. Assessment of dental caries with digital imaging fiber-optic transillumination (DIFOTI): in vitro study. Caries Res 1997;31:103–10.

43. Boston DW, Graver HT. Histological study of an acid red caries-disclosing dye. Oper Dent 1989;14:186–92.

44. List G, Lommel TJ, Tilk MA, Murdoch HG. The use of a dye in caries identification. Quintessence Int 1987;18:343–5.

45. Fusayama T. Two layers of carious dentin: diagnosis and treatment. Oper Dent 1979;4:63–70.

46. Kuboki Y, Liu CF, Fusayama T. Mechanism of differential staining in carious dentin. J Dent Res 1983;62:713–4.

47. Fusayama T. Clinical guide for removing caries using a caries-detecting solution. Quintessence Int 1989;19:397–401.

48. Styner D, Kuyinu E, Turner G. Addressing the caries dilemma: detection and intervention with a disclosing agent. Gen Dent 1996;44:446–9.

49. Anderson MH, Charbeneau GT. A comparison of digital and optical criteria for detecting carious dentin. J Prosthet Dent 1985;53:643–6.

50. Kidd EA, Joyston-Bechal S, Smith MM, et al. The use of a caries detector dye in cavity preparation. Br Dent J 1989;167:132–4.

51. Boston DW, Graver HT. Histobacteriological analysis of acid red dye-stainable dentin found beneath intact amalgam restorations. Oper Dent 1994;19:65–9.

52. Yip HK, Stevenson AG, Beeley JA. The specificity of caries detector dyes in cavity preparation. Br Dent J 1994;176:417–21.

53. Kidd EA, Joyston-Bechal S, Beighton D. The use of a caries detector dye during cavity preparation: a microbiological assessment. Br Dent J 1993;174:245–8.

54. Ashley PF, Blinkhorn AS, Davies RM. Occlusal caries diagnosis: an in vitro histological validation of the Electronic Caries Monitor (ECM) and other methods. J Dent 1998;26:83–8.

55. Eggertsson H, Analoui M, van der Veen M, et al. Detection of early interproximal caries in vitro using laser fluorescence, dye-enhanced laser fluorescence and direct visual examination. Caries Res 1999;33:227–33.

56. Ross G. Caries diagnosis with the DIAGNOdent laser: a user's product evaluation. Ont Dent 1999;76:21–4.

57. Shi XQ, Welander U, Angmar-Mansson B. Occlusal caries detection with KaVo DIAGNOdent and radiography: an in vitro comparison. Caries Res 2000;34:151–8.

58. Lussi A, Imwinkelried S, Pitts N, et al. Performance and reproducibility of a laser fluorescence system for detection of occlusal caries in vitro. Caries Res 1999;33:261–6.

59. Calvo P. Treatment of sensitive dentin. Dent Cosmos 1884;26:139–41.

60. Johnson DC. Innervation of teeth: qualitative, quantitative, and developmental assessment. J Dent Res 1985;64(Spec Issue):555–63.

61. Gysi A. An attempt to explain the sensitiveness of dentin. Br J Dent Sci 1900;43:865–8.

62. Kleinberg I. Dentinal hypersensitivity. Part I: the biologic basis of the condition. Compend Cont Educ Dent 1986;7:182–7.

63. Anderson DJ, Ronning GA. Dye diffusion in human dentin. Arch Oral Biol 1962;7:505–12.

64. Pashley DH. Dentin–predentin complex and its permeability: physiologic overview. J Dent Res 1985;64(Spec Issue):613–20.

65. Berman LH. Dentinal sensation and hypersensitivity: a review of mechanisms and treatment alternatives. J Periodontol 1985;56:216–22.

66. Brännstrom M. A hydrodynamic mechanism in the transmission of pain producing stimuli through the

dentin. In: Anderson DJ, ed. Sensory mechanisms in dentin. Oxford: Oxford Press, 1962:73–9.

67. Nahri MVO. The characteristics of intradental sensory units and their responses to stimulation. J Dent Res 1985;64(Spec Issue):564–71.

68. Absi EG, Adams D, Addy M. The patency of dentinal tubules in hypersensitive and nonsensitive cervical dentine [abstract]. Br Soc Dent Res 1986.

69. Flynn J, Galloway R, Orchardson R. The incidence of 'hypersensitive' teeth in the West of Scotland. J Dent Res 1985;13:230–6.

70. Graf H, Galasse R. Morbidity, prevalence, and intraoral distribution of hypersensitive teeth [abstract]. J Dent Res 1977;56(Spec Issue):A162.

71. Jensen AL. Hypersensitivity controlled by iontophoresis: double-blind clinical investigation. J Am Dent Assoc 1964;68:216–25.

72. Orchardson R, Collins WJN. Clinical features of hypersensitive teeth. Br Dent J 1987;162:253–6.

73. Brännstrom M, Astrom A. A study on the mechanism of pain elicited from dentin. J Dent Res 1964;43:619.

74. Mjor IA, Pindberg JJ. Histology of the human tooth. Copenhagen: Langkjaers Boytrykkeri, 1973.

75. Brännstrom M, Linden LA, Astrom A. The hydrodynamics of the dentinal tubule and pulp fluid: a discussion of its significance in relation to dentinal sensitivity. Caries Res 1967;1:310–7.

76. Anderson DJ, Matthews B. An investigation into the reputed desensitizing effect of applying silver nitrate and strontium chloride to human dentin. Arch Oral Biol 1966;11:1129–35.

77. Pashley DH, Depew DD. Effects of the smear layer, Copalite, and oxalate on microleakage. Oper Dent 1986;11:95–102.

78. Chan DCN, Jensen ME. Dentin permeability to phosphoric acid: effect of treatment with bonding resin. Dent Mater 1986;2:251–6.

79. Sandoval VA, Cooley RL, Barnwell SE, Dale RA. Evaluation of potassium oxalate as a cavity liner [abstract]. J Dent Res 1989;68(Spec Issue):208.

80. Pashley DH, Livingston MJ, Reeder OW, Horner J. Effects of the degree of tubule occlusion on the permeability of human dentine in vitro. Arch Oral Biol 1978;23:1127–33.

81. Cooley RL, Sandoval VA. Effectiveness of potassium oxalate treatment on dentin hypersensitivity. Gen Dent 1989;37:330–3.

82. Hoyt WH, Bibby BF. Use of sodium fluoride for desensitizing dentin. J Dent Res 1943;22:208.

83. Lefkowitz W, Bodecker CF. Sodium fluoride: its effect on the dental pulp. Ann Dent 1945;3:141.

84. Hodosh M. A superior desensitizer—potassium nitrate. J Am Dent Assoc 1974;88:831–2.

85. Jensen ME, Doering JV. A comparative study of two clinical techniques for treatment of root surface hypersensitivity. Gen Dent 1987;35:128–32.

86. Fusayama T. Etiology and treatment of sensitive teeth. Quintessence Int 1988;19:921–5.

87. Knewitz JL, Drisko CL. Anorexia nervosa and bulimia: a review. Compend Cont Educ Dent 1989;9:244–7.

88. Levinson N. Anorexia and bulimia: eating functions gone awry. N Y J Dent 1986;56:90–4.

89. Brown NW. Medical consequences of eating disorders. South J Med 1985;78:403–5.

90. Clark NP, Schumancher JL. Bulimia nervosa: recognition and dental treatment. Fla Dent J 1986;57:17–9.

91. Hellstrom I. Anorexia nervosa—odontologic problem. Swed Dent J 1974;67:253–69.

CHAPTER 3

GLASS IONOMERS

The scientific mind does not so much provide the right answers as ask the right questions.

Claude Lévi-Strauss

THE FIRST DENTAL CEMENTS

The development of amalgam, gold, and porcelain restorative materials in the mid-1800s stimulated the creation of dental cements. In 1855, Sorel introduced zinc oxychloride cement, the first popular dental cement. In 1875, Pierce and Flagg originated zinc oxide eugenol cement, which became popular because of its improved effect.

Zinc phosphate cement

In 1870, Pierce introduced zinc oxide–phosphoric acid cement, which replaced oxychloride and oxysulfate cements, because it caused less irritation to the pulp and had greater durability.[1] The work of Ames and Fleck established the modern-day zinc phosphate cement.[2,3] By the turn of the century these cements were used to lute gold and porcelain crowns and inlays to teeth, in addition to serving as temporary filling materials and cavity bases.

In 1907, Taggart introduced the cast gold restoration; its widespread use popularized dental cements. In 1873, Thomas Fletcher introduced the first tooth-colored filling material, silicate cement. This cement did not become popular until 1904, however, when Steenbock introduced an improved version (Steenbock P. Improvements in and relating to the manufacture of a material designed for the production of cement. British Patents 15176, 15181. 1904). In 1908, Schoenbeck developed silicate cement that contained fluoride.[4]

By about 1925, three basic types of cement were widely available: zinc phosphate, zinc oxide eugenol, and silicate, all of which mechanically attached inlays, crowns, posts, bridges, and orthodontic bands. They were also used under amalgams as liners and bases. Over the next 50 years, these materials remained relatively unchanged.

Although as early as 1902 Fleck remarked, "The ideal cement will be found outside the phosphate class,"[3] it took 60 years to improve on the existing preparations.

Polyacid cements

In 1963, Dennis Smith, a British researcher, developed the first polyelectrolyte cement that set by the reaction of metal oxides and acidic water-soluble polymers.[4,5] The first such cement, now known as zinc polycarboxylate cement, used a polyacrylate liquid and a zinc oxide powder. The first commercial polycarboxylate was Durelon®, developed by Dr. Robert Purmann of ESPE (ESPE Dental-Medizin, Seefeld, Germany).

Polyacrylic acid was chosen because of its ability to bind to calcium and to hydrogen bond with organic polymers such as collagen.[6,7] In addition to their low toxicity and good physical properties, a major feature of the polyacrylate cements was adhesion to tooth structure.

Glass-ionomer cements

Although they provided improved properties, zinc polycarboxylate and zinc phosphate cements were opaque and unesthetic. The British Laboratory of the Government Chemist (BLGC), which is the British equivalent of the United States National Institutes of Health (NIH), proceeded to improve on the properties of the dental silicate cement. In 1965 and 1966, Alan Wilson and his colleagues at BLGC examined cements prepared by mixing dental silicate glass powder with aqueous solutions of various organic acids, including polyacrylic acid. Formulations using zinc-containing glass ceramics and silicate cement powders were investigated for years. Wilson and Brian Kent established that the setting mechanism for these materials was an acid–base reaction between the glass powder and phosphoric acid, which formed a salt. With this knowledge, they worked with Smith's adhesive polyacid liquid and the more esthetic silicate powder to develop a glass-ionomer cement. Simply put, today's glass-ionomer cements combine polyacrylic acid liquid with silicate cement powder, yielding a material that demonstrates the best properties of both (Table 3–1).

In 1972, Wilson and Kent produced more reactive glasses.[8] By adding tartaric acid accelerators and by modifying the ratio of aluminum oxide to silicon dioxide (Al_2O_3:SiO_2) in the silicate glass, they made the first glass-ionomer cement.[9] However, the liquid's short shelf life, due to gelation, was a major problem. The following year, Jurecic discovered that the gelation was caused by intrachain hydrogen bonding, which could be prevented by using acrylic acid-itaconic acid copolymers.

The first commercial cement, aluminosilicate polyacrylate-1 (ASPA-1) was clinically tested by British dentist John McLean. He waited 20 minutes for the material to set hard.[10] In addition, because of its high fluoride content, the cement was extremely opaque and had poor esthetics; but, it was a start. Despite its clinical shortcomings, ASPA-1 was well retained in Class V erosion lesions without need for a cavity preparation. McLean developed the clinical techniques for the material and was the first to demonstrate the caries resistance of the enamel margins around ASPA-1 restorations. Later versions of ASPA contained tartaric acid and a synthesized copolymer of acrylic and itaconic acid that proved stable in a 50% aqueous solution. This material was first marketed in 1975.

In 1979 and 1980, there was a steady flow of new products, including Fuji Ionomer (GC International, Tokyo, Japan), Chemfil (Dentsply International Inc., Konstanz, Germany), and Ketac-fil (ESPE). ESPE washed the glass powder with acid to remove calcium ions from the surface, thus delaying initial set and giving excellent working and setting characteristics. ESPE was also the first company to use copolymers of acrylic and maleic acid, which is a stronger and more reactive acid, to accelerate setting. With these improved glass ionomers, the dental profession began to use these cements routinely.

GLASS-METAL IONOMER MIXTURES

In 1957, Massler published an article about using a restorative of amalgam powder mixed with zinc phosphate cement for pulp capping.[11] In 1962, Mahler and Armen showed that adding amalgam alloy to zinc phosphate cement improved the transverse strength, solubility, and disintegration of the resulting material compared with using zinc phosphate cement alone.[12]

In the early 1980s, prior to the introduction of radiopaque glass ionomers, lucent glass ionomer powders were mixed with amalgam powders to produce glass-metal ionomer mixtures that are radiopaque yet maintain many of the favorable properties of the glass ionomers.[7] Generally, this is done by mixing amalgam powder (12 to 14% by volume) into a glass-ionomer restorative powder. These restoratives are called admixtures. In the United States, some clinicians call this combination "miracle mix" and have made metal-ionomer mixtures popular as core buildups, bases, retrofills, endodontic sealers, and crown repairs.

Some laboratory studies indicate that adding alloy powder to the glass-ionomer cement improves compressive strength, tensile strength, cohesive bonding strength to teeth, and solubility.

The major material disadvantage of the glass-metal ionomer mixture is the difficulty of achieving a homogeneous mix of silver and glass throughout the restorative. In addition, the metal particles are not well bonded to the set material, which results in erosion and increased wear as the poorly

Table 3–1. Components of Conventional Acid–Base Cements

	Phosphoric Acid Liquid	Polyacrylic Acid Liquid
Zinc oxide powder	Zinc phosphate cement	Polycarboxylate cement
Silicate glass powder	Silicate cement	Glass-ionomer cement

attached metal particles are plucked from the surface. Clinical problems also result from moisture contamination during setting.

Glass-metal ionomer mixtures are contraindicated for large posterior restorations in adult teeth since these admixtures undergo heavy wear and fatigue fracture. These materials are available in both powder-liquid and capsules.

CERAMIC-METAL GLASS IONOMERS

In 1987, the first cermet (ceramic + metal) glass ionomer, Ketac-Silver® (ESPE), was introduced. ESPE researchers McLean and Gasser developed these ionomers filled with sintered metal and glass compositions.[13] Their intention was to improve the bond between the metal filler and the glass cement powder and produce a material with better wear properties. Using a silver-impregnated coating around the aluminosilicate glass powder lowered the coefficient of friction, thereby significantly improving abrasion resistance.

Cermet ionomers are prepared by sintering (at 800°C) compressed pellets made from a mixture of fine metal powders and ion-leachable glass fillers.[13–15] The sintered metal and glass frit is then ground into a fine filler, which results in ceramic-metal particles of fused metal and ground glass. The bond between these metals and glass particles results in a seal that is similar to that of a porcelain-fused-to-metal restoration. The resulting metal-fused-to-glass filler particles can be reacted with polyacid copolymers to form an ionomer restorative. The most suitable metals for these cermet ionomers are gold and silver.

Ketac-Silver, which has pure silver powder fused to a 3.5-μm (average size) ion-leachable calcium aluminum fluorosilicate glass powder, is mainly available in capsules. The silver content, by weight, is 50% in the powder and 40% in the set material. In addition, 5% titanium dioxide by weight is added to improve the color. However, the silver discolors the surrounding tooth structure, posing a major clinical problem. Discoloration results from migration of the free photographic emulsion silver particles out of the material to penetrate the surrounding tooth structure. After a period, these free silver particles form silver oxide, which blackens tooth structure. This discoloration is inorganic and cannot be bleached out. In anterior teeth, this discoloration could be so severe as to require full-coverage restoration.

Silver cermets have also been used as a buildup or core material; however, because of their low fracture toughness, they often fail in stress-bearing areas. These materials should be reserved for non–stress-bearing buildups in posterior teeth that are to be treated with full-coverage restorations. These materials have poor esthetics when used to build up teeth prior to partial coverage restoration, because the darkness of the material, like amalgam, causes the color value of the tooth to drop greatly. Gold cermet cements were also made; however, the high cost of these materials made them unmarketable. The gold cermet behaved clinically like silver cermet except that it did not discolor the tooth and instead looked like a gold foil.

RESIN-MODIFIED GLASS IONOMERS

Resin-modified glass-ionomer materials attempt to combine the best properties of composite resins and glass ionomers. They have some cariostatic properties, a low thermal expansion, and the hydrophilic qualities of the glass-ionomer cements. The polymerizing resin matrix of resin-modified glass ionomers improves the fracture toughness, wear resistance, and polish of these materials compared with conventional glass ionomers.

Antonucci and co-workers introduced the light-cured glass-ionomer cements in 1988. Vitrebond, the first commercially viable cement of this type, was developed by Mitra in 1989. These early modified resin ionomers had two setting mechanisms: a light-intiated polymerization reaction and a glass ionomer acid–base reaction. In 1992, Mitra added the first autocured resin capabilities to resin-modified glass-ionomer cements. These cements contained additional chemical initiators to allow the resin to polymerize without light. These materials are available in auto- and dual-cure forms. The dual-cured materials have three setting reactions: photocure, autocure, and acid–base reaction between the glass-ionomer powder and the polyacid.

Regardless of their curing mechanism, the resin-modified glass-ionomer cements develop strength more rapidly because of the resin polymerization component of their setting reaction. One problem with these materials is that the modified polyacrylic acid is less soluble in water. Therefore, hydroxyethyl methacrylate (HEMA) must be added as a co-solvent to avoid phase separation of the resin from the glass-ionomer components. When HEMA and similar hydrophilic monomers are added to these materials, the set material can swell in water, increase in volume, and weaken.[16] In general, the greater the amount of HEMA incorporated into a material, the greater the swelling and, usually, the greater the reduction in strength.[17] These materials have been improved to the point that their mixtures are now stable in the mouth.

CLASSIFICATION OF GLASS IONOMERS

Glass ionomers are part of a large group of materials that set through an acid–base reaction in the presence of water. Historically, these materials have been referred to as cements, and they are involved in a variety of powders and liquids. Glass ionomers originally got their name from the glass filler and ionic polymer matrix used to make them. They have a unique matrix that forms ionic bonds to the glass filler and tooth structure. A number of classification systems have been proposed for ionomers. For the sake of simplicity, just two are explored here.

Traditional classification

When glass ionomers were first introduced, the most common classification was an application-oriented I-to-IV numbering system for autocured glass ionomers,[18] with an additional class V to represent light-cured glass ionomers. Type I, for luting inlays, onlays, crowns, and bridges, has a film thickness of 20 μm or less. Type II, for restorations in low–stress-bearing areas, has a film thickness up to 45 μm. Type III, for sealing pits and fissures, has a film thickness of 25 to 35 μm. Type IV, which includes metal-reinforced ionomers, is used for high–stress-bearing areas; film thickness is 45 μm and over. The advantage of this classification system is that it is simple; the disadvantages are that it is limited descriptively and leaves out a variety of products.

Classification by use

Alternatively, if ionomers are classified by use, eight classes are formed.

1. Glass-ionomer luting cements are used as luting agents. They are autocured.
2. Glass-ionomer restoratives are used as restorative materials. The major difference between luting and restorative glass ionomers is that the restorative is available in more shades, has a higher filler load, and has a much higher film thickness. They are autocured.
3. Glass-metal ionomer mixtures are intended for bases and buildups. These are sometimes called admixtures. They are autocured.
4. Cermet-ionomers are ionomers containing metal-fused-to-glass particles. Neither the glass-metal nor the cermet-ionomers are tooth-colored. They are autocured.
5. Glass-ionomer liners are rapid-setting radiopaque materials for dentin liners under composites and amalgams. They are light-cured.
6. Glass-ionomer bases are intended as bases under other restoratives. These materials are generally stronger but sometimes pulpally compatible than lining cements. Glass-ionomer bases are often recommended when a bulk of material is needed in stress-bearing restorations. They are autocured.
7. Glass-ionomer sealants are for sealing pits and fissures. They are autocured.
8. Resin-modified glass ionomers include light- and dual-cured glass ionomers. The term light-cured ionomer is technically incorrect, since an acid–base reaction like that of a glass ionomer cannot be light-cured or polymerized.

In dental literature, the term glass-ionomer cement frequently refers to all eight types of materials. For clarity, the term is used here when these materials are discussed as a class.

COMPONENTS OF IONOMER SYSTEMS

Glass-ionomer cements are among the most useful and versatile of conventional luting agents. Early glass ionomers contained only two components: polyacrylic acid dissolved in water and a calcium aluminosilicate glass powder. Newer materials contain acid accelerators and hardeners in the liquid, and metal additives in the powder, which alters their clinical properties.

Glass-ionomer liquids

The major component of all glass-ionomer liquids is water, usually in an aqueous solution of polyacid copolymer. Because of their water content, glass ionomers are always susceptible to desiccation. The liquids in glass-ionomer cements belong to the chemical family of organolithic macromolecular materials, a component of other cements (eg, as concrete use in construction).

The liquid of most glass ionomers is a 35 to 65% aqueous solution containing copolymers of polyacrylic acid. The early liquids were made solely of a 50% aqueous solution of polyacrylic acid. These solutions were unsatisfactory because they gelled in 10 to 30 minutes. Scientists thought the liquid formed hydrogen bonds between the polyacid chains.

It was later discovered that using copolymers containing acrylic and itaconic acids improved both stability and shelf life. Copolymers containing acrylic, fumaric, and maleic acid have also been used. Many of these polyacid chains have a molecular weight of about 56,000 (Figure 3–1).[18]

Because conventional glass ionomers use the polyacid in liquid form, they are hydrous. These large molecular weight liquids can form complexes and thicken in the bottle, which reduces their shelf life. Later materials used freeze- or vacuum-dried polyacid to improve shelf life. These dried polyacid powders are usually added to the glass fillers. Since the polyacid is stored in dried form, the materials are anhydrous. Materials using both hydrous and anhydrous forms of polyacid in the same product are called semihydrous. This combination provides intermediate liquid viscosities for luting and speeds the initial slow set associated with the anhydrous materials. As expected, the shelf life is somewhere between the hydrous and anhydrous forms.

Some manufacturers refer to anhydrous glass ionomers as water-hardened, and hydrous as conventional. Clinicians are often confused by these terms because they are not descriptive of formulation or intended use. In addition, the terms wrongly imply superiority for the former. Both have similar physical properties. In this text, the terms hydrous, anhydrous, and semihydrous are used to describe how the polyacrylic acid is stored. *Warning: Leaving the top off a bottle of an anhydrous or semihydrous glass-ionomer cement powder can cause moisture contamination and initiate a partial setting reaction.*

How glass-ionomer cement liquids work

Polyacid copolymer liquids are thought to bond by an ionic interaction between the negatively charged polyacid chains of the ionomer matrix and the positively charged calcium on the tooth surface. Polyacids also form hydrogen bonds and undergo ion exchange in the collagen and inorganic components of the tooth structure, particularly to calcium, carboxylate, and phosphate; they chemically bond to the restorative material and the tooth structure.[9] The hypothesized mechanism is illustrated in Figure 3–2.[9,18,19] Unlike most resin bonding systems, these polyacid-based systems are hydrophilic and can maintain their bond in the presence of moisture.

Mono-acid accelerators

One of the problems with the early glass ionomers was their slow set. Some smaller molecular weight organic acids (eg, salicyclic acid, citric acid, and tartaric acid) were found to act as accelerators. Of these, the stereo isomer D-tartaric acid (the optically active, naturally occurring form) was the most effective (Figure 3–3). Used alone, none of these acids forms a cement.[20]

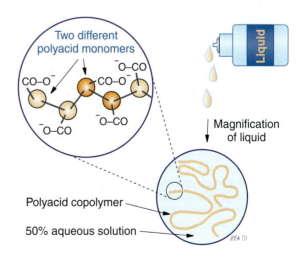

Figure 3–1. Schematic illustration of an aqueous polyacrylic acid copolymer liquid with thousands of carboxyl groups (MW = 56,000) reacting with the glass-ionomer powder.

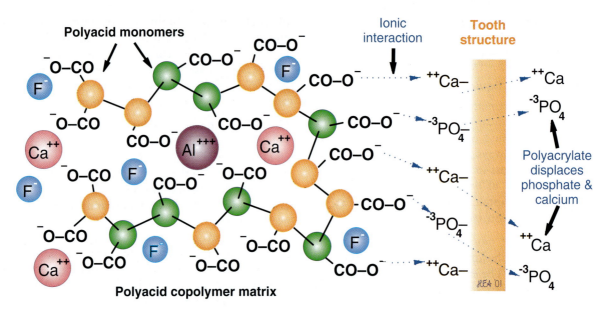

Figure 3–2. Mechanism by which polyacid copolymers ionically bond to glass fillers and tooth structure.

Currently, almost all polyacid liquids commercially available contain D-tartaric acid (usually 5 to 10%) to shorten the setting time (but not the working time). Tartaric acid also acts to harden and improve compressive and tensile strengths.[9] Tartaric acid can be freeze-dried and placed in glass powder. The resulting powder is mixed with distilled water or a dilute 30% solution of tartaric acid (eg, Ketac-Cem®, ESPE). These anhydrous ionomers have an unlimited shelf life.

Tartaric acid is thought to work by actively removing aluminum and calcium ions (in that order) from the glass. Since tartaric acid is a free bimolecular acid, it is not sterically hindered, as is the polyacrylic copolymer; that is, it can bridge the gaps between the unreacted metal ions to help cross-link and stabilize the matrix gelation. Smaller polyacids are thought to aid in bonding to any trivalent ion, such as aluminum, that might have difficulty attaching to the larger polyacid chain at three points.

Glass-ionomer powders

Early glass powder
Efforts were directed toward mixing the polyacrylic acids used in polycarboxylate cements with conventional silicate glass powder. Silicate powder has poor reactivity, since it was designed for use with orthophosphoric acid, which is highly reactive. The result was a weak, slow-setting cement. The development of more reactive glass powders made the early glass ionomers viable restoratives.

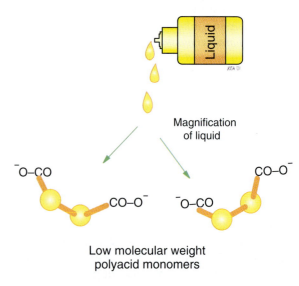

Figure 3–3. Tartaric acid has only two carboxyl groups to react with the glass-ionomer powder.

The typical glass in a glass ionomer is made by fusing quartz, alumina, cryolite, fluorite, aluminum trifluoride, and aluminum phosphate. Glass-ionomer fillers typically contain by weight 15.7 to 20.1% calcium fluoride (CaF_2), 35.2 to 41.9% silicon dioxide (SiO_2), 20.1 to 28.6% aluminum oxide (Al_2O_3), 3.8 to 12.1% aluminum phosphate ($AlPO_4$), 1.6 to 8.9% aluminum fluoride (AlF_3), and 4.1 to 9.3% sodium fluoride (NaF). The material is about 20% fluoride by weight.

The reactivity of the glass is partly related to the temperature to which it is raised during fusion. Generally, the quartz, alumina, metal fluorides, and metal phosphates are heated together to 1100° to 1300°C for 40 to 150 minutes (Figure 3–4, A).[9]

The melt is then poured onto a steel tray to cool. When the melt is dull red, the mixture is quenched in water and becomes a milky white glass (Figure 3–4, B). This frit is converted into cement powder by ball milling, then passing through a number of meshes, typically 45 μm for restorative materials and 20 μm for luting materials. The average glass particle size is well under 20 μm for the glass-ionomer luting agents.[9,19]

Volume changes in powders

To measure a consistent amount of glass-ionomer powder, it is important to establish a consistent routine of shaking and tapping, or both, because the powder settles. Figure 3–4, C and D, illustrate that the volume of a single bottle of glass-ionomer powder nearly doubles after gentle shaking.

Powder:liquid ratios

The ratio of powder to liquid of ionomers is critical to strength and solubility. The mix should be thick, shiny, and provide adequate working time before setting (Figure 3–5). Because of the difficulty of getting a consistent mix, a number of clinicians prefer using glass ionomer packaged in capsules. Capsules also allow a higher ratio of powder to liquid (typically 4.5:1 for capsules, compared to 4:1 for hand mixing).

THREE PHASES OF GLASS-IONOMER SETTING

Glass ionomers undergo three distinct and overlapping setting reactions (Figure 3–6). They are the immediate ion leaching phase (immediately after mixing), the hydrogel phase (initial set), and the polysalt gel phase (final set).[20] Once set, a glass ionomer consists of three components: a matrix, a filler, and a salt that attaches the filler to the matrix (Figure 3–7).

Ion-leaching phase

Ion leaching occurs when the powder and liquid are first combined. The aqueous solutions of polyacid copolymers and tartaric acid accelerators attack the ion-leachable aluminofluorosilicate powder and dissolve the outer glass surface. The hydrogen ions from the polyacid and tartaric acids cause the release of metal cations, such as Ca^{2+} and Al^{3+}, from the glass-powder surface. These initially react with fluoride ions to form CaF_2, AlF_2^-, and larger complexes. As the acidity continues to increase, the unstable CaF_2 breaks down and reacts with the acrylic copolymer to form a more stable complex. Heat of 3° to 7°C, depending on the ratio of powder to liquid, is liberated by the chemical reaction. The higher the ratio, the more vigorous the reaction and the more heat is liberated.

Appearance

During this early phase, the glass ionomer adheres to the tooth structure. It appears shiny or glossy from the unreacted matrix. Placement should be completed in the early part of this phase, because the maximum amount of free polyacid matrix is available for adhesion. At the end of this phase, as the material loses its shine, the free matrix reacts with the glass and is less able to bond to the tooth or any other surface. Glass ionomers should not be manipulated once the initial gloss is gone.

Hydrogel phase

The hydrogel phase, which begins 5 to 10 minutes after mixing, causes the initial set. During this phase, the positively charged calcium ions are released more rapidly and react with the negatively charged aqueous polyanionic polyacid chains to form ionic cross-links. The hydrogel phase reduces the mobility of the aqueous polymer chains, causing initial gelation of the ionomer matrix. During this phase, the ionomer should be protected from moisture and desiccation.

Appearance

The glass ionomer at this stage is rigid and opaque. The opacity is attributable to the large difference

50 Tooth-Colored Restoratives

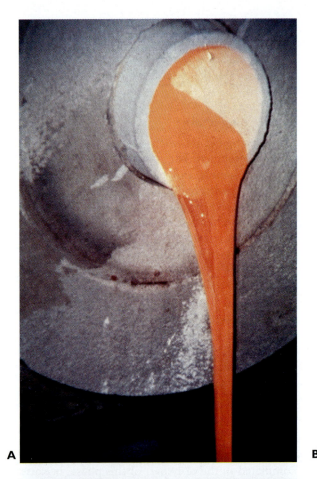

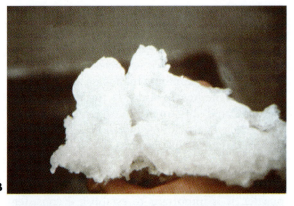

in the index of refraction between the glass filler and the matrix. This opacity is transient and should disappear during the final setting reaction.

Polysalt gel phase

The polysalt gel phase, which occurs when the material reaches its final set, can continue for several months. The matrix matures when aluminum ions, which are released more slowly, help form a polysalt hydrogel to surround the unreacted glass filler.

Appearance

The glass ionomer now looks more tooth-like because the index of refraction of the silica gel sur-

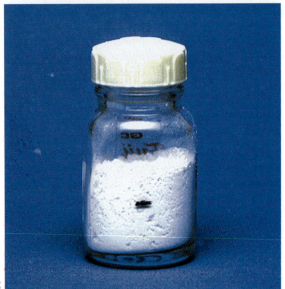

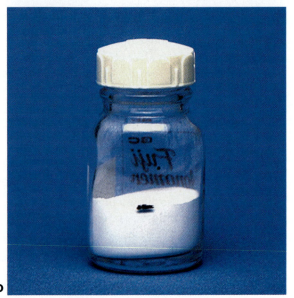

Figure 3–4. *A*, Glass-ionomer fillers are complex glasses made at high temperature. *B*, The glass is supercooled in water to produce highly reactive flake-like plates that settle. *C*, A typical bottle of glass-ionomer powder before and, *D*, after shaking. Since these materials are dispensed with a scoop, mix accuracy is affected.

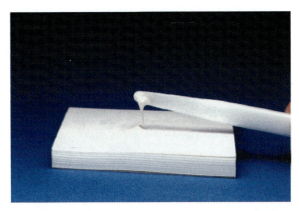

Figure 3–5. A typical mix of glass-ionomer cement. Notice the shiny surface and stringiness of the mix.

rounding the glass filler is more similar to the matrix. This reduces light scattering and opacity. *Note: If the ionomer retains the opaque appearance of the hydrogel phase, this indicates the polysalt gel did not form properly, possibly because of water contamination early in the process. If this occurs, the restoration may fail prematurely.*

Desiccation

Glass ionomers must be protected from desiccation. Hence, they may not perform well when used internally in nonvital teeth where it may not be possible to maintain adequate moisture.

PROPERTIES OF GLASS IONOMERS

The early conventional glass-ionomer materials were technique sensitive, slow setting, considerably opaque when set, and sensitive to both desiccation and hydration during setting. This led to early loss of material from the surface. All of these problems have been alleviated in newer materials. Modern glass ionomers are fast setting and more esthetic, and hydration and sensitivity problems are relatively limited. However, unlike composites, they still should not be used as stress-bearing restorations.

The newer highly filled, packable, and quick-setting glass-ionomer materials include Fuji IX GP (GC International) (called Fuji IX in Europe), Ketac Molar (ESPE), and Shofu Hi-Dense (Shofu Dental Corp., Kyoto, Japan). These radiopaque, tougher glass-ionomer cements are useful for non–stress-bearing buildups, root caries, tunnel restorations, and long-term provisional restorations in primary and adult dentitions. Their opacity makes them less desirable in esthetically sensitive areas.

The following list summarizes the characteristics of traditional glass-ionomer materials:

Advantages

- Form a rigid substance on setting
- Good fluoride release (bacteriostatic, inhibit caries)
- Low exothermic reaction on setting
- Less shrinkage than polymerizing resins
- Coefficient of thermal expansion similar to dentin
- No free monomers
- Dimensional stability at high humidity
- Filler–matrix chemical bonding
- Resistant to microleakage
- Nonirritating to pulp
- Good marginal integrity
- Adhere chemically to enamel and dentin in the presence of moisture
- Rechargeable fluoride component
- Good bonding to enamel and dentin
- High compressive strength

Disadvantages

- Susceptible to dehydration over lifetime
- Sensitivity to moisture at placement
- Poor abrasion resistance
- Average esthetics
- Less tensile strength than composites
- Technique sensitive powder-to-liquid ratio and mixing
- Less color-stable than resins
- Contraindicated for Class IV or other stress-bearing restorations
- Poor acid resistance

Generally, glass ionomers demonstrate lower tensile strength and higher wear properties than either

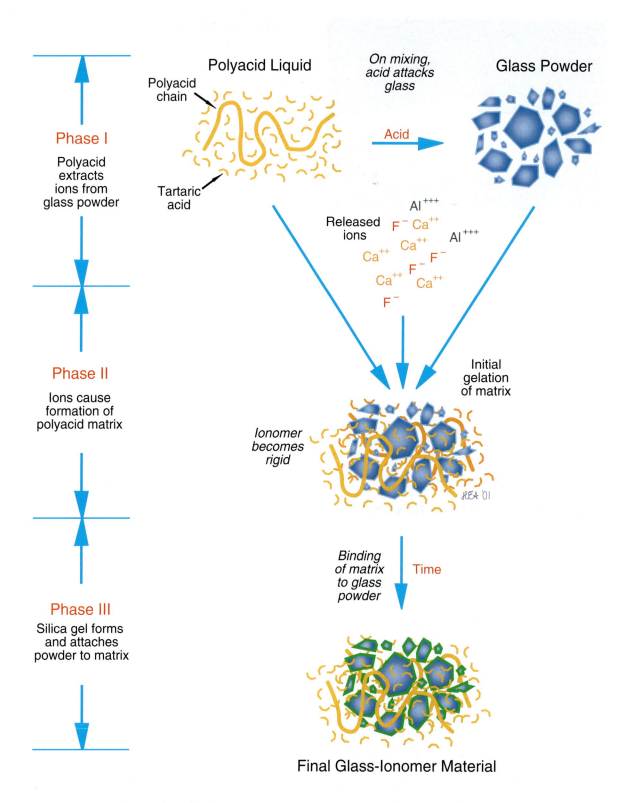

Figure 3–6. The three phases of glass-ionomer setting.

Glass Ionomers 53

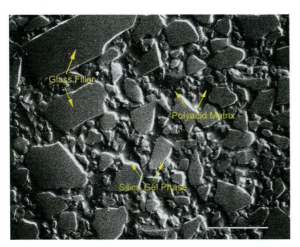

Figure 3–7. Microscopic cross-section showing the three components of a fully set glass-ionomer cement.

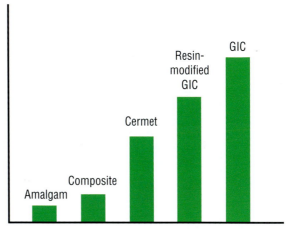

Figure 3–9. Bar graph illustrating the difference in simulated occlusal wear between amalgam, a composite, a resin-modified glass-ionomer cement, a glass-ionomer cement, and a silver cermet. GIC = glass-ionomer cement.

amalgam or composite (Figures 3–8 and 3–9). Resin-modified glass ionomers vary enormously but their properties fall in the range between composites and conventional glass ionomers.

Recharging glass-ionomer cements

Toothpaste with fluoride and topical neutral fluoride solutions can replenish the fluoride in glass ionomers (Figure 3–10).[21,22] The potential to recharge glass ionomers has been referred to as the "reservoir effect." Glass ionomers release fluoride from a reservoir contained in the unreacted glass-ionomer filler of the matrix. Once the reservoir is depleted, it can be recharged, typically with a topical application of fluoride in a gel, rinse, or toothpaste. Clinicians have had long-term success using frequent neutral fluoride applications to replenish the fluoride in glass-ionomer restorations of individuals at high risk for caries.

The fluoride content of a glass ionomer is much higher than the normal fluoride content of a tooth. Through ion exchange, fluoride ions diffuse from the area of high concentration (in the cement) to the area of lower concentration (the tooth). In the process, some of the hydroxyapatite in the tooth is permanently transformed into fluoroapatite. In time, the fluoride content of the tooth and glass ionomer reach equilibrium. Because of its high fluoride content, the tooth surface under a glass ionomer is likely to remain caries free for the lifetime of the restoration.

At the tooth surface, glass ionomers release fluoride into the saliva. Since equilibrium of fluoride between the glass-ionomer cement surface and oral fluids is not possible, most of the fluoride from the ionomer's surface is lost to the oral fluids. Only some of this fluoride is available to the 1- to 3-mm periphery around the restoration. This means fluoride-induced caries inhibition at the restoration

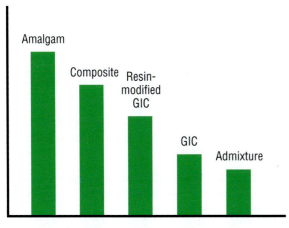

Figure 3–8. Average tensile strengths of crown buildup materials. GIC = glass-ionomer cement. (Modified from Chaine J Dent Res 1985;64(Spec Issue).

54 Tooth-Colored Restoratives

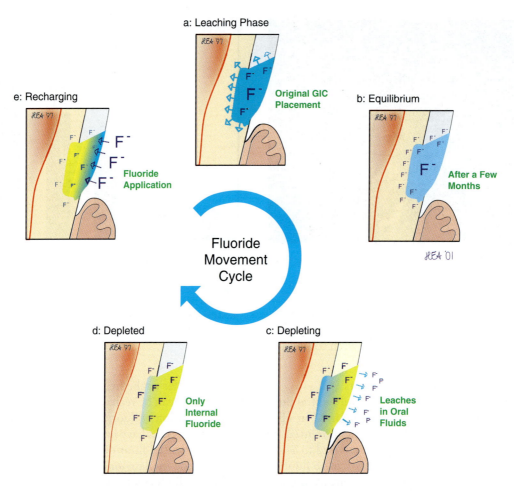

Figure 3–10. Fluoride balance between glass ionomer and tooth. *A*, Fluoride ions from a glass ionomer leach into the tooth. *B*, Fluoride in the restoration and tooth reach equilibrium. *C*, Saliva draws fluoride from the tooth and restoration. *D*, Both tooth and restoration are depleted of fluoride. *E*, A topical application of fluoride recharges the cement.

margins decreases over time. This is of particular concern for patients with high caries susceptibility, such as the elderly and patients who have undergone radiation treatment.

REFERENCES

1. Pierce CH. Discussion, Pennsylvania Association of Dental Surgery. Dent Cosmos 1879;21:696.

2. Ames WVB. A new oxyphosphate for crown setting. Dent Cosmos 1892;34:392.

3. Fleck DJ. The chemistry of oxyphosphates. Dent Items Int 1902;24:906.

4. Smith DC. A new dental cement. Br Dent J 1967;123:540–1.

5. Smith DC. A new dental cement. Br Dent J 1968;124:381–4.

6. Wall FT, Drenan SW. Gelation of polyacrylic acid by divalent cations. J Pol Sci 1951;7:83–90.

7. Leach SA, Puttnam NA. Infrared studies of the interaction of weak acid anions with hydroxyapatite. J Dent Res 1962;41:716.

8. Peters WJ, Jackson RW, Iwano K, Smith DC. The biological response to zinc polyacrylate cement. Clin Orthop 1972;88:228–33.

9. Wilson AD, McLean JW. Glass-ionomer cement. Chicago: Quintessence, 1988.

10. McLean JW. The evolution of glass ionomer cements: a personal review. In: Hunt PR, ed. Glass

ionomers: the next generation. Philadelphia: International Symposia in Dentistry, 1994:61–73.

11. Massler M, Berman DS, James VE. Pulp capping and pulp amputation. Dent Clin North Am 1957; Nov:797.

12. Mahler DB, Armen GK. Addition of amalgam alloy to zinc phosphate cement. J Prosthet Dent 1962;12:157–64.

13. McLean JW, Gasser O. Glass-cermet cements. Quintessence Int 1985;16:333–43.

14. McLean JW. Alternatives to amalgam alloys. 1. Br Dent J 1984;157:432–3.

15. McLean JW. New concepts in cosmetic dentistry using glass ionomer cements and composites. CDA J 1986;14:20–7.

16. Nicholson JW, Anstice HM, McLean JW. A preliminary report on the effect of storage in water on the properties of commercial light-cured glass-ionomer cements. Br Dent J 1992;173:98–101.

17. Anstice HM. Studies on light-cured dental cements. PhD thesis. London, UK: Brunel University, 1993.

18. Albers HF, ed. ADEPT Report 1990;1:1.

19. Crisp S, Wilson AD. Reactions in glass ionomer cements: I. Decomposition of the powder. J Dent Res 1974;53:1408–13.

20. Crisp S, Pringuer MA. Reactions in glass ionomer cements: II. An infrared spectroscopic study. J Dent Res 1974;53:1414–9.

21. Hatibovic-Kofman S, Koch G, Elkstrand J. GICs ionomer materials as a rechargeable F-release system [abstract]. J Dent Res 1994;73:134.

22. Alvarez AN, Burgess JO, Chan DCN. Short-term fluoride release of six ionomers: recharged, coated, and abraded. J Dent Res 1994;73:134.

Chapter 4

Resin Ionomers

Conversation would be vastly improved by the constant use of four simple words: "I do not know."

André Maurois

RESIN-IONOMER CLASSIFICATION

This chapter introduces resin ionomers, which have been adapted for numerous clinical uses ranging from luting agents to restoratives. Resin ionomers evolved from manufacturers' efforts to improve on traditional glass ionomers by adding resin components. These new materials have better initial esthetics; improved physical properties, such as greater tensile strength and fracture toughness; set on demand through light-curing; and have fewer desiccation and hydration problems. Because they are stronger, they have a stronger bond to tooth structure when conventional bonding precedes application. In addition, the resin can form a chemical bond with tooth structure. It is unknown whether this has any clinical significance.

Resin-modified glass-ionomer cements

Resin-modified glass-ionomer cements, also known as glass-ionomer hybrid cements, set through a combination of acid–base reaction and photochemical polymerization. "Resin-modified" refers to all cements in which the acid–base reaction of true glass-ionomer cements is supplemented by a light-cure polymerization reaction.[1] This is achieved by adding a water-soluble monomer, such as hydroxyethyl methacrylate (HEMA), to the liquid of a water-soluble polyacrylic acid. The term resin-modified can also imply materials in which the resin component sets via a chemically induced polymerization (ie, not via light-cure). This text uses the term resin-modified glass ionomer instead of the more precise chemical nomenclature, which is resin-modified glass-polyalkenoate cement.[1]

The term glass-ionomer cement is reserved exclusively for the simple acid–base material. For the term glass ionomer to be applicable, the acid–base reaction must contribute to setting of the material, and there should be a pH change on setting as neutralization takes place. Thus, an essential feature of glass-ionomer cements is that they set on their own after mixing, without the addition of light initiation. Failure to set in the dark is sufficient proof that a material does not contain a glass ionomer.

Understanding the timing of the various setting reactions in resin ionomers is of critical importance. The light-curing reaction is first and cures the surface layer closest to the light. Since these materials shrink considerably, the initial layer, which can be considered the bonding layer, should be no more than a thin wash on the tooth surface. This layer must be light-cured before more material is added in multiple layers of no more than 1 mm each. Air inhibition at the surface is achieved by overfilling or by placing a thin coating of resin over the surface. Although the material appears set after light-curing, it becomes harder over time, owing to the acid–base setting reaction between the acidic polyacids and the basic glass-ionomer filler particles. Early finishing can damage the immature bonds to the tooth structure as well as weaken the material so that unreacted glass-ionomer components wash out.

Polymerization

Conventional glass ionomers do not include a polymerizing resin; therefore, the strands in their polyacid matrix cannot covalently cross-link.

Figure 4–1 shows a cross-sectional view of the relation between the polyacid polymer and the glass filler of a conventional glass ionomer in which the only setting mechanism is an acid–base reaction. Resin-modified glass ionomers entail polymerization, because their liquid contains HEMA and polyacrylic acid (or an analogue), with or without pendant methacrylic groups.[1,2] Bis-GMA, PMDM, PMGDM, BPDM, and many other commonly used large molecular weight monomers (used to control composite shrinkage) cannot be used in resin-ionomer materials, because they are not water soluble. Some resin-ionomers have free-radical polymerizable side chains grafted onto their main polyacid molecule. Examples of these materials are Vitrebond and Vitremer (3M Dental Products, St. Paul, Minnesota). Figure 4–2 shows a single-polymer resin-modified glass ionomer. Other materials use smaller polyacid glass polymers combined with larger, water-soluble methacrylate polymers (called oligomers) that contain pendant methacrylate groups. These are multipolymer resin-modified glass ionomers (eg, Fuji II LC, Fuji Duet, GC, Tokyo, Japan, and Photac-Fil, ESPE, Seefeld, Germany). Figure 4–3 illustrates a multipolymer cross-linked material.

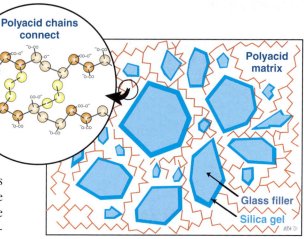

Figure 4–2. Schematic representation of the relation between a polyacid polymer and a glass filler of a single-polymer resin-modified glass ionomer (cross-sectional view). Note that the polymers are covalently cross-linked. 3M Dental Products (St. Paul, Minnesota) makes products that use this system.

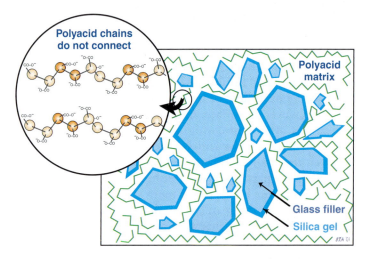

Figure 4–1. Schematic representation of the relation between a polyacid polymer and a glass filler of a conventional glass-ionomer cement restoration (cross-sectional view). Note that the polymers remain individual and are not covalently linked.

After setting, both of these systems form a large amount of poly-HEMA polymer that can interact either mechanically or chemically (by covalent bonding) to pendant methacrylate groups. HEMA is the major monomer used in these systems.

Photocured systems

A photoinitiated setting reaction occurs when methacrylate groups graft onto the polyacrylic acid chain and methacrylate groups of the HEMA. The setting reaction begins when the powder and liquid are mixed and exposed to light. In other words, two separate setting reactions occur: one common to conventional glass ionomers and the other common to photoinitiated resin composites. The photoactivation may affect the material's final properties, depending on the strength of the glass-ionomer cure. The setting reaction sequence of resin-modified glass ionomers is shown in Figure 4–4. Commercially available materials produce varying degrees of polymerization through each setting mechanism.

Dual-cured systems

Dual-cured systems are similar to light-cured systems, except they have additional chemical initiators to polymerize their methacrylate components. This allows them to undergo polymerization with-

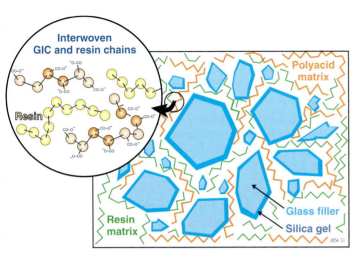

Figure 4–3. Schematic representation of the relation between a polyacid polymer and a glass filler of a multipolymer resin-modified glass-ionomer system (cross-sectional view of a dual polymer system). Note that the polyacid polymers remain individual and are intertwined with the covalently cross-linked methacrylate polymer. GC (Tokyo, Japan) and ESPE (Seefeld, Germany) make materials that use this system.

out light. These materials are most commonly used as luting agents.

Polyacid-modified resin composites

Polyacid-modified resin composites, which are more widely known by the name "compomers," attempt to combine the best properties of glass ionomers and composite resins. A major reason for their success is that they are user friendly: they are soft, nonsticky, do not need to be mixed, and are easy to place. They are easy to inject into a cavity, simple to shape, quick to cure, and readily polished after curing. They are used in anterior proximal restorations and in cervical restorations. In almost all other areas, composites and glass ionomers are preferred.

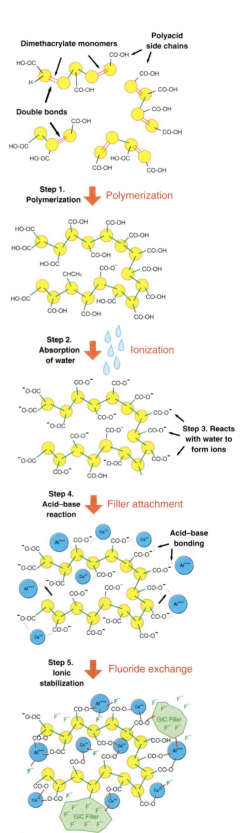

Figure 4–4. Schematic representation of the chemical relation in the setting reaction sequence of a resin-modified glass-ionomer system. The resulting polyacid-methacrylate polymer is covalently cross-linked. Note the steps in the setting reaction with this type of resin-modified glass ionomer. *Top,* The methacrylate-containing polyacid polymer in the liquid prior to mixing with the powder and resin and curing. *Steps 1 to 5,* The five-step setting reaction of this type of resin-modified glass ionomer.

Compomers have nominal adhesion to tooth structure and, therefore, are always attached with resin–dentin bonding agents. They are made of an acid-functionalized dimethacrylate resin that can undergo an acid–base reaction with a glass-ionomer powder, which may also contain conventional composite glass filler (see Figure 4–4). They work by absorbing water, which expands the restoration over time. This absorbed water can then cause an acid–base reaction between the polyacid side chains of the resin matrix and the glass-ionomer filler. This results in fluoride release at a level about 20% that of a conventional glass ionomer. The more acidic carboxyl groups a compomer contains, the more hydrophilic and ionic the matrix becomes, which results in greater water absorption. Unlike those of glass ionomers, the physical properties of a compomer decrease as water is absorbed. With some materials, this decrease can be as much as 50%, leaving an inferior material in terms of strength.

Compomers provide less fluoride release than glass ionomers, and the small amount they do release may be of limited value, since the resin-bonded interface prevents the fluoride from entering the tooth. Nevertheless, surface fluoride release from compomers can affect the surrounding tooth structure.

History
The first compomer, introduced in 1993, was Dyract (Dentsply, Konstanz, Germany). It was first introduced in Europe, then Canada, and then in the United States. Although many European clinicians felt positive about these materials, researchers and educators in the American academic community were less optimistic. Dyract has undergone a few formulation changes. One was the addition of fluoride, and the other was use of a smaller particle.

The next such material introduced was Compoglass (Vivadent, Amherst, New York), and other manufacturers followed shortly with similar products, including Hytac (ESPE). Each of these materials is completely different, and none underwent clinical trials prior to introduction. What they have in common is light-initiated polymerization and water absorption after placement. They are also softer than composites and can be more easily flexed. Their other physical properties generally do not measure up to conventional composites.

Chemistry
The compomers are hydrophobic resins by definition that contain polyacid side chains that are attached to one or more of their methacrylate monomers. They rely primarily on the light-initiated free-radical polymerization mechanism for curing. These materials can be thought of as low–fluoride-releasing composite resins. The fillers include a reactive aluminofluorosilicate glass (used in glass ionomers).

The monomer ionizes by absorbing water during the days and weeks after it is light-cured. The hydrogen ions that are released then react with the glass filler to initiate an acid–base reaction. Ionic cross-linking also occurs, and fluoride is released.

The advantages of compomers include the following characteristics:

- No mixing required
- Easy to place
- Easy to polish
- Good esthetics
- Excellent handling
- Less susceptible to dehydration
- Radiopaque
- Higher bond strengths than resin-modified glass ionomers
- Stronger than glass ionomers

The disadvantages of compomers include the following characteristics:

- Bonding agent required
- More leakage than resin-modified glass ionomers
- Expand from water sorption over time
- Wear more easily than composites
- Longevity difficult to predict because of enormous variation of products
- Physical properties weaker than those of composites, and they decrease over time
- Limited fluoride uptake

Ionomer-modified resins
Ionomer-modified resins, or fluoride-containing composite resins, are materials that contain glass-ionomer fillers but no polyacids. They have been on the dental market for a long time and represent

the first attempt to impart to composite resins the beneficial effects of glass ionomers. They suspend ionomer-glass or reacted glass-ionomer components in a resin system, and hence are also known as suspension systems (Figure 4–5). Unfortunately, whereas compomers absorb water, which gives them the potential for acid–base reactions and significant fluoride release, suspension systems have no such potential. The only avenue for fluoride release from an ionomer suspension system is diffusion of ionomer particles entrapped in voids that fill with water after placement.

The distinction between compomers and ionomer-in-resin suspensions is very fine. Many materials marketed as compomers are mainly suspension systems. There is no definitive test to differentiate the two materials. There is no proof that compomers do better clinically than suspension systems or composite resins, since little clinical testing has been done comparing these restorative systems.

Ionomer-modified resins exhibit almost no traditional glass-ionomer-like properties. Hence, materials called compomers (a term that presently sells materials in the marketplace) that are really suspension systems may be clinically disappointing. In fact, the clinical superiority of either compomers or suspension systems has yet to be determined.

Examples of these products include Resin-Ionomer (Bisco, Schaumburg, Illinois) and Geristore (Den-Mat Corp., Santa Maria, California).

Both are fluoride-containing composite resins that are filled about 50% by volume with barium fluorosilicate glass (particles averaging 3 to 4 μm).

Summary of terms

Resin ionomers is an umbrella term for materials that contain glass-ionomer and resin components.

Glass-ionomer cements are materials that contain water, a basic decomposable glass, and an acidic polymer; they set by means of an acid–base reaction between components in the presence of water.

Resin-modified glass ionomers (sometimes called hybrid materials) are glass ionomers in which the matrix portions of the materials undergo both an acid–base reaction and a polymerization reaction.

Polyacid-modified resins (compomers) are materials that do not contain water but have some of the essential components of a glass-ionomer cement—at levels insufficient to promote an acid–base cure reaction in the dark.

Ionomer-modified composite resins or *fluoride-containing composite resins* contain fluoride but do not fit into other ionomer classes. These materials are also known as suspension systems.

HISTORY OF RESIN-MODIFIED GLASS IONOMERS

Resin-modified glass ionomers were introduced as liners. The first methacrylate-modified glass ionomer introduced was Vitrebond Liner/Base (3M Dental Products) as a two-part powder-liquid system. The powder is a photosensitive aluminofluorosilicate glass. The filler is a typical glass-ionomer powder that imparts the usual fluoride release through a water-soluble polyacrylic acid matrix. The liquid contains 25% HEMA, a polyacrylic acid copolymer to which pendant methacrylate groups have been attached, additional photoaccelerators, and water. After mixing, the liquid and powder contain only about 9% HEMA. Both powder and liquid are sensitive to light, so the material must be dispensed just before mixing.

After mixing and light initiation, the water-soluble methacrylate HEMA copolymerizes with the modified polyacrylic acid polymer through the attached methacrylate group. This causes an initial covalent (rather than ionic) binding between the long polyacid chains forming the glass-ionomer

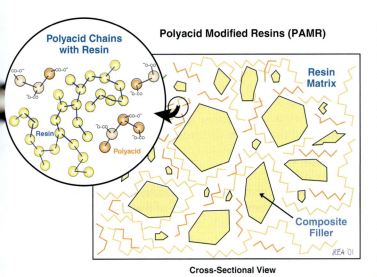

Figure 4–5. Polyacid-modified resins (PAMR).

matrix. This bond is possible since the carboxylic groups of the polyacid are not involved in the light-initiated polymerization reaction. This matrix makes a durable liner that bonds ionically to a tooth.

Currently available light-cured resin-modified glass ionomers, such as Vitrebond, Fuji Lining LC, and Photac-Bond, can be used in most areas where a thin, strong liner is required. These materials are well suited for blocking out minor undercuts and protecting the dentin. In deep areas, light-cured resin-modified glass ionomers can be placed over a small calcium hydroxide liner.

Chemistry of current resin-ionomer liners

Vitrebond

Vitrebond contains a single copolymer that can undergo two competing reactions on the same chain. These polymers contain carboxylic groups, which are the main component in glass-ionomer bonding, and active polymerizable methacrylate groups on the same polymer (mixed in with about 20% HEMA). This creates a more durable material as a result of cross-linking of the resin matrix.

In the polymer phase, the first setting reaction is rapid; later, when the glass-ionomer phase takes over, the polymer is already rigid, limiting the activities of the second phase. In other words, after polymerization, the cross-linked polyacid strands cannot move to form optimal bonds to the pieces of silica glass filler. Once polymerized, the matrix strands are literally tied in place—there is a double bond every 5 to 10 carbon molecules.

The resulting chain has less than 10% cross-linking with the polymer. The HEMA, which is in the liquid, can directly react with the noncrosslinked members of the polymer chain. The end result is a material that is mostly dependent on resin polymerization for its integrity and requires light-curing. If it is mixed and not light-cured, there is too little acid–base glass-ionomer reaction to form a clinically suitable material. Vitrebond does dual-cure, but the self-cure mechanism is clinically unacceptable.

Fuji Lining LC

In both Fuji Lining LC and Fuji II LC, GC used two separate polymers with two separate setting reactions. One polymer (in the powder) is a long polymerizable chain of high molecular weight, including polymerization methacrylate groups. GC put the HEMA in the water component with chains of polyacrylic acid. The carboxylic group component is the same as in traditional ionomers but it has a lower molecular weight, to allow it more mobility after the first phase of polymerization.

Light-curing causes the long methacrylate polymers to immediately bind with HEMA, resulting in a relatively rigid material. In the second phase, the polycarboxylic members are more free to bind with the glass particles in the matrix.

Combining two polymers in the same system provides slightly better physical properties, because the slower ionomer reaction can proceed with less interference from the earlier polymerization reaction. This is the key difference between Vitrebond and Fuji Lining LC.

The glass ionomer–resin balance

Glass-ionomer cements and composite resins can be considered on a continuum. At one extreme are traditional glass ionomers that set via acid–base reaction; at the other extreme are materials similar to composite resins, which cure almost exclusively through chemical- or light-initiated free-radical polymerization. Between these two points are materials in which an initial polymerization of resin components is combined with a chemical cure typical of conventional glass ionomers (Figure 4–6).

The physical properties of these materials vary greatly according to where they fall on this continuum of acid–base to polymerization setting reactions. Materials on the glass-ionomer end have low thermal expansion and high fluoride release and require only polyacid conditioning treatments for surface cleaning. Materials on the composite-resin end have increased thermal expansion and decreased fluoride release and, because they exhibit little adhesion to dentin, require dentinal bonding agents.

Fluoride release

The glass-ionomer acid–base reaction releases a large amount, or "burst," of fluoride, followed by a more diffuse long-term release of fluoride. Glass ionomers also have an advantage in that they are in direct contact with the tooth structure; whereas a resin-based system requires a resin bonding layer, which bars fluoride diffusion into the tooth, even if it is present in the restorative material.

Resin Ionomers 63

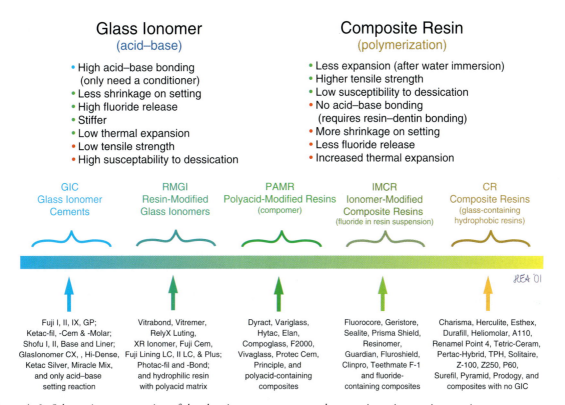

Figure 4–6. Schematic representation of the glass-ionomer cements and composite resins continuum. At one extreme are traditional glass ionomers that set via acid–base reaction; at the other extreme are materials similar to composite resins, which cure almost exclusively through free-radical polymerization.

The glass-ionomer fluoride-release curve shows an initial spike followed by a nearly flat but steadily declining release. The farther a material moves along the spectrum from glass-ionomer to resin polymerization, the less fluoride is available. Moreover, the fluoride in glass ionomers can be replenished by external sources, such as fluoride rinses, gels, and toothpastes.

Esthetics
Composite resins have by far the best esthetics. Resin-ionomers look equally good initially but discolor over time. Compomers and ionomer suspension systems have good initial esthetics but are unlikely to demonstrate the long-term stability common to composite resins.

Adhesion
All of these technologies have the potential of developing a bond to both enamel and dentin. With resin systems, a linkage to the tooth requires acid etching and a bonding agent. With glass ionomers, an inherent ionic bond develops from the restorative material to the tooth structure. Pretreating the tooth surface with polyacrylic acid cleansing agents can enhance this bond.

When glass ionomers are used correctly they have excellent long-term retention rates, including systems with relatively low bond strength measurements.

Finishing
Glass ionomers can be carved when the setting reaction has neared completion. Any of the light-cured resin-based systems set hard on curing. In general, the hardness and toughness of a material increases in the direction of resin systems. The compomers, being somewhat softer than composites, can be carved with a sharp instrument. Contouring and finishing procedures are easier with softer materials. However, the final finish of any system is ultimately controlled by the size of the filler particles.

Surface smoothness does not necessarily correlate with plaque retention; the chemical composition of the material is also important. Resin-based systems have residual components that seem to attract plaque, whereas glass ionomers release fluoride, which is toxic to plaque.

Resin-modified glass-ionomer materials are unique in that their properties span the gulf between the two traditional materials. Overall, the esthetic outcome with these materials is equal to most and better than that achievable with some composite resins, and is superior to that of almost all conventional glass ionomers. Their characteristics of adhesion to tooth structure, translucency, and fluoride release give them great potential as prototypes for future material development.

Changes in the glass ionomer–resin balance greatly alter the properties of these materials. The optimal balance for particular clinical situations is not yet known. Only long-term clinical results can determine the best means to tailor these materials for specific patient treatment needs.

CLINICAL USES OF RESIN IONOMERS

Resin ionomers are appropriate for use as liners, bases, luting agents, restoratives, and bonding agents. Since they have long-term fluoride release, they are particularly useful for Class V restorations and for older patients and those at high risk for caries. Resin ionomer materials are excellent for restoring geriatric dentition and may reduce caries in saliva-deficient patients. Their major limitations are reduced stiffness and high wear, as well as poor dimensional and color stability. When these limitations are weighed against good adhesion and good caries inhibition properties, resin ionomers offer good service for treating the aging dentition in non–stress-bearing areas.

One unusual benefit of resin ionomers is their capacity to take up topically applied fluoride. Both toothpaste with fluoride and topical neutral fluoride solutions have been proven to recharge the fluoride depleted from glass ionomers.[3,4] Clinicians who are aware of this function have had success using frequent neutral fluoride applications to replenish the fluoride in glass ionomers in the treatment of individuals at high risk for caries. The pH of topical fluoride is critical. Acidulated phosphate fluoride solutions and other acidified fluoride preparations should be avoided, since they alter the surface of conventional glass-ionomer restorations.[5] For example, one study showed the surface of glass ionomers is rougher after the application of a topical fluoride solution.[6,7] Acid phosphate solutions produced the greatest increase in surface roughness, and the neutral sodium fluoride produced the least. The study also demonstrated that resin-modified glass ionomers were more resistant to surface degradation than conventional glass ionomers. This was expected since the polysalt matrix found in conventional glass ionomers is less resistant to acid attack than the polyHEMA or methacrylate resin-containing matrices found in resin-modified glass ionomers.

Physical properties of resin ionomers

In addition to having the properties of conventional glass ionomers (bonding to tooth structure and metal, fluoride release, biocompatibility, and thermal insulation), the resin ionomers have significantly greater early compressive and diametral tensile strengths, are more resistant to moisture and desiccation, and are easier to finish.

Shear bond strength

The shear bond strength of conventional glass-ionomer cements is low, varying from 3 MPa to 5 MPa.[8–10] When these materials fail, they usually fail within the material, so the bond strength is actually a measure of cohesive strength. The shear bond strength of resin-modified glass ionomers is usually greater than that of conventional glass ionomers; however, this is mostly attributable to the increased cohesive strength of the materials and not to increased adhesion to tooth structure. Depending on the material evaluated, shear bond strength values for resin ionomers vary from 0.7 MPa to 12 MPa.[11–16] Use of the specific conditioner or primer the manufacturer supplies with its resin ionomer is essential. The bond strength decreases if the material is not light-cured (except for dual-cured systems) or if no conditioner or primer is used. Bonding to deep dentin also decreases the bond strength of some materials (eg, Photac-Fil, ESPE, and Variglass, LD Caulk) compared with bonding to superficial dentin.[16]

As with all ionomers, isolation is required to ensure that saliva does not contaminate the dentin surface; contamination greatly reduces bond strength. If conditioned dentin is contaminated before the material is placed, it must be rinsed and reconditioned, and a new glass ionomer mix must be applied.

Coefficient of thermal expansion
The coefficient of thermal expansion is thought to explain much of the clinical effectiveness of conventional glass-ionomer restorations. Although the shear bond strength of a glass-ionomer restoration is less than that of current dentin bonding agents, glass ionomers placed in Class V preparations have better longevity than composite resins used in these areas.

Measurement of the thermal expansion of glass ionomers and modified resin ionomers shows that even though resin-modified glass ionomers have a higher coefficient of thermal expansion than tooth structure, their thermal expansion compares more favorably with tooth structure than does that of composite resins.[17,18] In general, the more a material moves from an acid–base glass ionomer to a methacrylate polymerizing resin system, the higher the thermal expansion.

Volume stability
Resin-modified glass ionomers generally expand after setting, which can alter a restoration's contour and stress crowns that are cemented with these materials.

Effects of fluoride release
Many in vitro and in vivo studies have examined the effect of fluoride released from glass ionomers on plaque and bacteria.[3,4,11,19–29] The release is initially great but quickly decreases to a lower but steadier long-term release. Studies show this long-term release inhibits bacterial growth. Over time, the release is thought to accelerate the remineralization of carious tooth structure. However, one 5-year clinical study reported similar rates of recurrent caries around Class V composite resin and glass ionomer restorations.[30] Unfortunately, the large number of clinical variables in such a study make it difficult to draw firm conclusions about these materials.

Fluoride treatments increase the fluoride content of glass ionomers but not of composites. Many dentists note a clinically significant improvement over a 5- to 10-year period in the performance of glass ionomers compared with composite resins when placed in Class V restorations with dentin margins. In Class V restorations with all-enamel margins, however, composite resins appear to have better longevity.

Resin ionomers vary greatly in their fluoride release.[6] For example, one study showed the fluoride release of Photac-Fil and Vitremer was significantly higher than that of Fuji II LC. Others show the differences are small and may not be clinically significant. Fluoride release from compomers has proven to be significantly lower than from resin-modified glass ionomers.

Many manufacturers recommend finishing resin ionomers and placing a varnish or unfilled resin over the finished restoration. This decreases the initial fluoride release from the surface. However, once this layer wears away, fluoride release from the material continues as normal.

Color stability
Composite resins are hydrophobic and set via polymerization reaction. They have the best long-term color stability of any direct placement material. Traditional glass ionomers are hydrophilic and set via acid–base reactions. They have moderate color stability. However, resin-modified glass ionomers, which set through a polymerization reaction (usually with polyHEMA) and an acid–base reaction (with polyacid and glass particles) have poorer color stability than either of the original materials. In this context, current resin-modified glass ionomers have poor color stability. This should be considered prior to their use. In gingival root areas, discoloration of the material over time, which may be self-limiting, may have little clinical significance. However, in Class V restorations on maxillary central incisors, color stability may be a major concern.

Experience suggests that the long-term postoperative discoloration of resin-modified glass ionomers is related to placement technique. When these materials are properly placed in 1-mm increments, immediately covered with an unfilled resin, cured, and left undisturbed for 10 minutes before finishing with a safe-end 20-μm diamond bur in a water spray, postoperative discoloration is greatly reduced (but not eliminated).

Another option is to add an outer, 1-mm layer of composite over a resin ionomer restoration. This combination provides the benefits of the ionomer internally and the color stability of the composite externally. This procedure is recommended for anterior teeth susceptible to caries and desiccation.

Finishing

In general, resin ionomers are smoother when finished than conventional glass ionomers.[6,7] Ideally, a resin ionomer should be left undisturbed for 10 minutes after the initial set to allow the silicate gel setting reaction to progress far enough to stabilize the filler and the polyacid components of the polyacid matrix. Since resin-modified glass ionomers are still susceptible to dehydration, they should be finished with a water spray after setting is complete.

Although resin ionomer restorations are more water stable than conventional glass ionomers, coating the resin ionomers with an unfilled resin fills small defects. Unfortunately, this also decreases fluoride release and may inhibit later fluoride uptake by the resin ionomer. Therefore, applying unfilled resin to the surface is recommended only for patients with a low risk of caries.[6]

If there is a void in a resin-ionomer restoration, material added within 15 minutes after placement chemically bonds to the underlying material. At subsequent appointments, the restoration can be repaired further with a similar material, but the repair will have a lower bond strength.

To make this kind of repair:

1. Roughen the material with a diamond bur.
2. Etch with phosphoric acid for 20 seconds, rinse, and dry until the material has a matte appearance (do not desiccate to the point at which the margins begin to degenerate).
3. Place dentin bonding agent.
4. Cure for 20 seconds.
5. Place the freshly mixed glass ionomer onto the prepared surface in 1- to 2-mm increments.
6. Light-cure each layer for 40 seconds.
7. Slightly overbuild the material to compensate for air inhibition.

Allow to rest for 10 minutes, then finish with a 20-μm diamond bur and a water spray. Since composite resin bonds to resin ionomers, composite resin can also be used to repair resin ionomers.

REFERENCES

1. McLean JW, Nicholson JW, Wilson AD. Proposed nomenclature for glass-ionomer dental cements and related material. Quintessence Int 1994;25:587–9.

2. Hammesfahr PD. Variglass: product profile. Technical perspectives. Milford, DE: LD Caulk, 1992:1–3.

3. Alvarez AN, Burgess JO, Chan DCN. Short-term fluoride release of six ionomers: recharged, coated, and abraded [abstract]. J Dent Res 1994;73:134.

4. Hatibovic-Kofman S, Koch G, Elkstrand J. GICs ionomer materials as a rechargeable F-release system [abstract]. J Dent Res 1994;73:134.

5. Tyas MJ. Cariostatic effect of glass-ionomer cement: a five-year study. Aust Dent J 1991;36:236–9.

6. Burgess J, Norling, Summitt J. Resin ionomer restorative materials: the new generation. Glass ionomers: the next generation. In: Hunt P, ed. Proceedings of the 2nd International Symposium on Glass Ionomers. Philadephia, PA: International Dental Symposia, 1994: 75–86.

7. Todo A, Hirasawa M, Tosaki S, Hirota K. The surface roughness of glass ionomer cement for restorative filling [abstract]. J Dent Res 1996;75(Spec Issue).

8. Hotz P, McLean JW, Sced I, Wilson AD. The bonding of glass-ionomer cements to metal and tooth substrates. Br Dent J 1977;142:41–7.

9. Powis DR, Folleras T, Merson SA, Wilson AD. Improved adhesion of glass ionomer cement to dentin and enamel. J Dent Res 1982;61:1416–22.

10. Aboush Y, Jenkins CBG. An evaluation of the bonding of glass-ionomer restoratives to dentin and enamel. Br Dent J 1986;161:179–84.

11. Mitra SB. In vitro fluoride release from a light-cured glass-ionomer base liner. J Dent Res 1991;70: 75–7.

12. Burgess JO, Burkett L. Shear bond strength of four glass ionomers to enamel and dentin [abstract]. J Dent Res 1993;72:388.

13. Pawlus MA, Swift EJ, Vargas MA. Shear bond strengths of resin-ionomer restorative materials [abstract]. J Dent Res 1994;72:328.

14. Bell RB, Barkmeier WW. Shear bond strength of glass ionomer restoratives and liners [abstract]. J Dent Res 1994;72:328.

15. Cortes O, Garcia-Godoy F, Boj JR. Bond strength of resin-reinforced glass-ionomer cements after enamel etching. Am J Dent 1993;6:299–301.

16. Friedl KH, Powers JM. Bond strength of ionomers affected by dentin depth and moisture [abstract]. J Dent Res 1994;73:183.

17. Stattmiller SP, Burgess JO. Shear bond strength of two glass ionomers to contaminated dentin [abstract]. J Dent Res 1994;72:328.

18. Cardenas L, Burgess JO. Thermal expansion of glass ionomers [abstract]. J Dent Res 1994;73:220.

19. Mitra S, Conway WT. Coefficient of thermal expansion of some methacrylate-modified glass ionomers [abstract]. J Dent Res 1994;73:219.

20. Burkett L, Burgess JO, Chan DCN, Norling BK. Fluoride release of glass ionomers coated and not coated with adhesive [abstract]. J Dent Res 1993;72:258.

21. Momoi Y, McCabe JF. Fluoride release from light-activated glass ionomer restorative cements. Dent Mater 1993;9:151–4.

22. Cranfield M, Kuhn AT, Winter GB. Factors relating to the rate of fluoride-ion release from glass-ionomer cement. J Dent 1982;10:333–41.

23. Forsten L. Short- and long-term fluoride release from glass ionomers and other fluoride-containing filling materials in vitro. Scand J Dent Res 1990;98:179–85.

24. Forsten L. Fluoride release from a glass ionomer cement. Scand J Dent Res 1977;85:503–4.

25. Swartz ML, Phillips RW, Clark HE. Long-term F release from glass ionomer cements. J Dent Res 1984;63:158–60.

26. Forss H, Nase L, Seppa L. Fluoride and caries associated microflora in plaque on old GIC fillings [abstract]. J Dent Res 1994;73:410.

27. DeSchepper EJ, Thrasher MR, Thurmond BA. Antibacterial effects of light-cured liners. Am J Dent 1989;2:74–6.

28. Forss H. Effects of glass-ionomer cements in vitro and in the oral environment. Kuopio, Finland: Kuopio University Printing Office, 1993:1–344.

29. Benelli EM, Serra MC, Rodregries AL, Cury JA. In situ anticariogenic potential of glass ionomer cement. Caries Res 1993;27:280–4.

30. Hatibovic-Kofrnan S, Koch G. Fluoride release from glass ionomer cement in vivo and in vitro. Swed Dent J 1991;15:253–8.

CHAPTER 5

USES OF IONOMERS

When the only tool you own is a hammer, every problem begins to resemble a nail.

Abraham Maslow

INTRODUCTION TO CEMENTATION

This section reviews the clinical aspects of cementation with ionomer cements. The information provided will assist a clinician in deciding when to use these materials to cement conventional crowns and bridges.

The cement selected for a restoration can affect both the longevity of the restoration and the tooth's pulpal health. There are five common types of cements:

- Zinc phosphate cement has established long-term clinical success.
- Zinc oxide and eugenol cements are sedative and may give good results when moisture is inevitable.
- Zinc polycarboxylate cements are adhesive and extremely kind to the pulp.
- Glass-ionomer cements offer low solubility, good adhesion, and long-term caries inhibition.
- Resin cements have the lowest solubility and the highest tensile strength and bond strength to etched enamel of all available cements. They are ideal for shallow, partial-coverage restorations.

All but the resin cements set via acid–base reaction and use two types of powders and liquids (Table 5–1).

Cement powders

Zinc oxide

Zinc oxide has many medical applications. It is bactericidal, enhances wound healing, and is radiopaque. The major disadvantage is that it is relatively soluble in oral fluids. Dental cements use zinc oxide with one of three liquids: eugenol, phosphoric acid, or polyacrylic acid.

Glass powders

Aluminofluorosilicate glass powders are relatively strong, contain and release fluoride, and are relatively insoluble in oral fluids. They are not bactericidal and have no wound healing properties. However, when used in a cement, they can have bacteriostatic effects, owing to their fluoride release.

Cement liquids

Eugenol

The cements formed from eugenol mixed with zinc oxide are used mainly as interim and so-called sedative cements (eg, zinc oxide-eugenol [ZOE]; intermediate restorative material [IRM]; Temp-Bond, Kerr Corp., Romulus, Michigan). Because they are highly soluble, they are a poor choice for final cementation. Some materials (eg, ethoxy benzoic acid [EBA]) are intended for final cementations and are appropriate where moisture control is impossible. Since eugenol can inhibit resin polymerization, all eugenol-based materials are contra-

Table 5–1. Powder and Liquid Components of Different Glass-Ionomer Types

	Acid Liquid		
Basic Powder	Eugenol	Phosphoric Acid	Polyacrylic Acid
Zinc oxide	ZOE, IRM, EBA cements	Zinc phosphate cement	Polycarboxylate cement
Glass powder	None	Silicate cement	Glass-ionomer cement

ZOE = zinc oxide-eugenol; IRM = intermediate restorative material; EBA = ethoxy benzoic acid.

indicated where resin bonding will be used as a permanent restoration. Eugenol does not react with glass powders.

Phosphoric acid
Phosphoric acid reacts with many powders and can etch and remove any soluble bacterial film on teeth (the smear layer), thus opening dentin tubules to increase dentin permeability. This provides a pathway for bacteria with potentially adverse pulpal effects. It does not adhere to tooth structure. Phosphoric acid reacts with glass powders to form silicate cement, or with zinc oxide powder to form zinc phosphate cement.

Polyacrylic acid
Polyacrylic acid, which has less effect on dentin permeability and is, therefore, less likely to have adverse pulpal effects, is unique in its ability to adhere to tooth structure. It reacts with zinc oxide powder to form polycarboxylate cement, or with glass powders to form glass-ionomer cement.

CLASSIFYING GLASS-IONOMER CEMENTS

The three types of glass-ionomer luting agents, classified by the form of premixed polyacid, are hydrous, anhydrous, and semihydrous.

Hydrous
In hydrous glass ionomers, all of the polyacrylic acid is in the liquid component of the glass ionomer material. This is how glass ionomers were first introduced. These cements are highly viscous, have less initial acidity, and are rarely associated with tooth sensitivity, as compared with other ionomers. Examples of these materials are older versions of Fuji Type I (GC International, Tokyo, Japan), Glass Ionomer Cement Type I (Shofu, Dental Corp., Kyoto, Japan), and Chembond (Dentsply De Trey, Konstanz, Germany).

Advantages: less pulpal sensitivity (less initial acidity), faster initial set, lower solubility.

Disadvantages: thicker, therefore, more difficult to seat castings, long-term solubility is greater, powder-to-liquid ratio is lower (which may result in poorer physical properties), and shelf life is shorter than for other ionomers.

Anhydrous
In anhydrous glass ionomers, the polyacrylic acid is freeze- or vacuum-dried and added to the glass powder component, then mixed with water or tartaric acid to reconstitute the polyacrylic acid. This gives the cement a longer shelf life. The resulting mix is also thinner and can be mixed to a higher powder-to-liquid ratio, which can improve physical properties. However, the resulting cement has higher initial acidity and is associated with a higher incidence of postoperative sensitivity and pulpal death.[1] Some operators (many of whom use higher powder-to-liquid ratios than manufacturers recommend) report no increase in sensitivity with anhydrous formations. This leads to the conclusion that placement technique affects the clinical performance of anhydrous glass ionomers.

Anhydrous glass-ionomer material was first available in 1981 as Chemfil (Dentsply DeTrey). Some anhydrous glass ionomers use a 30% tartaric acid liquid (eg, Ketac-Cem, ESPE Dental-Medizin, Seefeld, Germany) whereas others include 5 to 10% tartaric acid in the freeze-dried portion of the powder (eg, Bio-Cem, LD Caulk, Milford, Delaware).

Advantages: less viscous, which makes crown seating easier, has the least long-term solubility, has an improved shelf life, and has higher powder-to-liquid ratios (which can result in better physical properties).

Disadvantages: less pulpally kind (more acidic), slower initial set (with increased potential for early marginal washout), and a higher associated incidence of pulpal irritation and pulp death.

Semihydrous
Semihydrous glass ionomers contain polyacrylic acid in both their liquid and their powder; they usually have an intermediate amount of tartaric acid in their liquid (eg, Fuji I and Fuji Cap I, GC; Maxicap, ESPE/Premier). They have a viscosity between that of hydrous and anhydrous glass-ionomer cements, have an intermediate initial acidity, and have been associated with a low to moderate amount of postoperative pulpal sensitivity.

Advantages: intermediate initial acidity and postoperative sensitivity; intermediate viscosity.

Disadvantages: higher initial acidity than hydrous systems, allowing more postoperative sensitivity, also slightly thicker than anhydrous cements.

All three forms of these ionomers, when mixed, create a fully hydrated polyacrylic acid copolymer that undergoes the same three-stage setting reaction described in Chapter 3. All three systems can have advantages in physical properties.

Effects of hydrosity on clinical properties

The term hydrosity refers to the extent a polyacrylic acid matrix is hydrated before mixing in glass-ionomer cement components. (Although not yet an accepted scientific term, it helps describe the clinical properties of glass-ionomer systems.)

Study group evaluations have evidenced some clear clinical trends. Hydrous materials have generally been associated with lower initial acidity and less postoperative pulpal sensitivity (less than 3 incidences per 100 cementations based on long-term study group evaluations). Anhydrous materials are associated with higher initial acidity and a higher incidence of postoperative sensitivity (8 to 10 per 100 cementations). Semihydrous materials show rates of acidity and pulpal kindness somewhere between the other two materials (3 to 6 sensitive pulps per 100 cementations).

These numbers should be compared with data related to polycarboxylate cement, which has the lowest incidence of postoperative sensitivity (less than 1 per 100 cementations). Unfortunately, polycarboxylates are more soluble than glass-ionomer cements and have limited fluoride release.

SELECTING A CEMENT

Selecting a luting agent for crown cementation can be difficult. Some short crown preparations and bridge abutments need optimal strength, whereas single crowns on patients with long preparations require minimal strength.

Teeth also vary in their need for a pulpally kind cementing material. Young teeth with deep porcelain-fused-to-metal preparations require a very kind material, since they have less dentin thickness to protect the pulp. Many conservative partial-coverage restorations on mature patients do well with a less kind cement, owing to increased dentin thickness and fewer open tubules. Endodontically treated teeth can tolerate a harsh cement.

Classifying cements by pulpal kindness

Study group participants have divided cementing agents into three classes: most pulpally kind, moderately pulpally kind, and least pulpally kind. The most pulpally kind class includes polycarboxylate cement and hydrous glass ionomers. The moderately kind class includes semihydrous glass ionomers and zinc phosphate cement with a protective varnish. The least kind class includes the anhydrous glass ionomers, zinc phosphate without a varnish, and the resin cements. As a general rule, the most pulpally kind cements are the weakest and most soluble, whereas the least pulpally kind cements are the strongest and least soluble. The type of cement used for placement of a temporary influences the sensitivity of the tooth; therefore, use of a pulpally kind temporary cement provides the greatest flexibility of choice of a final cementing agent (Tables 5–2 and 5–3).

Table 5-2. Physical Characteristics of Common Types of Temporary Cement

Agent	Strength	Solubility	Tooth Adhesion	Fluoride Release	Pulpal Kindness	Technique Sensitivity
Antibacterial ointment	Very low	Very high	None	None	Good	High
Calcium hydroxide	Low to moderate	High	None	None	Excellent	Low
Eugenol	Moderate	Moderate	None	None	Good	Moderate
Noneugenol	Low to moderate	Moderate	None	None	Moderate	Moderate
Dilute polycarboxylate	High	Moderate	Yes	None	Good	Moderate
Zinc phosphate	High	Low	None	None	Low	Moderate
Dual-cure composite	High	Very low	None	None	Low	High

72   Tooth-Colored Restoratives

Table 5-3. Properties of Common Types of Final Cementing Agents

Cementing Agent	Strength	Solubility	Tooth Adhesion	Fluroide Release	Pulpal Kindness	Technique Sensitivity
Zinc phosphate	Moderate	Moderate	No	No	Moderate	Moderate
Polycarboxylate	Moderate to low	High	Yes	No	Very high	Low
Glass ionomer						
Hydrous	Moderate	Pre-set: moderate Post-set: low	Yes	Yes	High	Moderate
Semihydrous	High	Pre-set: high Post-set: low	Yes	Yes	Moderate	Moderate
Anhydrous	High	Pre-set: very high Post-set: very low	Yes	Yes	Low	Very high
Resin-modified glass-ionomer	Moderate	Low	Yes	Yes	High	Low
Polyacrylic acid-modified composite	High	Low	Some	Some	Moderate	Moderate
Composite resin	Very high	Very low	Some	No	Low	High

Classifying prepared teeth by sensitivity

Teeth can be categorized as very sensitive, moderately sensitive, and slightly or not sensitive. The time to determine tooth sensitivity is when the temporary crown is removed from an unanesthetized tooth, just prior to cementation (Figure 5–1; Table 5–4).

Very sensitive teeth

A very sensitive tooth is a tooth that a patient reports is painful when air is drawn over it after removal of a temporary restoration. This is often found with full-coverage restorations in young patients or whenever the remaining dentin is very thin.

Moderately sensitive teeth

A tooth is considered moderately sensitive if it does not hurt and the patient can draw in a slight to moderate amount of air without pain, but cold air from a syringe causes discomfort. Most patients with typical crown-and-bridge preparations are in this class.

Slightly and nonsensitive teeth

This describes a tooth that gives little discomfort in relation to air, even from a moderate blast of air from an air syringe. Such nonsensitive teeth are commonly found in very mature patients with receded pulps, or in teeth with large buildups where little dentin is exposed on the axial walls.

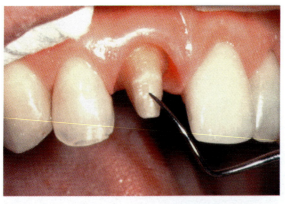
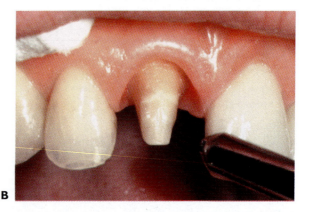

Figure 5–1. Testing tooth sensitivity. *A,* air test; *B,* touch test.

Table 5-4. Determining Tooth Sensitivity

Sensitivity	Air test	Touch test
Slight to none	Minimal discomfort to air syringe	No response
Moderate	Moderate discomfort to air syringe	Some discomfort to explorer
High	Responds to room air with lips open	Large response to slight touch

Another way to evaluate sensitivity is to touch an uncovered prepared tooth with a dry cotton pellet or the tip of an explorer. A very sensitive tooth reacts very strongly; moderately sensitive teeth feel the gentle rubbing but little pain; and the least sensitive group feels no sensation from forceful rubbing with either apparatus.

Though these sensitivity classes leave room for interpretation, they can guide a dentist in cement selection. Very sensitive teeth should be treated with the most kind cements, and least sensitive teeth could benefit from the less soluble least kind or moderately kind cements. If cement strength is a major concern, a dentist should weigh the importance of each factor. Moving up one class in "kindness of cement" can be tolerated by most patients, even though there is increased risk that sensitivity and pulpal death could result.

That being said, it is generally inadvisable to use one of the least kind cements on sensitive teeth. In these cases, pulp sensitivity and death is much more common in study group evaluations. Ideally, a dentist should be familiar with one material in each class to provide the most flexibility in meeting patient needs (see Table 5–3).

IONOMER CEMENT SENSITIVITY

A number of factors can affect marginal sensitivity. Studies show that properly placed glass ionomers protected by a varnish have no more marginal leakage than other cementing systems. Without a varnish, cement washout can occur. An alternative to varnish is to leave a 1-mm bead of cement past the margins until the material has fully set, usually 10 minutes (Figure 5–2). The disadvantage of this technique is that the excess cement is difficult to remove. Either method works well.

Hydraulic pressure from cementation and the low pH of some cements during initial set can also contribute to postoperative sensitivity.[2] However, the main cause of postcementation sensitivity is thought to be dessication.

Postoperative sensitivity with glass ionomers may be attributable to washout and open margins from early saliva contamination. If the smear layer covering the dentin tubules has been removed with conditioning liquids, early cement loss can permit bacteria access to the exposed and opened tubules.

Air entrapment prior to cementation

Air entrapment at the dentin–cement interface has long been suspected in postoperative cementation sensitivity. According to this theory, when a preparation is dried, air can be entrapped in the dentin tubules. It is difficult for any tissue to resorb air, and it can take considerable time for dentin tubules to absorb air. Despite the slowness of this process, retained air space is usually self-correcting. Changes in air pressure alter the hydrodynamics of dentin and the pain fibers. Pain on biting is a major symptom, since biting compresses air, which stimulates C-fiber pain.

The typical symptoms of postoperative sensitivity from entrapped air include:

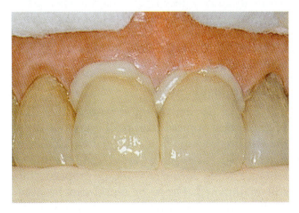

Figure 5–2. Cementation of crowns on two central incisors, showing use of a 1-mm cement bead to prevent washout prior to setting.

- Sensitivity to biting
- No sensitivity to hot or cold
- No signs of pulpitis

Endodontic evaluations

Sensitivity on biting is also associated with an abscessed tooth. This discomfort can be as much as with pulpitis but usually does not result in acute pain on tapping; instead, it responds mainly to steady loading. When endodontics is mistakenly done on these teeth, they are vital.

Because of the potential for misdiagnosis, it is important to obtain a patient history to assist in a proper diagnosis of reversible pulp disease. If all other symptoms and tests are negative, it is highly likely that the symptoms will self-correct, but it can take 1 to 12 months for them to completely resolve.

Prevention

A hydration period of 2 to 10 minutes prior to cementation can greatly reduce the risk of postoperative sensitivity.

Treatment

The best thing to do for a symptomatic tooth is to wait for the situation to resolve. If the symptoms continue to improve, the prognosis is good. Alternatively, in cases with severe pain, an opening should be made in the unit just into the dentin but not near the pulp. Then this opening is hydrated for 10 minutes with a topically applied local anesthetic and sealed with traditional glass-ionomer cement. The sensitivity usually goes away in days following this procedure, even when it has lasted for over a year.

CLINICAL CONCERNS WITH IONOMERS

Powder-to-liquid ratios

The correct powder-to-liquid ratio is important since physical properties drop off exponentially as the mix becomes too fluid. Generally speaking, as much powder as possible should be mixed into an ionomer while adequate working properties are still maintained. Drops of liquid can be accurately dispensed slowly; increased speed makes larger drops. The components should be mixed on glass, plastic, or a waxed pad—untreated paper may absorb some of the liquid and alter the powder-to-liquid ratio.

Glass-ionomer powders can change volume by as much as 50%, depending on how long they have been on the shelf and how long it has been since they have been shaken or tapped. The amount of glass-ionomer powder should be calibrated to a special scoop-to-drop ratio. Packed powders are more consistent than fluffed powders, although either can be used. The mix can be adjusted, depending on the intended use. Encapsulated systems are the most accurate.

Adhesion to casting and tooth structure

Polyacrylic acid-based systems, including glass ionomers and polycarboxylate cements, can bond to tooth structure and metal castings.

The oil in eugenol-based cements (eg, TempBond, IRM, and ZOE) can inhibit glass-ionomer bonding and, in excess, can inhibit setting. Noneugenol temporary cements are recommended for cases in which an ionomer is to be used for final crown cementation. Some popular noneugenol cements are TempBond NE (Kerr, Corp., Romulus, Michigan), Freegenol (GC), Nogenol (GC America Inc., Chicago, Illinois), Zone (Cadco, Dental Products Inc., Los Angeles, California), and Varibond (Van R Dental Products, Oxford, California).

Polyacrylic acid-based cements bond well to clean oxidized metals and only slightly to nonoxidized metals. For maximum retention, the crown should be sandblasted, tin-plated, and scrubbed with a toothbrush, water, and mild detergent before bonding.

Remaining dentin thickness

A critical determinant of good pulpal health and reduced postoperative pulpal problems is remaining dentin thickness, especially when virgin teeth are prepared for full-coverage all-porcelain or porcelain-fused-to-metal restorations. Radiographs can help estimate remaining dentin thickness proximally.

GLASS-IONOMER CEMENTATION TECHNIQUE

Following is a recommended technique for ionomer cementation.

Step 1. Isolate the tooth as well as possible using cotton rolls, dry angles, or a rubber dam. Place a dry retraction cord in the sulcus of all restorations with subgingival margins; this stops hemorrhage or oozing of gingival fluid.

Step 2. Clean the tooth thoroughly with pure pumice mixed with water, or a water- or air-abrasion unit. Be sure no saliva, blood, or intersulcular fluid contaminates the tooth before cementation.

Step 3. Select the cement and the correct amount of powder. (Calibrate with each new bottle of cement.)

Step 4. Hydrate the tooth for 2 minutes with a damp gauze or cotton pellet before cementation. With sensitive teeth, topically apply a saline solution to the desiccated tooth as a local anesthetic. Just before cementation, dry the tooth with a cotton pellet to remove any pooled moisture. The dentin should not look chalky white before cementation.

Step 5. Mix cement rapidly (follow manufacturer's recommendations), coat all crown walls with 1 mm of cement, and start to seat within 30 seconds after mixing. Slowly press the crown in place (about 10 seconds), allowing excess cement to extrude around all margins. This eliminates the need for a varnish coating at this point. Floss each contact once, to remove the marginal portion of cement. Leave in place until after the initial set. Setting time is temperature-dependent. Use a cold glass slab below the dew point if more working time is needed.

Step 6. Maintain isolation. Keep the cemented crown totally isolated until it reaches its initial set (usually 2 to 5 minutes). A damp (not wet) gauze can be placed over the tooth to establish 100% humidity until the cement reaches a more final set, at least 10 minutes. Hardness can be verified with an explorer.

Step 7. Remove excess cement bead from margins with a sharp instrument. Removing the retraction cord removes much of the proximal cement.

Step 8. Protect margins from early cement loss by covering with methyl cellulose or other suitable varnish. Some clinicians prefer unfilled resin for this step. Varnish is recommended since the excess removes itself in a few days.

Step 9. Do not adjust the occlusion for at least 10 minutes after the set.

Cements are initially highly soluble; following these steps reduces excessive penetration of cement into the dentin tubules or washout at the margins during the early phases of cementation. This cementation technique has a less than 2% incidence of pulpal sensitivity or death when teeth are matched to cement by sensitivity and type as previously described.

Dentin conditioners

A number of conditioners can be used to remove the smear layer and prime the surface before cementing with a glass ionomer. Most are 10 to 25% solutions of polyacrylic acid. Studies show these conditioners result in a more consistent ionomer bond strength to dentin. Used properly, they do not increase tooth sensitivity. Conditioners are generally indicated before Class V glass-ionomer restorations are placed.

GLASS-IONOMER RESTORATION

Glass ionomers have many clinical uses. Experience shows that they constitute the best restorative for Class V lesions, for Class III lesions involving dentin margins, for repair of crown margins, and for root caries. They are contraindicated for stress-bearing restorations (Figure 5–3). They are the most cost-effective restorative materials in dentistry, primarily because they are quick and easy to place, are self-adhesive, last a long time, and are anticariogenic. Their placement requires only three steps: (1) tooth conditioning, (2) mixing of material, and (3) placement of material. One drawback is that mixing can be technique sensitive; this difficulty is eliminated with encapsulated systems. Resin ionomers require light curing and, therefore, placement in layers. Autocured materials are placed in bulk but take longer (2–5 min) to set.

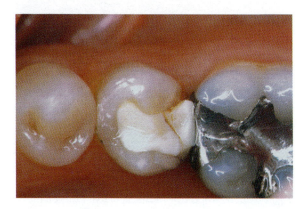

Figure 5–3. Fracture of a 2-year-old glass-ionomer provisional restoration because of occlusal function.

76 Tooth-Colored Restoratives

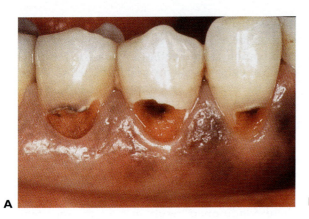 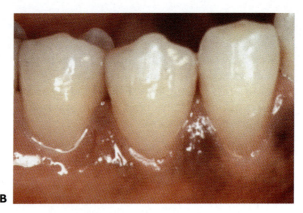

Figure 5–4. Treatment of significant Class V caries with a resin ionomer: *A*, preoperative. *B*, postoperative. (Courtesy of GC America Inc.).

Resin ionomers perform well in Class V restorations because they bond equally well to enamel and dentin, their thermal coefficient of expansion is similar to that of tooth structure, and they maintain marginal integrity long term (Figure 5–4). Over time, however, resin ionomers tend to expand and, therefore, require trimming at a later appointment. Expansion is most severe when materials are not adequately mixed or are contaminated with water during placement (Figure 5–5). Large Class V restorations are subject to the stress of tooth flexure, which can break the bond and dislodge the whole

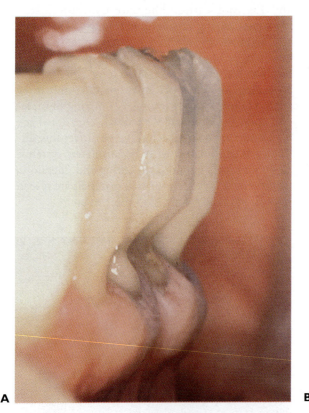 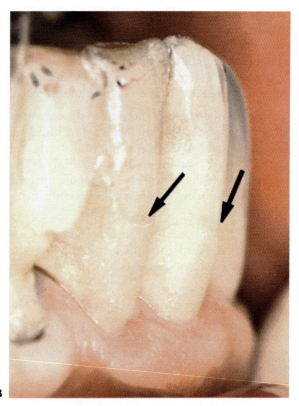

Figure 5–5. *A*, Preoperative treatment of root caries on the mandibular right central and lateral incisors. *B*, Two years after treatment, resin ionomer expansion is obvious. The excess material is easily trimmed with a fine diamond. The restoration on the mandibular right canine was lost owing to tooth flexure.

Uses of Ionomers 77

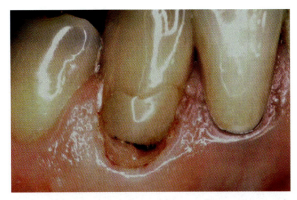

Figure 5–6. Two years after treatment of root caries with composite the marginal seal of this restoration is chipped and stained.

restoration. Retention grooves are advisable to reduce the potential for such peeling during flexure. The alternative restorative material, composite resin, does not maintain a good gingival seal and has a higher incidence of marginal staining of the dentin (Figure 5–6).

Any Class III carious lesion involving a dentin margin is best restored with a glass ionomer (Figure 5–7). Fluoride release from a glass-ionomer restoration can be maintained by recharging the ionomer through topical fluoride application or fluoride gel in a polyethylene splint (which would increase contact time) to reduce caries recurrence. This is particularly important for patients who

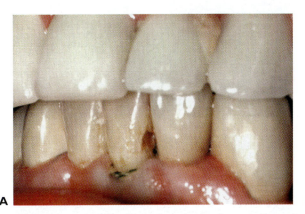
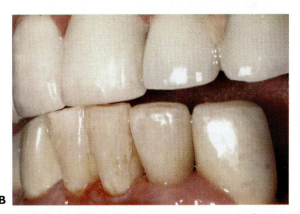

Figure 5–7. Proximal restorations at the dentin–enamel margin are well suited to glass-ionomer restoration. *A*, A gingival retraction cord is used to enhance tooth isolation, contain the glass ionomer to the preparation, and assist in finishing. Removal of the cord after ionomer setting creates a gap that provides access for a finishing instrument. *B*, Immediate postoperative appearance.

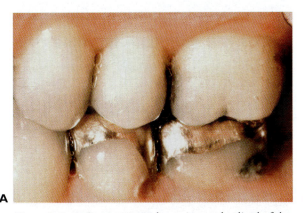
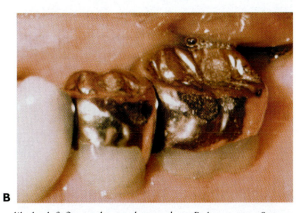

Figure 5–8. *A*, Carious gingival margins on the distal of the mandibular left first and second premolars. *B*, Appearance 8 years after treatment with traditional glass ionomer. Note the color stability and good marginal seal.

78   Tooth-Colored Restoratives

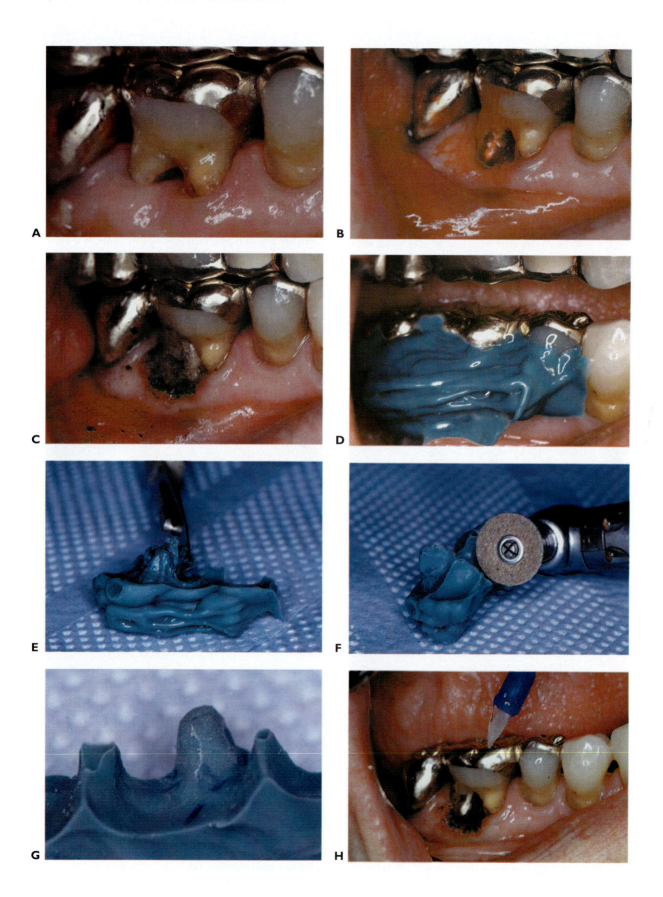

Uses of Ionomers 79

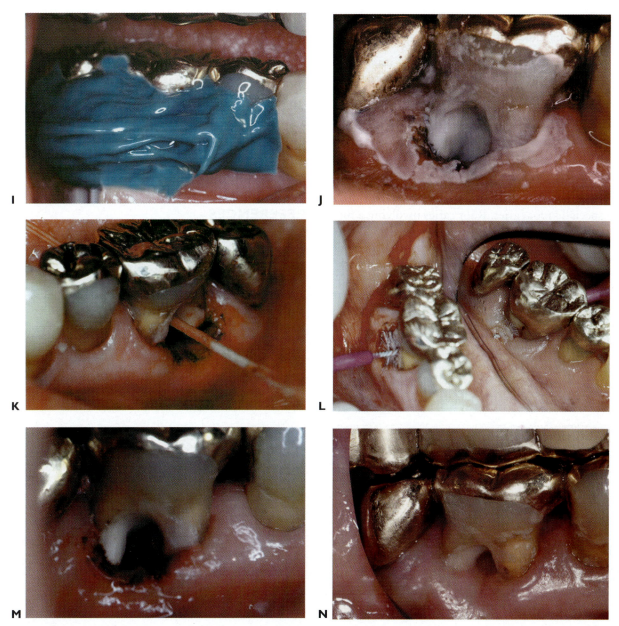

Figure 5–9. *A*, A severely carious furcation in an 87-year-old male with a heart condition. The tooth has had endodontic therapy and would normally be extracted. *B*, The tissue has been trimmed away and all caries removed. *C*, Hemorrhage is controlled by the use of ferric sulfate on a cotton pellet, electrosurgery, superoxol, or an astringent paste (eg, Eposyl, Kerr Corp.). *D*, A light-bodied impression material is injected into the furcation and around the adjacent teeth to make a mold of the tooth structure. *E*, Excess impression material is trimmed with a Bard Parker blade. *F*, The internal aspects of the template are smoothed. *G*, Finished template. The template should be tried in the mouth to ensure it fits passively with a predictable route of insertion. *H*, Lubricant is applied sparingly with a brush to coat adjacent teeth, internal aspects of the template, and other areas not to be restored. *I*, The autoset glass ionomer is injected into the furcation, and the template is placed gently, without pressure. The material is left to set. *J*, Once the material has set, the template is removed and the tooth inspected for adequate bulk of restorative. Additional material can be added, as necessary, to complete the contours (water soluble lubricant must first be washed away). *K*, Excess material is chipped away, and the restoration is contoured. Material is trimmed to allow a floss threader to fit through the furcation. *L*, The furcation is contoured from buccal and lingual to allow access with a proxy brush. The patient is instructed to clean the furcation from both sides with a proxy brush dipped in fluoride gel. *M*, The final finish is achieved with a rubber point. No effort is made to achieve a high polish. *N*, Appearance 3 months after treatment. Note the health of the surrounding tissues. This is largely attributable to daily application of topical fluoride with a proxy brush.

have xerostoma, such as individuals who have undergone radiation therapy for oral cancer.

Glass-ionomer material can greatly extend the life of a crown, because the restoration maintains its margin seal (Figure 5–8). This is of enormous benefit when a bridge abutment is carious; the option to repair the caries with glass ionomer is significantly less invasive and less expensive than replacing the entire prosthesis.

Traditional autoset glass ionomers are among the most common restoratives for aging dentition, especially root caries. Root caries involving a furcation is particularly difficult to restore. Untreated, this type of caries causes tooth loss. Root caries is easily restored when it occurs in accessible areas. Glass ionomers can be used with a template to restore even nonaccessible areas, such as caries at the center of a furcation. This technique is indicated for older patients who are medically compromised and would not easily tolerate an extraction, bridge, or implant. Fluoride recharging of these restorations is accomplished with a proxy brush dipped in fluoride gel. Figure 5–9 shows a challenging root caries treatment that involved use of a template to facilitate placement. Performing the same restoration with resin would be difficult because composite, unlike glass ionomer, cannot be trimmed with a blade after initial setting.

REFERENCES

1. Council on Dental Materials, Instruments, and Equipment. Reported sensitivity to glass-ionomer luting cements. J Am Dent Assoc 1984;109:476.

2. Smith DC, Ruse ND. Acidity of glass-ionomer cements during setting and its relation to pulp sensitivity. JADA 1986;112:654–7.

CHAPTER 6

RESIN POLYMERIZATION

It takes less time to do a thing right than it does to explain why you did it wrong.

Henry Wadsworth Longfellow

HISTORY OF DIRECT DENTAL POLYMERS

Self-curing acrylic resins were developed in 1941 by German chemists. They used tertiary amines with benzoyl peroxide to initiate methacrylate polymerization reactions. Their discoveries led to the development of acrylic filling materials (eg, Sevriton) in 1948. The major problems with these materials were high rates of polymerization shrinkage (about 20 to 25%), poor color stability, limited stiffness, high thermal expansion, and lack of adhesion to tooth structure. Polymerization shrinkage itself resulted in leakage and bacterial penetration, prompting a high incidence of dental caries. Many of these problems are still encountered.

Early attempts to reduce polymerization shrinkage and improve resin physical properties involved incorporation of fillers. This approach had worked to improve acrylic denture-base materials. Acrylic filling materials containing alumino silicate glass fillers were formulated in the 1950s.[1] Improved properties were obtained with these materials when the silicate glass particles were precoated with polymer or primed with silane.[2] These materials were difficult to handle, however, and were superseded by Bowen's Bis-GMA composites. Present-day composites generally consist of a resin matrix, filler particles, initiators of polymerization, and coupling agents.

COMPOSITION OF RESIN MATRIX

Currently, manufacturers use resin matrices composed of a wide variety of mono- and difunctional acrylates. This composition allows them to formulate composites that have specific properties.

The majority of resins are long hydrophobic dimethacrylate copolymers, chosen because they reduce shrinkage, are more color stable, and have better physical properties owing to cross-linkage.

Fundamentals of polymerizing resins

Polymerization yields three types of polymer structures: linear, branched, or cross-linked. *Linear polymers* are long chains, usually formed of a monofunctional monomer, for example, the polymethacrylates. *Branched polymers* have a second monomer that contains attached, branching side groups, such as ethyl methyl methacrylate. Both linear and branched polymers are used in temporary materials. *Cross-linked polymers* have a difunctional monomer with double bonds on both ends that can connect two linear branches. Two connecting branches are called a cross-link. Cross-linked polymers are typically more viscous and have better physical properties than other types of polymers; hence, they are used in restorative materials. Generally, the shorter the monomer, the greater the polymerization shrinkage, and the poorer the physical properties.

Chemical compositions

One of the most popular dimethacrylate resins used in dentistry is synthesized by the reaction between bisphenol A and glycidyl methacrylate. It is 2,2-bis[4-(2-hydroxy-3-methacryloxy-propoxy)-phenyl]-propane, referred to as Bis-GMA. Bowen introduced this resin in 1962. Bis-GMA is a relatively long and rigid difunctional monomer that allows for a cross-linked polymer and low shrinkage (about 4 to 6%). The structure of this resin is illustrated in Figure 6–1. The structure of methyl methacrylate is shown for a size comparison.

82 Tooth-Colored Restoratives

Methyl methacrylate (MMA)

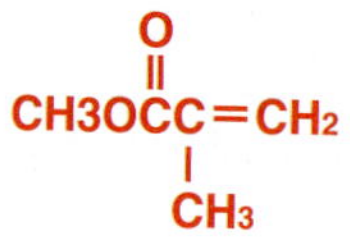

$$CH_3OCOC(CH_3)=CH_2$$

Bis-GMA

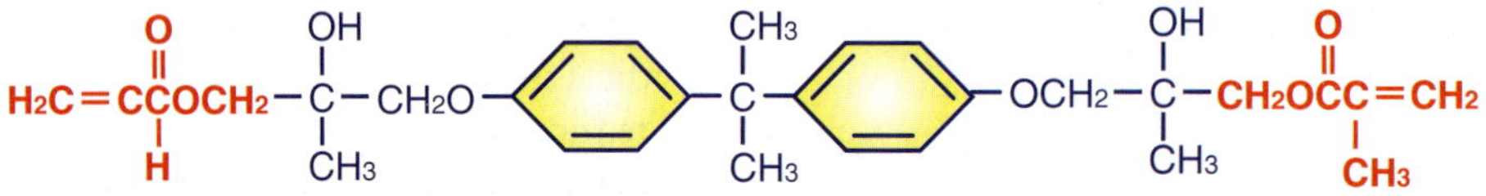

Figure 6–1. Bis-GMA. The chemical structure of Bis-GMA, a resin invented by Ray Bowen. It also is referred to as Bowen's resin.

Since Bis-GMA is viscous, it helps to strengthen the resin matrix. It is usually mixed with a resin of lower molecular weight, such as TEGDMA (triethylene glycol dimethacrylate), to reduce its viscosity and enable filler loading. TEGDMA has two reactive double bonds on both ends, as does Bis-GMA, but its shorter length increases shrinkage; TEGDMA shrinks about 15%. Varying the mixtures of these two difunctional monomers allows manufacturers to control the viscosity of the resulting composite resin. These two monomers are used in the majority of composite resins. The typical Bis-GMA-TEGDMA resin system shrinks about 3 to 5%. This high rate of shrinkage is the reason composite resins are usually placed in layers.

In 1974, Foster and Walker introduced another difunctional resin, urethane dimethacrylate (UDM). The major advantage of this resin is its low viscosity, which facilitates filler loading without the need to add low molecular weight monomers. The major disadvantages of this resin are that it is more brittle and it undergoes more polymerization shrinkage than Bis-GMA, shrinking about 5 to 9%. These properties may be attributable to its shorter molecular length. The structure of the urethane dimethacrylate is illustrated in Figure 6–2. This molecule is similar to one used in the Vivadent (Amherst, New York) resins. LD Caulk Co. (Milford, Delaware) uses a large monomer that is a combination of urethane and Bis-GMA; it shrinks about 7%. ESPE uses a patented tricyclo dimethacrylate resin with fewer hydroxy groups (–OH); it has lower water sorption and shrinks about 7%.

Manufacturers prefer Bis-GMA resins because they have an aromatic structure that increases stiffness and compressive strength and lowers water

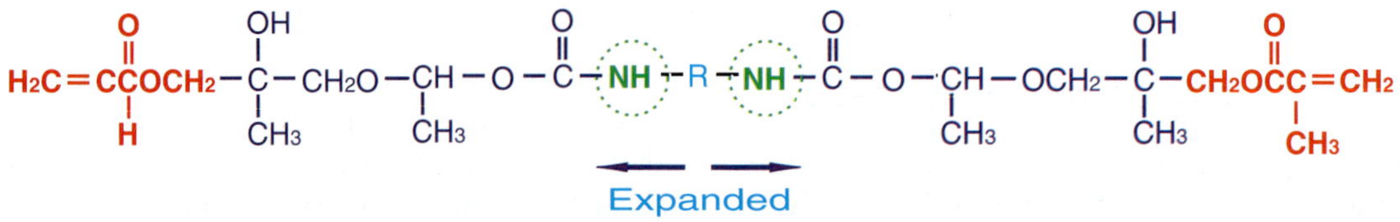

Figure 6–2. Urethane dimethacrylate. The chemical structure of popular difunctional urethane resins. R = a number of carbon compounds that can be used to lengthen or alter the properties of the monomer. Nitrogen in the form of NH–R–NH is the urethane component.

absorption. (Water is a plastizer that softens resins and decreases their color stability.) These larger molecules also undergo less polymerization shrinkage than smaller methacrylate-based monomers. Currently, one of the important areas of research is the development of new resins with stiffer and longer molecules. This would improve future composite materials.

Viscosity controllers

Many dimethacrylate resins, such as Bis-GMA, are highly viscous liquids. If very small monofunctional monomers (eg, methyl methacrylate) were used to lower viscosity, these more volatile components could shorten the shelf life of the composite, as well as increase polymerization shrinkage. Because of this, monomers that are less volatile are typically used to control viscosity. TEGDMA, urethane dimethacrylate, and EDMA (ethyleneglycol dimethacrylate) are commonly used to lower the viscosity of composite resins. Of these, TEGDMA is the most common and comprises 10 to 35% of most macrofilled composites and 30 to 50% of most microfilled composites. TEGDMA is a smaller and more flexible difunctional resin than Bis-GMA. Using TEGDMA makes the resin more flexible and less brittle, improves its marginal edge strength, and reduces the resin's resistance to abrasion. Since TEGDMA is smaller than Bis-GMA, it shrinks more when polymerized.[3] The chemical structure of TEGDMA is illustrated in Figure 6–3.

Resin materials stored in non-airtight containers (eg, as single-dose capsules) or in tubes missing their tops will dry out and deteriorate. The surface of an unpolymerized composite material should appear moist. If it is dry or crumbles when dispensed, it should be discarded.

Inhibitors and stabilizers

Inhibitors

To prevent premature resin polymerization, compounds such as 4-methoxyphenol (MEHQ) and 2,6-di-tert-butyl-4-methyl phenol or butylated hydroxytoluene (BHT) are generally added in amounts of about 0.1%.

Color stabilizers

Chemically cured composites may contain compounds such as benzophenones, benzotriazoles, or phenylsalicylate that absorb ultraviolet (UV) light and act as color stabilizers. These materials are not found in the UV light-polymerized systems because they can inhibit polymerization. The inhibitor BHT adds color stability.

COMPOSITE FILLERS

Filler particles provide dimensional stability to the soft resin matrix. The filler particles used in composite resins vary in size from less than 0.04 μm to over 100 μm. Filler particles reduce polymerization shrinkage, decrease the coefficient of thermal expansion, and increase hardness. Common filler particles are crystalline quartz; pyrolytic silica (such as in Aerosil®, Degussa Corp., Ridgefield Park, New Jersey); and glasses such as lithium aluminum silicate, barium aluminum silicate, and strontium aluminum silicate. All of these materials have excellent hardness, chemical inertness, and a refractive index similar to that of commonly used resin

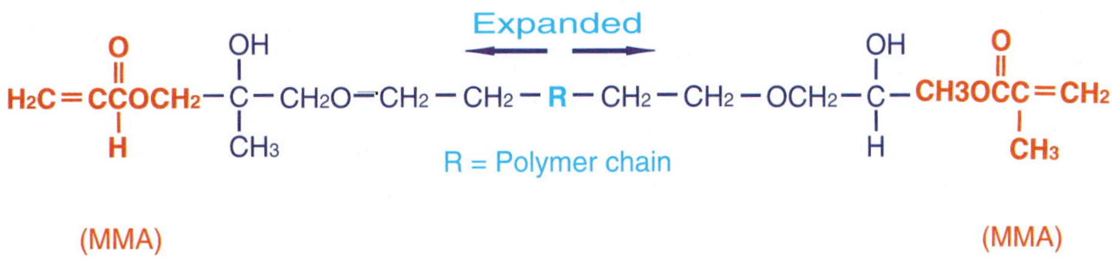

Figure 6–3. TEGDMA. The chemical structure of triethyleneglycol dimethacrylate (TEGDMA, which is also abbreviated TEDMA and TEGMA). The structure of methyl methacrylate (MMA) is shown for comparison.

matrices. Opacity is controlled by adding titanium dioxide pigments, and color is achieved by adding metal oxides of iron, copper, magnesium, and others. Unfortunately, many of these radiopaque glasses are susceptible to erosion. With some composites, the flexural strength and the flexural modulus are reduced by up to 45% after being in water for 3 months.[3]

Quartz and heavy-metal glass are commonly used fillers in conventional macrofilled composites. Submicron silica is the predominant filler in microfilled composites. Quartz is twice as hard as and is less susceptible to erosion than most glass fillers. Quartz is so hard it is difficult to grind into small particles, and composites made from quartz are more difficult to finish. However, silanes (discussed below under coupling agents) bind to quartz fillers better than any of the glass fillers. This may be why quartz-filled composites are so color-stable in clinical studies, compared with more soluble glass-filled composites of similar loading and particle size. A major limitation is that quartz fillers are radiolucent.

Silica dioxide and agglomerated submicron silica are used in making microfilled composites or are added to glass-filled composites to produce hybrids. Silica dioxide particles (0.04 μm) are made from silicon through a heating process that results in a fine ash. Agglomerated silica is made by precipitation of silica dioxide particles; this increases their size, which reduces surface area and increases filler loading.

Owing to the clinical need for radiopacity, radiopaque heavy-metal glass fillers have replaced quartz in most new macrofilled composites. The most common elements added to increase radiopacity are barium, strontium, zinc, zirconium, and ytterbium.[4] Bowen and Cleek invented barium glass fillers in 1969.[5] Barium fillers have a number of advantages: (1) good radiopacity; (2) fine particle size (average 0.4 to 0.6 μm; the size of enamel crystals, which makes them more polishable and wear-resistant); (3) good index of refraction relative to resins (increases esthetics); (4) lower cost; and (5) ready availability in pre-ground fillers. The disadvantages of barium glass fillers are that they are more soluble, softer, and more difficult to attach to the resin matrix than some other fillers.

Bowen invented strontium glass filler in 1980 (United States Patent No. 4,215,033, July 29, 1980). Compared with barium glass, it is stronger, less soluble, harder and more abrasive to enamel, and more difficult to grind into fine particles. Zirconium is harder than heavy-metal glass but not as hard as quartz. The zirconium fillers used in the product Z250 (3M Dental Products, St. Paul, Minnesota) are made through a priority precipitation process. Zirconium fillers can also be coated with silica to improve attachment to the matrix (eg, Palfique Estelite, J. Morita, Tustin, California).

Methods of particle fabrication
Fillers larger than 0.1 micron are typically made by grinding larger particles of glass or quartz to size and, sometimes, by precipitating crystals out of a solution. Therefore, grinding of glass fillers has become one of the most important and most highly sophisticated procedures in the production of macrofilled composites. The ability to produce extremely small particles accounts for the development of composites that are both strong and polishable.

Mill grinding
Milling is the traditional method of grinding glass. In this process, glass particles are crushed between two harder and tougher surfaces. Mill grinding produces particles with sharp edges. The major limitation of this method is the impurities contributed by the grinding wheels. These impurities are difficult to remove and can destroy the esthetics of the final composite.

Air abrasion
In air abrasion, filler particles grind themselves as they collide and fracture in two forced streams of particles. In theory, this process is similar to blasting sand against itself or another more solid object. The difficulty with this technique is that as the particles get smaller they miss each other more often. Hence, it takes a long time to grind fine particles. The advantage is that larger particles are quickly eliminated since they readily collide with other particles. Particles created by fracture have sharp edges.

Ultrasonic interaction
In this method, glass particles collide in suspension in a solvent undergoing ultrasonic vibration. This method can produce small particles from almost

any filler. The disadvantage is that the process takes considerable time. Particles produced by this process have rounded edges because of the mechanical effects of particle-to-particle interaction. The process is similar to polishing rocks in a rotating can: they continually get smoother.

Erosion

Erosion grinding is based on the solubility of glass particles in acidic solutions. Erosion combined with vibration (usually ultrasonic) makes particles smaller at a rapid rate. The technique is similar to polishing rocks in a vibrating tumbler that contains chemicals to speed up the erosive process while the fillers are ground mechanically. These particles have rounded edges and, depending on the chemicals used, may have a porous surface.

Effects of filler loading on composite resins

Filler size and loading are associated with three trends in composite resin performance: (1) the ability to polish increases as filler particle size decreases, (2) wear resistance improves as filler particle size decreases, and (3) fracture durability generally increases as the percent of inorganic filler loading by volume increases (this is termed percent filled).

Fracture resistance increases as the interparticle distance decreases because less distance reduces the load-bearing stress on the resin and inhibits crack formation and propagation.[6] The formation of cracks and their enlargement (called propagation) are the initial events leading to composite failure. Composites with smaller particles and higher filler loading (less interparticle distance) are more resistant to cracks. In addition, particles with smooth and rounded edges distribute stress more evenly throughout a resin and perform with fewer cracks. Filler particles with sharp edges pack better but can cause cuts or cracks in the resin during loading unless packed very tightly. Similarly, there is a direct linear relation between the stiffness of a composite (Young's modulus) and the volume of filler used (Figure 6–4).[7]

Coupling agents

Coupling agents are used to help bond resin matrix and filler particles together; they are also sometimes called adhesives. In conventional composites, the matrix material and filler particles are different and

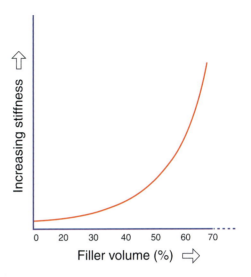

Figure 6–4. The relation between filler loading by volume and stiffness, as measured by Young's modulus. (Adapted from Braem M, Lambrechts P, Van Doren V, Vanherle G. The impact of composite structure on its elastic response. J Dent Res 1986;65:648–53.)

no chemical bond exists between them. Coupling agents reduce the gradual loss of filler particles from the composite surface. Commonly used coupling agents are epoxy, vinyl, and methyl silanes. The single most commonly used silane in dental composites is 3-(methacryloyloxypropyl) trimethoxysilane (Union Carbide).

Most silanes are difunctional molecules that, in theory, can ionically bond to the inorganic filler particles and simultaneously chemically bond to the organic matrix. In reality, silanes probably work mostly by reducing the surface tension between the inorganic filler and organic matrix. In simple terms, they act like a soap that increases the resin wetting of the filler. Silane-containing resins form a better physical bond because the resin can adapt to the irregularities of the filler particles. Though silanes help reduce wear, there is room for improvement in filler coupling-agent technology. Presently, silane coupling agents work best on quartz fillers, since silica is available in both materials to form bonds.

Microfills that use coupling agents coat the microfill or the prepolymerized resin particles. Coupling agents (eg, silanes) add little volume.

86 Tooth-Colored Restoratives

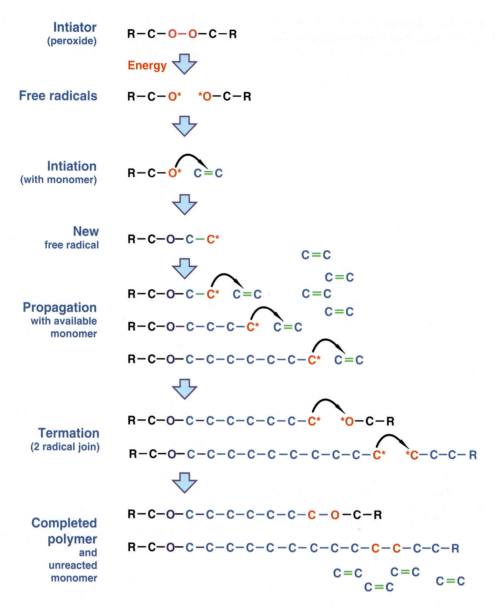

Figure 6–5. The chain reaction of a free radical continuing the polymerization process.

Most manufacturers include the weight of these materials in the figures quoted as percent filler. The filler coupling agents have a thin film thickness; generally, they add 1 to 6% to the weight of filler particles. Some microfills, such as those using Aerosil 200, do not have coupling agents. Since fillers are heavier than resin, percent filler by weight is a larger number than percent filler by volume, which is the clinically significant factor. For example, a typical composite filled 75% by weight is usually filled only 50 to 60% by volume.

INITIATORS OF POLYMERIZATION

Initiation systems start the polymerization process through the formation of a free radical, a compound with a reactive unpaired electron. When a free radical collides with a carbon double bond

(C=C) in the resin monomer, the free radical pairs with one of the electrons of the double bond, converting the other member of the pair to a free radical, and thus the reaction continues (Figure 6–5).

Generation of free radicals is brought about in four different ways. In heat-activated systems, benzoyl peroxide splits under heat exposure and forms free radicals. In chemically activated systems, a tertiary amine (that acts as an electron donor) is used to split the benzoyl peroxide into free radicals. In UV light-activated systems, a 365-nanometer (nm) UV light source splits benzoin methyl ether (in amounts of 0.2%) into free radicals without the presence of tertiary amines. In light-cured systems, a light source of 468 nm (±20) excites camphoroquinone (0.03 to 0.09%) or another diketone into a triplet state that interacts with a nonaromatic (referred to as aliphatic) tertiary amine, such as N,N-dimethylaminoethyl methacrylate (0.1% or less).[8] The camphoroquinone together with the tertiary amine starts a free radical reaction. Some manufacturers use an aromatic amine because it is more reactive and allows the use of less camphoroquinone. This combination results in less profound quinone lightening and resulting color changes during polymerization (Figure 6–6). No studies have been done to determine if this combination improves or has any long-term effects on color stability.

In chemically activated systems, the chemicals that initiate polymerization are usually separated into two pastes. When the pastes are mixed, polymerization starts. In light-activated systems, one paste contains all of the polymerization initiation chemicals, and polymerization is light-initiated (UV light in older systems and visible light in present-day systems). The four types of initiation reactions are summarized in Table 6–1.

INITIATION SYSTEMS

The polymerization process lasts until most of a resin's free monomers become polymerized. The amount of monomer converted into copolymer is called the conversion rate. Some initiation systems have a higher degree of conversion than others.

Measurements of polymerization rate (percent conversion)

The conversion rate of a composite is measured in a number of ways, typically by infrared (IR) spectroscopy. For a single material, a polymer's rate of conversion correlates with its hardness.[9] However, since hardness also increases with filler loading, differences in conversion rate among different materials do not necessarily translate into differences in hardness.[6] For a single material, conversion, hardness, and stiffness are directly related to the rate and amount of polymerization.[7]

Heat curing provides the highest conversion rate and results in a resin that is stiffer, more stain-resistant, and more fracture-resistant than resins cured by other methods. Heat curing is used to make prepolymerized filler particles for microfilled composites and indirect composite restorations, such as veneers, inlays, and onlays, and facings for crown-and-bridge restorations. The next most complete curing occurs with light-activation, which is preferred for direct composites. Light-curing is efficient and results in a uniform cure of the resin matrix. Autocuring can result in the least uni-

Table 6–1. Chemical Reactions that Produce Free Radicals*

Initiator	Chemical Reaction
Heat	Benzoyl peroxide + heat = free radical
Chemical	Benzoyl peroxide + 2% aromatic tertiary amine = free radical
UV light	0.1% benzoin methyl ether + 365-nm UV light source = free radical
Visible light	0.06% camphoroquinone + 0.1% aromatic or 0.04% aliphatic tertiary amine + 468-nm (±20) visible light source = free radical

*Once free radicals are formed, polymerization begins.

88 Tooth-Colored Restoratives

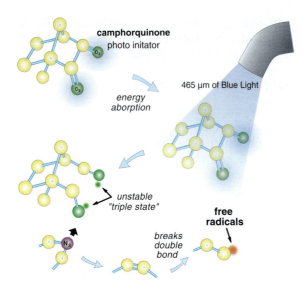

Figure 6–6. The free radical formation of camphoroquinone.

form cure, especially when thick composites are mixed, since the final mix lacks homogeneity on a molecular level. Another factor lowering the conversion rate is instability of the peroxide initiators used in autocured composites. Using very high amounts of autocuring chemicals can greatly increase conversion. However, this compromises color stability and is appropriate only for areas with low esthetic demands, such as core material.

Effects of oxygen incorporation
Mixing two composite pastes incorporates air into a restorative. Air inhibition reduces compressive strength by 30% in a macrofill and by 35% in a microfill. It also reduces fatigue strength by 20%.[10]

Color stability of initiator compounds
Two types of discoloration occur in resin systems: internal (intrinsic) and external (extrinsic).

Intrinsic stains
The aromatic tertiary amines are reactive compounds, and the oxidation of excess amine in a cured polymer is thought to be a major cause of intrinsic discoloration.[11] These amines are commonly used in large amounts in autocured systems, and in small amounts in some light-activated systems.

The tertiary amines are strong electron donors. In resin systems, the amine normally reacts with benzoyl peroxide during initiation. When amine and peroxide are present in equal amounts, both are consumed in the setting reaction and postoperative intrinsic discoloration is minimal. Severe discoloration is a result of the relative instability of benzoyl peroxide, which decomposes when stressed by heat or long-term storage. This peroxide breakdown disturbs the amine-to-peroxide balance, leaving excess amine. When curing, only a portion of the amine can react with the limited amount of peroxide remaining in the resin. The unreacted amine then oxidizes, and the composite discolors. Large concentrations ($\geq 2\%$) of amine compounds are needed to make autocure systems work. Hence, peroxide decomposition in these systems could result in large amounts of unreacted amine and would explain the relatively high incidence of intrinsic discoloration in these resins.[12]

Visible light-cured composite systems are efficient and, thus, require less tertiary amine ($\leq 0.1\%$). The color stability of light-cured composites is further improved by the use of aliphatic amines. These amines are nonaromatic and, therefore, considerably less reactive; they result in less intrinsic discoloration when they are left unreacted. A major cause of discoloration in light-cured systems is undercuring, which results in unreacted initiators as well as a porous and soluble material. Clinical studies have demonstrated that when autocured and light-cured materials are properly stored and used, they have comparable color stability after 3 years.[13]

Extrinsic stains
External discoloration is usually superficial and is associated with restoration roughness. However, water-soluble stains can discolor composite throughout a resin matrix. This is usually attributable to chemical degeneration of the filler–resin bond and solubility of the resin matrix.

Heat generated by chemical and light activation
Considerably less heat is generated by autocured systems than by light-cured systems. The type of light source also influences heat generation in light-cured systems. Heat adds kinetic energy to a curing system and increases conversion. Because light-cured systems produce heat faster than autocured systems, the temperature rise is more distinct. A

higher temperature increases the mobility of the monomers and leads to a higher reaction turnover.

CURING SYSTEMS

Autocured systems

Autocured (ie, chemically activated) systems, usually consisting of two pastes, dominated the tooth-colored restorative field for many years. They are still common in many parts of the world. Autocured systems generate small amounts of heat during curing and do not need a light source. Their disadvantages include: (1) a long setting time, (2) voids in the final restorative (voids caused by mixing typically account for 3 to 10% of the volume, inhibiting polymerization and increasing surface roughness), and (3) a higher probability of long-term discoloration after placement.[14]

Ultraviolet light-activated systems

The first light-activated systems, introduced in 1970, used UV light, which presented the advantages of rapid cure; indefinite working time, because no setting occurs until the light source is applied; and less composite waste. The disadvantages of UV light-activated systems include: (1) curing units require a 5-minute warm-up period, (2) depth of light penetration is 1 to 2 mm at best, (3) maintaining the light at 100% efficiency is difficult, and (4) UV radiation can cause corneal burns. Another difficulty is that the loss of UV efficiency cannot be determined by looking at the unit. Thus, a dentist cannot determine if a composite has adequately cured. The first product using UV light to cure composites was the Nuva System developed by LD Caulk, which also introduced acid etching.

Visible light-activated systems

Over the past 25 years, many visible light-cured composite resins and curing units have been introduced. The key advantages of visible light-activated composites are: (1) materials can be manipulated longer and still have a shorter curing time (20–40 seconds or less vs. minutes for autocured composites), (2) earlier finishing, and (3) better color stability. Other advantages include no lamp warm-up time; less chance of voids and air bubble incorporation; less waste of materials; and use of halogen bulbs, which maintain constant blue light efficiency for 100 hours under normal use. Halogen light is not without its problems: as with all incandescent bulbs, halogen bulbs gradually lose the higher energy wavelengths in their light output, which are needed for curing. Another problem is bulb silvering; that is, the bulb can blacken from the inside, thereby reducing the intensity of the light emitted.

The disadvantages of visible light-activated composites include: (1) possible eye damage (retinal burns with visible light systems), (2) a maximum depth of light penetration of about 3 mm, (3) heat generation that could harm the pulp, and (4) the high purchase and maintenance costs of curing lights. In systems using flexible fiber-optic bundles, it is difficult to maintain the efficiency of the light cord, which can result in a less effective depth of cure. Nevertheless, the advantages outweigh the disadvantages, making visible light-curing the preferred system.

The mechanism of visible light-curing uses a diketone, most commonly, camphoroquinone. When this photoinitiator absorbs blue light, the molecule forms a free radical and starts the polymerization process.

Configuration factor

The most important consideration a dentist has when placing a restorative that shrinks on setting, like composites, is the number of opposing walls facing the restorative since these margins can be opened when the material shrinks.

The c-factor (configuration factor) is a term used for the ratio of the number of walls bonded to unbonded. It is the reason different application sequences are used when placing composite resins. As the c-factor increases, ramp, step, and pulse curing become effective ways of reducing marginal openings and cuspal strain from polymerization shrinkage. The c-factor is illustrated in Figure 6-8A. This is explained more fully in Appendix A.

CURING TECHNIQUES

Historically, dentists have restored teeth by using conventional curing lights to cure layers of composites, typically at time intervals of 40 seconds per layer. Over the past few years, the industry has focused on reducing the resin curing time by using stronger curing lights or altering resin composition. The goal is to achieve restorations more quickly.

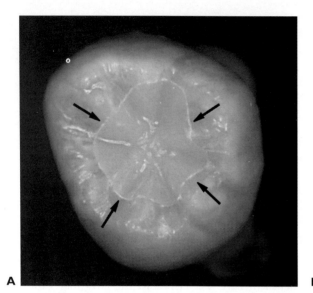 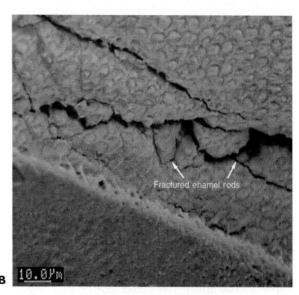

Figure 6–7. *A*, Photographic view of a white line margin in a Class I composite restoration. These typically occur on larger composites with opposing walls. *B*, Electron microscopic photograph of fractured enamel rods at the margin between enamel and composite on a Class I restoration—the same type as shown in *A*. (Courtesy of Bisco, Schaumburg, Illinois.)

Manufacturers have introduced new composites that yield a greater depth of cure. This assumes that one thick layer creates a superior restoration. In fact, a single, thick composite layer is a poor restoration because it increases the polymerization stress on the restoration margins. Stress from resin shrinkage results in white lines, which are cracked enamel rods or marginal gaps, and open margins (Figure 6–7). Hence, composites or curing units that provide larger depths of cure are of limited value, since composites must be layered to limit the effects of polymerization shrinkage. Careful attention to composite layering and curing technique can reduce the incidence of broken enamel margins.

A review of standard visible light-curing techniques helps to lay the groundwork for understanding where each type of curing unit fits into a dentist's armamentarium. Two categories of technique are commonly used in curing polymers: continuous and discontinuous. The continuous cure refers to a light-cure sequence in which the light is on continuously (Figure 6–8B). There are four types of continuous curing: uniform continuous cure, step cure, ramp cure, and high-energy pulse (Figure 6–9). Continuous curing is conducted with halogen, arc, and laser lamps. The discontinuous cure is also called soft cure, which commonly uses a pulse delay (Figure 6–10). This is similar to holding a halogen light at some distance from a tooth to initiate a cure, and then moving it close to the restoration for the duration of appropriate exposure. Soft-cure settings are available on some halogen curing lights.

Continuous curing techniques

Uniform continuous cure

In the uniform continuous cure technique, a light of constant intensity is applied to a composite for a specific period of time. This is the most familiar method of curing currently used.

Step cure

In the step cure technique, the composite is first cured at low energy, then stepped up to high energy, each for a set duration. The purpose is to reduce polymerization stress by inducing the composite to flow in the gel state during the first application. Theoretically, this practice reduces the overall polymerization shrinkage at the margin of the final restoration. The reduction in shrinkage, however, is small and results in less composite polymerization because the lower intensity light yields lower energy levels. In addition, this technique results in an uneven cure, since the top layer is more saturated with light and thus more highly cured. Step curing is possible only with halogen lamps; arc lamps and lasers cannot be used because

Resin Polymerization 91

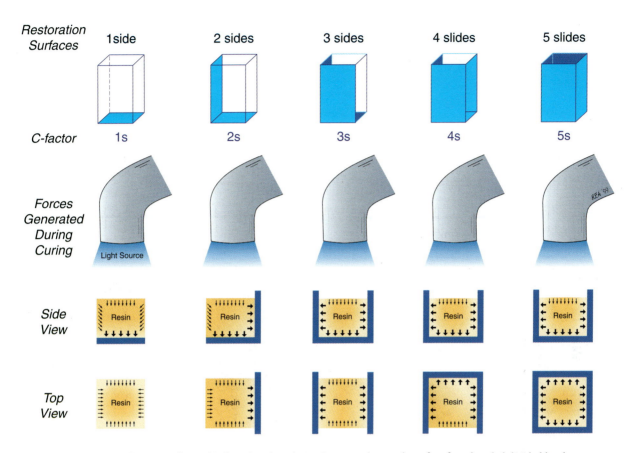

Figure 6–8A. The configuration factor (C-factor) is the relation between the number of surfaces bonded divided by the number of surfaces unbonded. As the configuration factor goes up, the effects of polymerization stress and strain become more significant in maintaining marginal seal. (Adapted from Feilzer AJ, de Gee AJ, Davidson CL. Relaxation of polymerization contraction shear stress by hygroscopic expansion. J Dent Res 1990;69:36–9.)

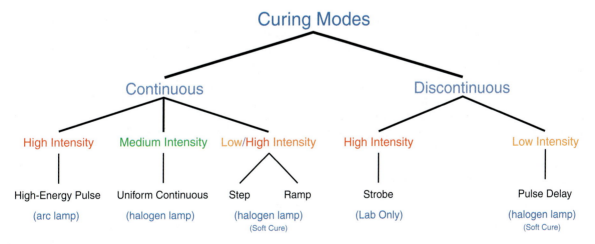

Figure 6–8B. A graphic depiction of common curing modes, also known as energy application sequences.

92 Tooth-Colored Restoratives

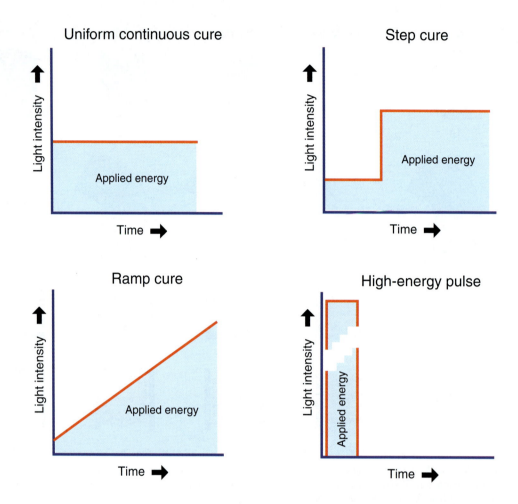

Figure 6–9. The four types of continuous curing techniques.

they work by applying large amounts of energy over short periods of time.

Ramp cure
In the ramp cure, light is initially applied at low intensity and gradually increased over time to high intensity. This allows the composite to cure slowly, thereby reducing initial stress, because the composite can flow during polymerization. Ramp curing is an attempt to pass through all of the different intensities in hopes of optimizing a composite's polymerization. Some studies indicate ramp curing causes polymerization with longer chains, resulting in a more stable composite. In theory, very high energy applied over a short period tends to cause dimethacrylate monomers to attach to themselves, resulting in shorter polymer chains and a more brittle material with higher polymerization shrinkage and more marginal gaps. Ramp curing, with its dependence on low intensity, is possible only with halogen lamps; arc and laser lamps can generate only large, nonvariable amounts of energy. It is possible to ramp cure manually by holding a conventional curing lamp at a distance from a tooth and slowly bringing it closer to increase intensity.

High-energy pulse cure
The high-energy pulse cure technique uses a brief (10 second) pulse of extremely high energy (1000–2800 mW per cm^2), which is three to six times the normal power density. This type of

Resin Polymerization 93

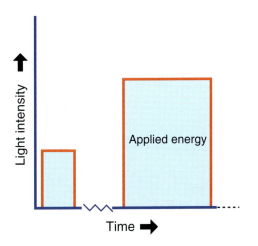

Figure 6–10. Pulse-delay cure. A plot of the pulse-delay discontinuous curing technique.

polymerization has not yet been adequately examined, and there are three areas of potential concern: (1) the rapid application of energy might result in a weaker resin restoration owing to the formation of shorter polymers; (2) it is possible that rapid applications of energy could reduce diametral tensile strength; and (3) there may be a threshold level at which a resin has good properties, and thus, higher energies would result in more brittle resins (Figure 6–11).

Discontinuous curing techniques

In the discontinuous or soft-cure technique, a low-intensity or soft light is used to initiate a slow polymerization that allows a composite resin to flow from the free (unbound) restoration surface toward the (bound) tooth structure. This reduces polymerization stress at the margins and could reduce "white line" or other marginal openings or defects. To complete the polymerization process, the intensity of the next curing cycle is greatly increased, to produce the needed energy for optimal polymerization.

Pulse-delay cure

In pulse-delay curing, a single pulse of light is applied to a restoration, followed by a pause and then by a second pulse cure of greater intensity and longer duration. It is best thought of as an interrupted step increase. The lower-intensity light slows the rate of polymerization, which allows shrinkage to occur until the material becomes rigid, and is purported to result in fewer problems at the margins (Figure 6–12). The second, more intense pulse brings the composite to the final state of polymerization. Pulse curing is usually done with halogen lamps.

CURING ENERGY

Composites are cured through photoinitiator energy absorption. Energy is a unit that includes the intensity of light and the duration of light application over a given area. For example, the typical composite requires a 40-second exposure to 400 mW of 400- to 500-nm light per square centimeter. The measure of energy is the joule. One joule is the energy generated from 1 watt for 1 second.

The typical composite needs 16 joules to polymerize properly. This is easily calculated by multiplying the power applied by the duration of application (time): 400 mW × 40 seconds = 16 joules. However, 16 joules could also be generated by curing at 800 mW for 20 seconds, or by curing at

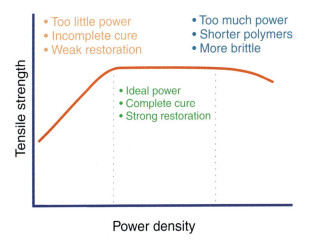

Figure 6–11. A plot of the theorized relation between power density and diametral tensile strength. This shows that there is a threshold at which a resin has good properties. Higher energies may result in more brittle resins. (Adapted from Kelsey WP, Blankenau RJ, Powell GL, et al. Power and time requirements for use of the argon laser to polymerize composite resins. J Clin Laser Med Surg 1992;10:273–8.)

94   Tooth-Colored Restoratives

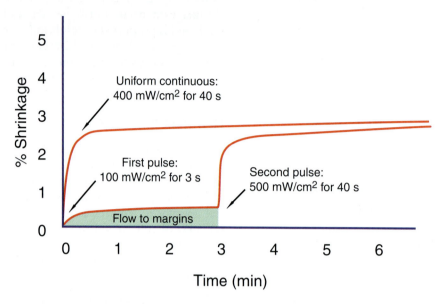

Figure 6–12. Plot of the typical reduction in strain from curing in two separate pulses over a 3-minute period. The first pulse is low energy to allow the composite to better remain attached to the margins. The second, delayed, pulse is high energy to complete the conversion of the composite. (Modified from information provided by Bisco, Schaumburg, Illinois.)

1600 mW for 10 seconds. Thus, curing times are dependent on light intensity. In addition, greater intensities increase curing depths.

Spectral overlap

The newer composites incorporate multiple photoinitiators to improve the polymerization properties of the restorative. This has implications for curing, because each initiator is activated at a different wavelength. It is important that the wavelength of the curing lamp include the photoinitiator's absorption wavelengths (ie, that there is spectral overlap between the wavelengths of the lamp and those of the photoinitiator). Figure 6–13 depicts the spectral overlap of three types of curing lamps.

Halogen lamps emit a large number of wavelengths of light (ie, they have a large bandwidth), which allows them to activate a wide range of photoinitiators. Laser lamps emit a narrow bandwidth, which enables them to activate only the photoinitiators that respond to those few bandwidths. These units do not fully polymerize many of the newer composites that include a variety of photoinitiators. Hence, an inferior composite restoration is most likely to result from use of laser curing devices. Arc lamps (also known as plasma arc curing [PAC] lamps) also have a relatively narrow bandwidth of curing wavelengths, although their span of activation is greater than that of laser units. However, since the plasma-filled cord filters the light, changing the cord can alter the bandwidth.

DENTAL TERMS FOR THE POLYMERIZATION OF RESINS

Discussion of the complexities of composite polymerization requires a common nomenclature that describes the various components and interactions involved in the process (see Appendix A). Eight leading manufacturers of dental polymers have agreed to adopt the nomenclature outlined here for reporting the results of polymer research as well as, potentially, for product labeling.

1. Wavelength requirements of the composite

   Spectral requirements (SR) for photopolymerization: the bandwidth of wavelengths necessary to activate the photoinitiator(s) in a specific composite; the bandwidths that absorb light energy and form the free radicals necessary for polymerization.

Resin Polymerization   95

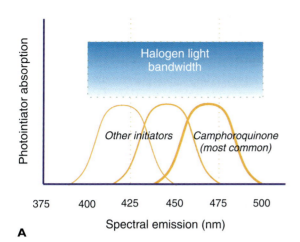

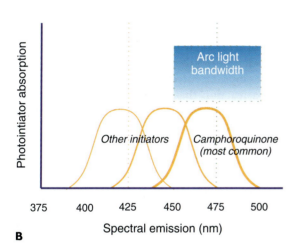

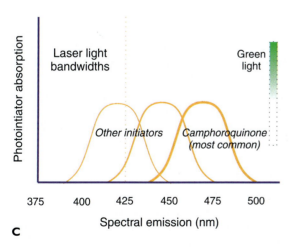

Figure 6–13. The spectral overlap showing the typical photoinitiator absorption curves for *A*, halogen, *B*, arc, and *C*, laser lamps.

Example: SR = 460 to 470 nm; specified by the composite manufacturer for camphoroquinone intitators.

2. Wavelength generated by the curing unit

   Spectral emission (SE) for photopolymerization: the effective bandwidth of wavelengths emitted by a curing unit for photopolymerization. The SE bandwidth should overlap or be congruent with the absorption range(s) of the photoinitiator(s) in the resin composite.

   Example: SE = 400 to 500 nm; specified by the curing-light manufacturer.

3. Intensity of wavelength the curing unit emits

   Power density (PD): the total power (units = mW or W) emitted by a curing unit within the stated effective bandwidth or SE, divided by the spot size of the curing tip (cm^2).

   Example: PD = 600 mW/cm^2 for an SE = 400 to 500 nm 1 mm from the surface. Specified by the curing-light manufacturer.

4. Total energy applied

   Energy density (ED): the power density (PD) multiplied by the exposure time(s).

   Example: ED = 800 mW/cm^2 × 30 s = 16 J/cm^2.

5. The energy the composite needs

   EOP@D = Energy density required for optimal polymerization at a specified depth.

   Example: 16 J/cm^2 @ 2 mm indicates that optimal polymerization can be achieved for a 2-mm increment with an ED of 16 J/cm^2; specified by the composite manufacturer.

6. How the energy is applied

   Energy application sequence (EAS): the way or sequence in which a clinician uses the curing unit to polymerize a composite. Since ED is the product of PD and exposure duration, the clinician typically chooses the highest power density and shortest exposure time necessary to reach the ED equal to the specified EOP@D. Unfortunately, the decrease or savings in exposure time is not inversely proportional to increases in PD; therefore, what is applied may be more intense than the composite can absorb. Variable energy

96 Tooth-Colored Restoratives

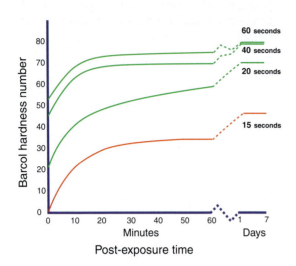

Figure 6–14. Composite continues to cure after the curing light is turned off. This plot illustrates the typical dark reaction (post-irradiation polymerization) of a light-cured composite resin. (Source: R. Leung, Fan P, Johnson W. Post-irradiation polymerization of visible light-activated composite resin. J Dent Res 1983;62:363–5.)

application sequences typically start with a low PD and then transition via a stepped or ramped increase to a higher PD. Some EAS use a pause between the initial low PD and the transition to a higher final PD. Whatever the EAS, the integrated area under the plot of PD versus time should result in an ED that is ideally one-third more than the EOP@D.

FACTORS THAT AFFECT LIGHT-CURING OF COMPOSITE

A review of light-curing basics is useful to understanding the pros and cons of the laser and arc lamps currently available for composite resin curing. The favorable properties of light-cured composites depend on achieving a complete cure of the resin matrix. Inadequate polymerization can result in loss of biocompatibility, color shifts, loss of retention, breakage, and excessive wear and softness.

Some of the most important factors to consider in using and maintaining a light-curing system are time, intensity, temperature, light distance, resin thickness, air inhibition, tooth structure, composite shade, filler type, accelerator quantity, heat, and room light. Following is a brief review of each of these factors.

Exposure

Light-cured composites polymerize both during and after visible light-activation. These two curing reactions are known as the "light" and "dark" reactions. The light reaction occurs while light from the curing unit penetrates the composite. The dark reaction, also called post-irradiation polymerization, begins immediately after the curing light goes off and continues for up to 24 hours, even in total darkness, but most of it occurs within 10 to 15 minutes post cure (Figure 6–14).[15]

The minimum curing time for a light reaction for most composites under a continuous curing mode is 20 to 40 seconds (using curing units with the normal 400 mW/cm^2 output). A classic study by Leung shows that traditional light-cured composites must be cured for at least 40 seconds to initiate a reaction that ensures the curing will continue to completion.[16] In all composites, maximum hardness is achieved within about 24 hours. Some newer composites have shorter light-curing times, but the total time required for the resin to completely set is about the same. Overcuring (curing for a longer time) is not harmful but does not improve a material's properties.

Regardless of how a composite is cured, the dark reaction takes time and greatly contributes to the overall strength of the material. Generally, waiting 10 to 15 minutes after curing before finishing a composite improves the hardness by 20 to 30%. A waiting period prior to finishing can improve wear properties significantly, because the finishing process damages the margins of a restoration. Damage to the margins is greatest when a composite is finished before it is fully polymerized. A good way to minimize finishing damage is to reetch and reseal the margins with a glaze after finishing.

Intensity

The curing intensity of a 468 ± 20 nm blue light has been about 400 mW/cm^2 for many years. This is the output of most curing units and is referred to as the "power density." Problems occur when the minimum intensity is not achieved. There are four common causes of decreased intensity: (1) as the bulbs in curing lamps age, the intensity of blue

Resin Polymerization 97

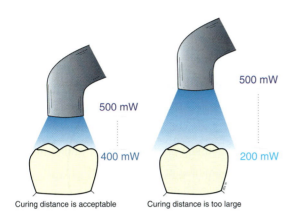

Figure 6–15. In deep restorations and those with poor access, the distance between the light guide and the composite can increase, which generally reduces the power density at the surface by over 70%.

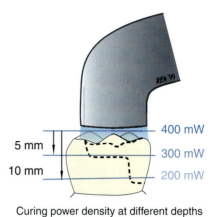

Figure 6–16. Schematic representation of a 50% reduction in light intensity in deeper areas of a preparation.

light can decrease, (2) voltage drops can affect blue light production, (3) sterilization of curing tips can reduce light transmission, and (4) filters to increase blue light transmission can degrade.

Light rods are available that can concentrate the light into a small spot size to increase the power density. A number of radiometer devices can measure blue light intensity, generally over 400 to 500 nm wavelengths (eg, Curing Radiometer, Demetron, Danbury, Connecticut, and Cure Rite, EFOS Inc., Williamsville, New York). Curing units should be checked every month with a radiometer to ensure production of adequate blue light intensity. When the intensity is low, replacing the bulb, filter, or curing tip usually returns the intensity to acceptable levels. Many curing lamps have radiometers built in. Newer curing units with a higher power density (600 to 1200 mW/cm^2) maintain acceptable output levels for a longer time.

Temperature

Light-cured composites cure less effectively if they are cold during application (eg, just taken out of the refrigerator). Composites at room temperature cure more completely and rapidly. Composites should be held at room temperature at least 1 hour prior to use.[17]

Most curing lamps produce heat, which speeds the curing process. However, excess heat can result in pulpitis and pulp death. The effect of heat from a curing lamp on a tooth is not fully understood, partly because there are so many variables.

Distance and angle between light and resin

The ideal distance of the light source from the composite is 1 mm, with the light source positioned 90 degrees from the composite surface.[18] Light intensity drops off rapidly as the distance from the light rod to the composite increases (Figure 6–15). If the base of a typical proximal box on a posterior composite is 5 mm from the tip of the light guide, adequate curing duration for a given intensity can be determined only by using a radiometer from the same distance. Distance can still be a problem if the lamp is placed against the tooth, since a deep box increases the distance the light must penetrate (Figure 6–16). This is a good reason to use a lamp that produces more than the minimum 400 mW/cm^2 power density. With many curing lamps, a higher power density (of about 600 mW/cm^2) is required to ensure that 400 mW/cm^2 reaches the first increment of composite in a posterior box. To compensate for the loss of intensity, cure for longer periods of time the layers of composite that are at a greater distance from the light rod. Further polymerization can be achieved by curing from the proximal surfaces after finishing.

Angle and path of the light

As the angle diverges from 90 degrees to the composite surface, the light energy is reflected away

98 Tooth-Colored Restoratives

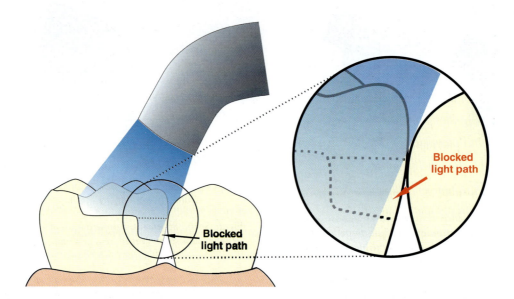

Figure 6–17. In deep restorations, particularly in posterior sites, a direct path of light to the entire restoration can be blocked. The critical area of the gingival margin is most commonly affected. Some light guides are not curved enough to allow a 90-degree angle of exposure on a molar tooth.

and penetration is greatly reduced. This can be demonstrated by angling the light rod against a radiometer and watching the intensity values shown on the meter drop. In molar preparations, the marginal ridge of the adjacent tooth blocks light when placed at an angle (Figure 6–17).

Thickness of resin

Resin thickness greatly affects resin curing. Optimum polymerization occurs at depths of just 0.5 to 1.0 mm, owing to the inhibition of air at the surface and the difficulty with which light penetrates a resin.

One classic study showed that 7 days after a 40-second curing cycle, a 1-mm deep composite (of light shade) is cured to 68 to 84% of optimum hardness, as measured by surface hardness.[19] At 2 mm, this same composite has only 40 to 60% of the desired hardness. At 3 mm, it has only 34% of the hardness. Thus, composites should be cured in increments of not more than 1 to 2 mm. This assumes an optimum light source and a composite that is light in shade (eg, A1, B1). In some studies, increasing the curing time to 2 minutes increased the depth of cure; however, additional curing time has limited effects on depth of cure (Figure 6–18). A manufacturer's statement that a composite has a 6-mm depth of cure is misleading. This implies that the composite can be placed in 6-mm increments, but doing so results in excessive polymerization shrinkage, open margins, and increased strain on the tooth.

Air inhibition

Oxygen in the air competes with polymerization and inhibits setting of the resin. The extent of surface inhibition is inversely related to filler loading. The under-cured layer can vary from 50 to 500 μm (or more), depending on the reactivity of the photoinitiators used. Unfilled resins should be cured, then covered with an air-inhibiting gel, such as a thin layer of petroleum jelly, glycerin, or commercial products, such as Oxyguard (J. Morita), and then re-cured. Some glazes have photoinitiators that are sufficiently reactive to make this unnecessary. In addition, curing through a matrix increases surface polymerization because the matrix reduces air inhibition.

Curing through tooth structure

It is possible to light-cure resin through enamel, but this technique is just one- to two-thirds as effective as direct curing and is appropriate only

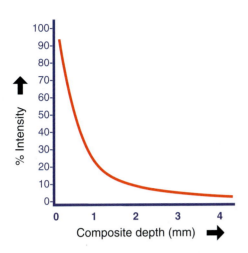

Figure 6–18. Typical light intensity drop at composite depth. Graphic illustration of the degree of resin polymerization at different resin depths (ie, the thickness of the resin) in relation to the duration of cure. Note that doubling the curing time from 1 minute to 2 minutes can double the depth of cure.

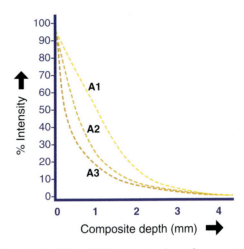

Figure 6–19. Typical light intensity drop of composites with darker shades and greater depth. Composite hardness based on shade and filler after a 40-second cure. Darker shades of composite cure more slowly and could benefit from the use of higher power densities. (Source: Swartz ML, Phillips RW, Rhodes B. Visible light-activated resins: depth of cure. J Am Dent Assoc 1983;106:634–7.)

when there is no alternative.[20] Such curing is possible through up to 3 mm of enamel or 0.5 mm of dentin, but the clinician should double or triple exposure times.[21] When light-curing through tooth structure, porcelain veneers, and other barriers, it is advisable to use a high-intensity light.

Shade of resin

Darker composite shades cure more slowly and less deeply than lighter shades.[22] At a depth of 1 mm, a dark composite shade achieves just two-thirds of optimum depth of cure achieved in translucent shades (Figure 6–19). A brighter light reduces the amount of time it takes to cure darker shades. Hence, when esthetics is not critical, the lightest shade should be used.

Type of filler

Microfilled composites are more difficult to cure than macrofilled composites, which have larger quartz and glass fillers. Generally, the more heavily loaded a composite is with larger inorganic fillers, the more easily the resin cures. However, extremely high loading can make a composite opaque, which actually increases the required duration of exposure. Manufacturers are well aware of this and load materials accordingly.

Amount of photoinitiator

Composites differ in the amount of photoinitiator they contain. Some manufacturers use less than the ideal amount of photoinitiator needed for maximum resin strength to increase the dentist's working time under the operatory light.

All photoinitiators deteriorate over time.[23] However, light-cured composites are more stable than chemically cured composites. Some light-cured composites lose about 10% of their physical properties when stored for 2 years at room temperature. The maximum usable life span of a light-cured composite is generally 3 to 4 years or more from the date of manufacture, if stored at room temperature. If contained in a sealed tube, they last much longer. The major cause of decreased shelf life for light-cured composite is evaporation of critical monomers from unidose containers. Autocured materials have shelf lives of 6 to 36 months. The key to longevity is the catalyst peroxide-containing paste; some are stabilized better than others. There are large variations in the shelf lives of various auto- and dual-cured composites. Most autocured composites have an extended shelf life if kept under refrigeration. Observing a manufacturer's product expiration date is important, especially with the shades used less frequently.

Heat generated by light-curing units

The heat given off by a curing light increases the rate of photochemical initiation and polymerization reaction and increases the amount of resin cured.[24] Excessive curing heat is thought to cause no photochemical damage to either the tooth or the composite. However, the heat generated in the tooth during light-curing results in higher intrapulpal temperatures, which could be harmful. Deep layers of resin should be cured thoroughly; cooling with a dry air syringe may be helpful.

Room-light polymerization

The working time of light-cured composites depends on the operatory light and the ambient room light to which the composites are exposed. Differences in these light sources can dramatically affect working time. Newer, faster-setting composites are even more sensitive.

Operatory lighting

Most operatory lights operate at high temperatures that produce spectrums in the blue range. This spectrum is included to improve the color selection of dental restoratives, but it initiates curing.

Incandescent lighting

Incandescent lights are low in blue light and provide the longest composite working time.

Fluorescent lighting

In general, fluorescent lighting has the shortest working time for light-cured composites, because it emits a large amount of blue light. Color-corrected tubes emit considerably more blue light and often have the shortest working time of all lighting systems.

Improving working time

Working time can be improved in two ways:

1. Place the operatory light further from the working field. Generally, doubling the distance of the operatory light from the patient greatly increases the working time while still providing adequate light for composite placement.

2. Place an orange filter over the operatory light. This can be held in place with Velcro®.

CURING UNITS

Almost all halogen visible light-curing units cure all visible light-cured composites. However, curing units differ in depth of cure, diameter of cure, number of available attachments, and heat generation. Many curing units use halogen bulbs, such as are found in standard slide projectors, as their light source. This light source produces many wavelengths of light. A special and complex dichroic filter separates the wavelengths to a narrow spectrum with a bandwidth of usable wavelengths of approximately 400 to 500 nm. For most composites, 470 nm is the optimal wavelength for polymerization, but this depends on the photoinitiators used in the resin. Some nonhalogen curing devices do not polymerize some composite resins. This is particularly true of lasers, because their wavelength spectrum is so narrow it may not include the optimal wavelength for some resins.

Some curing units contain better filters and light guides than others. Units with poor filters permit longer-wavelength energy to pass through the guide, resulting in higher temperatures at the curing tip or inadequate blue light output. The light from the curing tip should be uniform in intensity and wavelength to reduce internal stress during the polymerization process and to provide optimal stability to the cured resin. These factors are responsible for differences in curing ability among units using a similar light source. Studies show these differences can be large—up to 50% in depth of cure measurements,[25] even between identical units made by the same manufacturer.

There are basically three types of visible light-curing units: countertop units, gun-type units, and fiber-optic handpiece attachment units.

Countertop units

The countertop unit contains all the functional parts in one box. A fiber-optic or fluid-filled cord carries the light from the box to the patient.

Some of these units have a control switch at the end of the cord so the operator does not have to leave the operating field to activate the light source. Some of these units have a control switch at the end of the cord so the operator does not have to leave the operating field to activate the light source.

The advantages of countertop units are that the fan and working parts of the unit are out of the operating field and that they are generally less expensive than other designs. The disadvantages are that many units lack a switch at the cord end, and many models do not have wide-diameter curing tips. In addition, many countertop units have fiber-optic cords that need periodic replacement because of fiber-optic bundle break down.

Gun-type units

The second type of visible light-curing unit has its light source in a gun handle. The light passes through a small fiber-optic cord or glass rod that forms the barrel of the gun. Generally, these units are attached to an additional table-top or wall-mounted unit that contains the necessary transformers to operate the light.

This type of unit is activated at the operator site. They typically have large diameters of cure with good intensity and are generally small and easily made portable. Gun-type units have no fiber-optic cords to replace since the gun barrels are usually inflexible. The disadvantages of gun-type units are the fan in the handle, which can be noisy and become warm with extended use; gun bulk and weight (more bulky than fiber-optic cord ends); and higher cost.

Handpiece curing attachments

The third type, the fiber-optic handpiece curing attachment, is generally adapted to existing fiber-optic handpiece light sources. Attachment units have curing tips that are usually smaller than but similar to those in countertop units. Some of these units generate considerable heat in the tooth, owing to inefficient or missing blue light filters.

These units are less expensive, especially if the fiber-optic handpiece is already in place. They are small and require no additional counter space. Their drawbacks include, generally, a smaller diameter of cure, less intense light source, release of excessive heat (some units), and periodic need for replacement of fiber-optic cords.

Line voltage effects on intensity

The power density of many visible light-curing units depends on the plug-in line voltage, as measured at the electrical receptacle (electric plug). In most American communities, line voltage is kept constant at 120 volts. Within an office, however, voltage can fluctuate 10 or 15 volts off this norm. Voltage is difficult to maintain at a constant level since it decreases as distance from the street transformer to the office increases. Thus, homes or offices closer to a transformer have a higher voltage than sites farther away. Voltage is like water or air pressure: the longer the line, the lower the pressure at the far end.

As a general rule, the lower the voltage, the lower the amount and depth of composite cure.[26] A 10% drop in voltage can result in a 40% reduction in power density, sufficient to produce undercured restorations and a limited depth of cure. To alleviate this problem, most manufacturers build voltage regulators into their visible light-curing units. These units are especially important for dentists who practice in areas where the line voltage is not maintained at a constant 120 volts.

CURING LAMPS

Four types of lamps predominate in clinical practice: tungsten-halogen, plasma arc, laser, and light-emitting diode (LED). Halogen lamps have the flexibility to apply energy at a range from low to high and for various lengths of time. Although appealing in concept, arc and laser units invariably apply large amounts of light and are therefore appropriate only for continuous or pulse curing; this limits their flexibility for clinical applications.

Tungsten-halogen

Interestingly, many halogen curing lamps use a 50- to 100-watt bulb to produce 500 mW of light that peaks at 468 nm. This approach yields an efficiency rate of only 0.5%; the other 99.5% of the energy is simply given off as heat. Heat, unlike light, can be damaging to a tooth and needs to be controlled. Thus, more powerful curing lamps need measures that reduce the heat that can radiate from the tip of the light guide.

Plasma arc

The plasma arc lamps (short-arc xenon) used for pulse energy curing usually have a 5-mm spot size and a wide bandwidth covering 380 to 500 nm. They yield a power density up to 2500 mW/cm^2. This is a tremendously powerful light energy source that requires a wait time (minimum 10 seconds) after each use to allow the unit to recover. The high intensity of the lamp causes silver to precipitate on the lamp window, which degrades lamp output over time. Argon bulbs, therefore, have a relatively short shelf life. A large number of dental composite manufacturers recommend that dentists not use these lamps for curing because of poor curing outcomes.

Laser

Laser lights (argon-ion) emit specific bandwidths of light at about 454 to 466 nm, 472 to 497 nm, and 514 nm (usable blue light). Lasers produce little heat, because of limited infrared output. A major limitation of arc and laser lamps is that they have a narrow light guide (or spot size). This requires the clinician to overlap curing cycles if the restoration is larger than the curing tip. As soon as overlapping is required, the advantage of speed is greatly diminished since each overlap doubles the curing time. In addition, overlaps need to be at least 1 mm; so a 12-mm restoration (the typical central incisor is 9 × 12 mm) would have to be overlapped three times with a 5-mm spot size, and four times for a 3-mm spot size.

Holding the lamp farther way from the tooth can increase the spot size. However, this greatly reduces the power density, and the required increase in curing time negates the time saved by using a more powerful light for restorations that are larger than the spot size. Thus, a halogen lamp with an increased spot size and a lower power density can cure a larger restoration faster than an arc or laser lamp, both of which have small spot sizes.

The situation for which high-powered lamps with small spot sizes have potential in saving time is when curing a single proximal box in a posterior tooth. The appeal of both arc and laser lamps is a shorter curing time for placing composite resins. Despite common beliefs, arc and laser lamps cannot cure a composite any more rapidly than a halogen lamp—the newer halogen lamps, that is. The energy of early halogen lamps was about 400 mW/cm^2. Newer lamps can double and often triple this output, yielding a higher amount of energy than is available from either laser or arc lamps. To reap the benefit of higher energy requires appropriate application: although research is not yet conclusive, it is obvious that there is a saturation point beyond which applying increased power to a composite produces minimal benefit.

In regard to reducing curing time, increased lamp intensity does shorten curing time, but this is not a linear relation; that is, doubling the light intensity does not halve the curing time. The increased intensity of the curing lamp decreases the ratio of curing by about the inverse square, such that doubling the curing lamp intensity may only decrease the curing time by 30%.

Light-emitting diode

Light-emitting diode curing lamps offer many advantages over other curing lamps. Light-emitting diodes are special semiconductors that emit light when connected in a circuit. They are frequently used as pilot lights in electronic appliances to indicate whether a circuit is open or closed. They operate at 1 to 4 volts and draw a current of 10 to 40 milliamperes. Their low energy use makes them ideal for battery-operated curing lamps.

Unlike halogen lamps, LEDs emit a narrow bandwidth of light, around 468 nm, and have an efficiency of about 16%. Wavelength specificity means that an LED curing at 468 nm would have a considerably lower reading than a halogen lamp on a 400 to 500 nm radiometer, since less usable light in that range is emitted. In addition, the LED would use less power, about 6 watts rather than 100 watts, to achieve needed curing.

One weakness inherent to LEDs is that their heat reduces performance. Cooling is critical when these units are used for extended periods, since their effective output is reduced over multiple continuous curing cycles. In contrast, halogen lamps tolerate extended curing cycles with limited reduction in output. When all is considered, LED lights are ideal for battery-powered curing units that are not used for extended periods.

Heat generation

Although all visible light-curing units release heat, they vary in the amount of blue light and longer wavelength light they produce. Some units produce little heat even though they have high curing intensities. The amount of heat generated is related to the wavelength and intensity of the light emitted. Longer wavelengths produce more heat per unit area (intensity remains constant). This heat generation does not indicate the curing ability of the

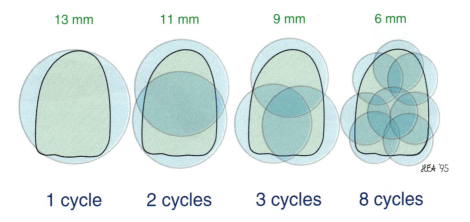

Figure 6–20. The number of overlapping cures required to polymerize a single layer of a full-surface restoration on a maxillary incisor. The average tooth requires a minimum of two or three 40-second curing cycles. Many complex restorations require many more curing cycles. For maximum efficiency, curing tip diameters should exceed 12 mm.

unit: the blue light that cures a composite gives off little heat. In addition, units vary in the amount their heat penetrates dentin.[27] Temperature differences across 2 mm of dentin can vary 1° to 8°F. More rapid curing with high-output units produces considerably more heat over a shorter period of time.

LIGHT GUIDES

When the area of composite to be cured is larger than the diameter of the light tip, composite sections must be overlapped at least 1 mm. Even in smaller restorations, studies show that wide curing tips provide better curing uniformity than narrow curing tips.[28] Failure to properly overlap during curing can result in poorly polymerized areas in the restoration (Figure 6–20). Curing time also must be increased to compensate for the increased area of resin.

To avoid the time-consuming and tedious process of overlapping, a number of wide-diameter attachments are available for many visible light-curing units. The attachments are particularly useful in curing composite veneers. Some wide-diameter curing attachments are adaptable to existing curing units and emit more light because of a larger curing tip on the unit connector. Others, however, spread the same narrow unit-connector light source over a larger diameter with the use of optics; most of these have reduced light intensity. This reduces the depth of cure, so composite must be cured in thinner layers. Examples of good wide-diameter systems are units from Demetron and Caulk that use a large-diameter entry port on the curing unit. Many wide-diameter attachments are available, and they cure from numerous angles.

Some manufacturers offer a number of light guides. Demetron, for example, offers 13 different light guides, each designed to optimize polymerization in a particular situation (Figure 6–21) One of these, the Turbo light guide, can concentrate the 13-mm light source of a Demetron curing lamp to a narrow 8-mm or 4-mm diameter, yielding 35 to 50% more intensity. These are useful for deep cavity preparations or cementing some indirect restorations with dual-cured cements. The Turbo tip can enhance the clinical life of a curing unit by maintaining its output above the required 400 mW/cm^2 (Figure 6–22).

LIGHT-CURING UNIT SELECTION AND MAINTENANCE

Selection

There is no one best visible light-curing unit, since different units work better for specific applications. The diameter of cure, for example, is not critical in the placing of only Class III, Class V, and Class IV restorations; whereas, a unit with a larger

104 Tooth-Colored Restoratives

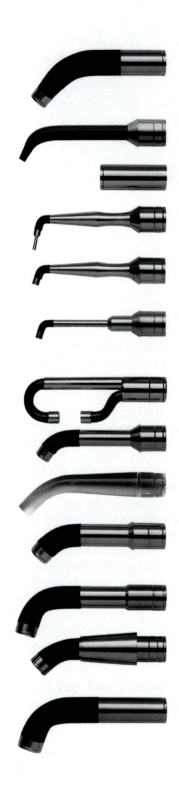

Figure 6–21. Examples of the large selection of light guides available from Demetron.

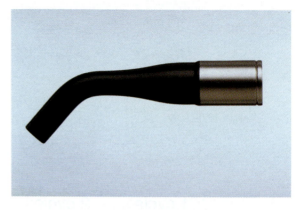

Figure 6–22. A Turbo light guide from Demetron. This unit reduces the diameter of cure but increases light intensity (by 34% on the Optilux 150 and by 50% on the Optilux 400 series curing lights). This increased intensity better activates the light portion of dual-cured resin cement.

diameter of cure saves chair time by curing larger portions of composites and veneers during each curing cycle. Dentists placing indirect veneers should have both a wide curing tip and a high-intensity light (as measured by a radiometer). The minimum intensity for light-cured cementing of lucent indirect veneers is usually 400 mW/cm^2 over the entire diameter of the curing tip.

To summarize, there are several factors that must be evaluated before purchasing a visible light-curing unit:

1. Power density
2. Maximum diameter of curing tip
3. Uniformity of power over the diameter of the curing tip
4. Longevity of adequate light spectrum once the unit is turned on
5. Heat generation within the tooth
6. Ease of use of controls and timer
7. Durability of curing tips to sterilization
8. Dependability of unit
9. Size and portability of unit
10. Voltage regulation
11. Price:performance ratio

A light-curing unit should be considered a long-term investment, like a handpiece that is used daily for many years. Owning more than one unit is recommended so that if one becomes inoperative, the other is available to complete procedures in progress.

Maintenance

A number of features must be checked to ensure that a visible light-curing unit is operating at full capacity.

Curing tip

Composite buildup on the curing tip can greatly reduce light intensity. Composite buildup occurs when the curing tip touches the composite during curing. *Note: The ideal curing distance is 1 mm.* At least one manufacturer, Demetron, offers a cleaning kit to eliminate buildup.

Fiber-optic cords

The fibers of fiber-optic bundles are brittle and break down if repeatedly bent. Procedures and storage that bends the cords unnecessarily should be avoided.

Light guides

Light-guide tips should be shiny and free of materials. Autoclaving can be used for cleaning most light guides but may eventually cause some degradation, observed as cloudiness at the ends of the fibers. "Boiler scale" results from repeated autoclaving of rigid light guides.[29]

Filters

Most curing units have a filter that selects out the appropriate wavelength to block glare, heat, light, and any energy not used in the curing process. This filter is usually located between the curing bulb and the cord tip or gun rod. Because the filters can pit, crack, or peel, they must be checked regularly and replaced as needed.

Fans

The fan should be kept clean by vacuuming the exhaust port where it is mounted.[29] It is not necessary to take the curing unit apart to do this. Clean fans run cooler and reduce the chance of heat damage to the housings or other electrical components. The smaller fans used in many gun-type units may need periodic replacement because of wear on the bearings. Worn bearings are noisy; noise is a warning of potential fan failure. A noisy fan should be repaired immediately by the manufacturer. Do not operate a unit if its fan stops working.

Problems with curing bulbs

Bulb frosting

Bulbs become frosted when the glass enclosing the filament becomes cloudy or white. This occurs as a result of either deposition of metal oxides, which vaporize and form a film on the glass bulb (which is called the envelope), or a process known as devitrification in which impurities in the glass-quartz envelope crystallize. Frosting can result in a 45% drop in curing light output.[30]

Bulb blackening

The deposition of silver and other metal oxides on the internal glass portion of a bulb causes black discoloration. Although the filament is still emitting light, the black oxide can result in a 74% drop in curing light output.[30]

Filament burnout

When the filament is broken, there is a complete loss of light output.

Reflector degradation

Reflector degradation occurs when there is a loss of the reflector film or a white or yellow coating of oxides develops over the reflector surface. This can result in a 66% drop in curing light output.[30]

Because of these problems, curing lights gradually lose intensity.[31] A dentist should have on hand two new replacement bulbs for each curing light operated, one for immediate replacement and a second in the event the primary backup bulb does not function. This is a small investment considering the considerable inconvenience of curing lamp failure.

Light-emitting diodes have fewer maintenance problems than halogen bulbs generally but must be checked for decreased power density owing to heat accumulation during long curing times. Heat also can result in LED degeneration over time.

Radiometers

A radiometer is a specialized light meter that quantifies blue light output; a radiometer determines the effectiveness of a curing unit by measuring the intensity of 468-nm light coming out of the tip of the light guide. Radiometers are sold as small handheld devices or may be built into curing units.

106 Tooth-Colored Restoratives

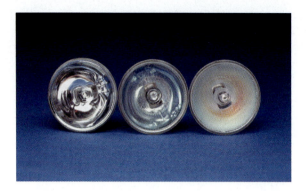

Figure 6–23. The bulb on the left is new and reads over 500 mW/cm². The bulb in the middle is 3 months old and reads 240 mW/cm². The bulb on the right is 9 months old and reads under 50 mW/cm². All three lamps were used in the same curing unit 5 days a week. The bulb that reads 240 mW/cm² (*middle*) was used approximately 30 to 120 minutes per day for about 3 months. The bulb that reads under 50 mW/cm² (*right*) was used approximately 30 to 120 minutes per day over 1 year. Note that the bulb on the right shows most of the features associated with bulb degeneration.

It is important to test a curing light when it is new to obtain a baseline for future reference. Most radiometers measure light in the 400 to 500 nm bandwidth. This is broader than is required by most photoinitiators and makes these units less reliable in evaluating curing units with narrower spectral outputs (ie, LEDs and lasers). This means the typical radiometer cannot be used to compare the efficiencies of LEDs and halogen curing units. A specialized radiometer capable of measuring a narrower bandwidth around 468 nm would give a more precise measurement of any unit's spectral bandwidth.

Ongoing testing of curing units is important, especially as the bulb approaches 50 hours of use. Disregard for light intensity could lead to restorations that discolor, leak, break, and prematurely wear away. Note that some radiometers (eg, the Heat Radiometer from Demetron) measure glare and heat at 520 to 1100 nm. This is useful in comparing units to ensure that the curing light is properly filtering out unwanted light wavelengths that can unnecessarily heat a tooth.

Bulb aging

Aging causes the light to change from a short wavelength blue to a longer wavelength yellow and reduces the available amount of 468-nm light (Figure 6–23). These changes are gradual and occur in all high-intensity lamps, including those

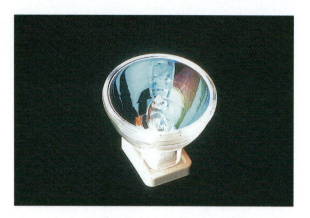

Figure 6–24. One of the newer curing bulbs that produce more 468-nm light. This bulb, from Demetron, also provides improved focus, better uniformity of light output, less energy consumption, and less heat production.

used for operatory lights. Although the output of LEDs drops over time, the wavelengths of that output remain more consistent.

Improved-output bulbs

When visible light-curing units were developed, the slide projector lamp was chosen as the light source because of its availability and small size. Most curing lights still use these bulbs. Unfortunately, their design frequently results in a spot of high intensity at the center of the light guide and less intensity at the outer edges. This drop off in intensity is more severe with large-diameter light guides. Projector lamps also have a silver reflective coating that reflects all visible light for correct color duplication. Only 468-nm light is useful in curing; the unnecessary wavelengths of light produce unwanted heat that stresses the filters. Currently, most curing lamps can accommodate specialized bulbs to improve their performance. In addition, curing tips that collimate the light down to a smaller spot size (eg, Turbotip, Dementron) can be used to further increase power density.

Customized bulbs have been developed (eg, the OptiBulb, Demetron, Figure 6–24) that offer the following important improvements over conventional bulbs:

1. The lamp distributes light uniformly for light guides of all diameters. The reflector has a deep-dish design, with a larger surface area, that collects more light than standard lamps. This results in higher efficiency and greater light output.

2. The reflector coating is optimized to reflect only the blue light energy that is useful for curing composite materials. Wavelengths of light other than 468 nm pass through the reflector and are removed.

OCULAR HAZARDS OF CURING LIGHTS

Ultraviolet light-curing units preceded those using visible light. Because UV light is harmful to human skin and eye tissues, the UV curing units included shielding, and manufacturers warned about the dangers of light exposure. Many dentists were concerned about using the lamps near patients and staff.

The introduction of the visible light-curing unit prompted great excitement. To many, the name implied that the light was harmless. How could visible light be harmful? The human eye is adapted to the diffuse light found in the forests where early man lived. Most of this light was in the yellow and green range; that is still the wavelength of light most suited for the human eye. The blue light used to polymerize composite is not well tolerated by the human eye. All light-cured polymerization systems use light that is harmful to vision. The human eye transmits 400 to 1400 nm of light to the retina. The visual range is 400 to 700 nm. As a lens ages it yellows and absorbs wavelengths between 320 and 400 nm.[32]

The high-energy blue light emitted from a composite curing unit initiates the curing process by splitting the double bonds of the camphoroquinone accelerators, thus forming free radicals that start resin polymerization. Of all visible light wavelengths, blue light is the least essential to vision. The macula lutea provides a yellow filter in the central area of the retina and absorbs short wavelengths of light. Vision is most acute in this central area, because the yellow filter enhances acuity. Marksmen, for example, wear yellow-tinted glasses to reduce blue blur and sharpen contrast. The eye's focal distance varies with the visible wavelengths because the lens refracts blue light differently than other wavelengths of visible light. Generally, blue light is not focused on the retina, since the eye needs to focus on the longer wavelength light reflected off objects. In addition, blue and other short wavelengths of light are subject to a phenomenon known as scattering. Blue light is scattered by the liquid media of the eye through which light is transmitted. This scattering reduces the acuity of vision. In older patients, who have a higher incidence of floating particles in the eye, blue light causes a blurring of vision.

A number of studies show that blue light is damaging to the retina of monkeys. It has been shown that blue light forms free radicals in the eye, just as it does in composite resins.[32,33,34,35] However, in the retina, these free radicals react with the water-content of cells, causing peroxides to form in the visual cells. These peroxides are reactive and denature the delicate photoreceptors of the eye. The results are harmful to vision. Researchers estimate that blue light is 33 times more damaging to the photoreceptors of the retina than is UV light.

Even small doses of blue light are thought to be damaging. Like the chemistry of composite curing, the biochemical mechanism of vision uses carbon–carbon double bonds. The active photoreceptors of the human eye are thought to depend on the rotation of a carbon–carbon double bond from a vitamin A molecule. A photoenzyme maintains vitamin A in an unstable, high-energy *cis* position. When a photon of light strikes this double bond, the vitamin A shifts to a low-energy *trans* position and triggers the process of vision. Adenosine triphosphate (ATP) energy is used to reposition the vitamin A back to the unstable, high-energy *cis* position so that it can again react to light. Even small amounts of blue light can damage or destroy these delicate photoreceptors, by splitting the high-energy double bonds of photoreceptors into free radicals.

HISTORY OF EYE DAMAGE RESEARCH

It took researchers in the dental profession a few years to realize that the light emitted from visible light-curing units is the blue light known to be harmful to human vision. Rhesus monkeys have been the subject of a lot of research in this field. They are excellent experimental models because their eyes are similar to human eyes.

The first researchers to study eye damage from blue light were Zigman and Vaugh.[36] They exposed mice to near-UV radiation and reported a thinning of photoreceptors after 10 weeks. After 16 weeks, this photoreceptor loss was accentuated. The destruction continued until all photoreceptors were lost after 87 weeks.

In 1978, Zuclick and Taboada exposed rhesus monkeys to blue light of 325 nm radiation and found that retinal damage occurred at exposures below those required to injure the cornea or lens.[32] Later, this work was expanded into the 400 to 500 nm range. Ham discovered that the damage caused from this light was photochemical rather than thermal or structural.[32]

The 468 to 480 nm wavelength of light that polymerizes composite resin is among the ranges of light most damaging to the eyes. The study by Ham showed that blue light causes retinal burns in monkeys after exposures of less than 1 second. As exposure duration increased, the burns became more severe. This damage has been named "solar retinitis." Retinal burns appeared 48 hours after light exposure and healing occurred in 20 to 30 days. The healed areas showed permanently degenerative tissues. These damaged tissues histologically have the appearance of senile macular degeneration. In other words, the light exposure rapidly aged the visual cells of the retina. Ham and Mueller showed that this damage to the retina is irreparable; the damaged rod and cone photoreceptors cannot regenerate (Figure 6–25).[37] Some laboratory studies indicate that exposures of under 2 minutes to visible light-curing units (total daily dose from 25 cm) may be safe.[38]

Researcher Ham considers 510 nm the minimal cutoff point for severe eye damage (Ham WT. Personal communication). Shorter wavelengths, those essential to cure composite, are exponentially more dangerous than longer wavelengths. For example, 441 nm, which is the most damaging wavelength, is 2.5 times more damaging than 488 nm.

Griess and Blankenstein have shown that repeated exposure to low levels of blue light produces cumulative retinal injury in rhesus monkeys.[39] They found that the additive effect of retinal damage from multiple exposures was 91% greater than single exposures when the interval between exposures was 1 day. Thus, repeated exposures to even low levels of blue light can be extremely damaging.

Younger eyes are more susceptible to blue light damage. It is important to educate staff about this so they can ensure that children are prevented from staring at curing lamps during treatment. The resulting damage could be profound and lifelong.

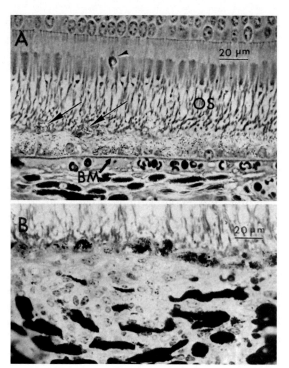

Figure 6–25. A histology slide showing the eye damage that can accompany large amounts of blue light exposure. *A*, the normal retinas of a Rhesus monkey; *B*, the retina of a Rhesus monkey at 30 days after a 30-second direct exposure to 475-nm light at close range. This would be similar to placing a curing lamp within 3 mm of the eye and exposing it to 1500 mW for 30 seconds. BM = basement membrane where the photoreceptors attach; OS = optical cells (rods and cones). (Reproduced with permission from Ham WT, Mueller Ruffolo JJ. Action spectrum for retinal injury from near-ultraviolet radiation in the aphakic monkey. Am J Ophthalmol 1982;93:299–306.)

EYE PROTECTION

In most clinical situations, the blue light in contact with the eyes is reflected light. Many scientists believe that reflected blue light is less harmful to the eye, but just how much safer it may be has not been established by research. In any case, scientists recommend that dentists wear protective eyewear or shields when working with visible light-curing lamps.[40,41] Any protective eyewear should transmit less than 1% of wavelengths below 500 nm.[42]

The best eye protection is to completely avoid looking at the curing light source. Covering the curing site with a dark object would be ideal. Some clinicians cover the curing site with their hand. This may prove an unsafe practice. In cell research, blue light is used to induce cancer growth; therefore, skin exposure is highly discouraged.

A simple yet effective way to provide shielding from curing lights is to cover the curing field with the reflective side of a mouth mirror. This prevents excess blue light from reflecting back against the restorative and improves curing. If the mirror is not large enough, a folded patient napkin easily covers most fields. A slight amount of brightness will show through the napkin and shows if the light is on or off.

If it is necessary to look at the light source for placement, eye protection is warranted. Unfortunately, most optical glasses and plastic contact lenses transmit blue light and near-UV light radiation with little attenuation. A number of colored plastic glasses and handheld shields are available.[43,44] Some of these plastics (usually red and orange) can block blue light. They can be cut and made into custom shields. Over time, they may need to be replaced, since the organic dyes used to color plastic fade with use. Colored protective lenses in glasses are another option. The drawback is that they require a 2- to 6-minute recovery period before normal color perception returns. This temporary distortion can interfere with the ability to judge shades.

It is easy to test the effectiveness of a light shield. The wavelengths that harm the eye are the same ones that cure composite. To test a shield (or pair of protective glasses), try to cure composite by shining the curing light through the shield onto composite. If the composite can be cured, the shield is ineffective for eye protection.

REFERENCES

1. Glenn JF. Composition and properties of unfilled and composite resin restorative materials. In: Smith DC, Williams DF, eds. Biocompatibility of dental materials. Vol. III. Boca Raton: CRC Press, 1982:97–130.

2. Carter JA, Smith DC. Some properties of polymer coated ceramics. J Dent Res 1967;46 (Spec Issue):1274.

3. Öysaed H, Ruyter IE. Composites for use in posterior teeth: mechanical properties tested under dry and wet conditions. J Biomed Mater Res 1986;20:261.

4. van Dijken JW, Wing KR, Ruyter IE. An evaluation of the radiopacity of composite restorative materials used in Class I and Class II cavities. Acta Odontol Scand 1989;47:401–7.

5. Bowen RL, Cleek GW. X-ray-opaque reinforcing fillers for composite materials. J Dent Res 1969;48:79–82.

6. Li Y, Swartz ML, Phillips RW, et al. Effect of filler content and size on properties of composites. J Dent Res 1985;64:1396–1401.

7. Braem M, Lambrechts, P, Van Doren V, Vanherle G. The impact of composite structure on its elastic response. J Dent Res 1986;65:648–53.

8. Shintani H, Inoue T, Yamaki M. Analysis of camphorquinone in visible light-cured composite resins. Dent Mat 1985;1:124–6.

9. Ferracane JL. Correlation between hardness and degree of conversion during the setting reaction of unfilled dental restorative resins. Dent Mater 1985;1:11–4.

10. McCabe JF, Ogden AR. The relationship between porosity, compressive fatigue limit, and wear in composite resin restorative materials. Dent Mater 1987;3:9–12.

11. Asmussen E. Clinical relevance of physical, chemical, and bonding properties of composites resins. Oper Dent 1985;10:61–73.

12. Wilder AD, May KN Jr, Leinfelder KF. Three-year clinical study of UV-cured composite resins in posterior teeth. J Prosthet Dent 1983;50:26–30.

13. Davis RD, Mayhew RB. A clinical comparison of three anterior restorative resins at 3 years. J Am Dent Assoc 1986;112:659–63.

14. Brauer GM. Color changes of composites on exposure to various energy sources. Dent Mater 1988;4:55–9.

15. Eliades GC, Vougiouklais GJ, Caputo AA. Degree of double bond conversion in light-cured composites. Dent Mater 1987;3:19–25.

16. Leung R, Fan P, Johnson W. Post-irradiation polymerization of visible light-activated composite resin. J Dent Res 1983;62:363–5.

17. McCabe JF. Cure performance of light-activated composites by differential thermal analysis (DTA). Dent Mater 1985;1:231–4.

18. Kelsey WP, Shearer GO, Cavel WT, Blankenau RJ. The effects of wand positioning on the polymerization of composite resin. J Am Dent Assoc 1987;114:213–5.

19. Onose H, Sano H, Kanto H, et al. Selected curing characteristics of light-activated composite resins. Dent Mater 1985;1:48–54.

20. Standlee JP, Caputo AA, Hokama SN. Light-cured composites. CDA J 1988;16:25–8.

21. Weaver WS, Blank LW, Pelleu GB. A visible light-activated resin cured through tooth structure. Gen Dent 1988;36:136–7.

22. Matsumoto H, Gres JE, Marker VA, et al. Depth of cure of visible light-cured resin: clinical simulation. J Prosthet Dent 1986;55:574–8.

23. de Lange C, Bausch RJ, Davidson CL. The influence of shelf life and storage conditions on some properties of composite resins. J Prosthet Dent 1983;49:349–55.

24. Stanford C. Sequential and continuous irradiation polymerization of photoactivated composites [abstract]. J Dent Res 1984;63(Spec Issue).

25. Lambert RL, Passon JC. Inconsistent depth of cure produced by identical visible light generators. Gen Dent 1988;26:124–5.

26. Fan PL, Worniak WT, Reyes WD, Stanford JW. Irradiance of visible light-curing units and voltage variation effects. J Am Dent Assoc 1987;115:442–5.

27. Tjan AHL, Dunn JR. Temperature rise produced by various visible light generators through dentinal barriers. J Prosthet Dent 1988;59:432–8.

28. Neo JC, Denehy GE, Boyer DB. Effects of polymerization techniques on uniformity of cure of large-diameter, photo-initiated composite resin restorations. J Am Dent Assoc 1986;113:905–9.

29. Friedman J. Care and maintenance of dental curing lights. Dent Today 1991;10:40–1.

30. Friedman J. Variability of lamp characteristics in dental curing lamps. J Esthet Dent 1989;1:189–90.

31. Antonson DE, Benedetto MD. Longitudinal intensity variability of visible light curing units. Quintessence Int 1986;17:819–20.

32. Ham WT. Ocular hazards of light sources: review of current knowledge. J Occup Med 1983;25:101–3.

33. Ham WT, Ruffolo JJ, Mueller HA, Guerry DK. The nature of retinal radiation damage: dependence on wavelength, power level, and exposure time. Vision Res 1980;20:1105–11.

34. Ham WT, Mueller H, Sliney D. Retinal sensitivity to damage from short wavelength light. Nature 1976;260:153–4.

35. Ham WT, Mueller HA, Ruffolo JJ, et al. Basic mechanisms underlying the production of photochemical lesions in the mammalian retina. Curr Eye Res 1984;3:165–74.

36. Zigman S, Vaugh T. Near-ultraviolet light effects on the lenses and retinas of mice. Invest Ophthalmol 1974;13:462–5.

37. Ham WT, Mueller Ruffolo JJ. Action spectrum for retinal injury from near-ultraviolet radiation in the aphakic monkey. Am J Ophthalmol 1982;93: 299–306.

38. Satrom KD, Morris MA, Crigger LP. Potential retinal hazards of visible-light photopolymerization units. J Dent Res 1987;66:731–6.

39. Griess GA, Blankenstein MF. Additivity and repair of actinic retinal lesions. Invest Ophthalmol 1981; 20:803–7.

40. Ellingson OL, Landry RJ, Bostrom RG. An evaluation of optical radiation emissions from dental visible photopolymerization devices. J Am Dent Assoc 1986; 112:67–70.

41. Counsel on Dental Materials, Instruments, and Equipment. Visible light-cured composites and activating units. J Am Dent Assoc 1985;110:100–3.

42. Counsel on Dental Materials, Instruments, and Equipment. The effects of blue light on the retina and the use of protective filtering glasses. J Am Dent Assoc 1986;112:533–4.

43. Berry EA, Pitts DG, Francisco PR, von der Lehr WN. An evaluation of lenses designed to block light emitted by light-curing units. J Am Dent Assoc 1986; 112:70–2.

44. Fan PL, Wozniak WT, McGill S, et al. Evaluation of light transmission characteristics of protective eyeglasses for visible light-curing units. J Am Dent Assoc 1986;115:770–2.

Chapter 7

Resins

Thinking is the hardest work there is, which is probably the reason why so few engage in it.

Henry Ford

HISTORY AND DEVELOPMENT

Filled resins, or composites, are reinforced with a variety of inorganic fillers. They were created to improve on the methyl methacrylate resins (eg, Sevriton™) that were based on amine-peroxide initiators developed in 1941.

In 1959, ESPE (Seefeld, Germany) introduced Cadurit, the first glass-reinforced methyl methacrylate composite restorative manufactured for dentistry. The epimine-based chemistry was then further improved to produce the commercial temporary crown and bridge product Scutan. Owing to clinical problems with technique, Scutan was removed from the market in 1964. In 1963, Addent™ (3M Dental Products, St. Paul, Minnesota) was the first composite restorative to use a Bis-GMA resin. The Bis-GMA component greatly improved polymerization shrinkage and color stability, since the resin was more hydrophobic. Both Scutan and Addent were chemically cured powder–liquid systems.

In 1969, the first two-paste Bis-GMA system, Adaptic (Johnson & Johnson) was introduced. Because it was easy to use and had favorable initial esthetic properties, Adaptic dominated tooth-colored restoratives within a few years. The typical relation between filler and resin is shown in Figure 7–1.

CLASSIFYING COMPOSITES BY FILLER TYPE

Current direct-placement composites have four major components: a *matrix phase* that usually contains a dimethacrylate resin; *polymerization initiators* that are activated either chemically (by mixing two materials) or by visible light (using a light-curing unit); a *dispersed phase* of fillers and tints; and a *coupling phase* that adheres the matrix to the filler particles (eg, silanes).

Composite resins are generally classified by the type of filler used (dispersed phase), since most employ similar resin matrices. Fillers are essentially of two types: large particles of glass or quartz (macrofiller) and small particles of silica (microfiller). Hybrid resins contain both.

If all other components are equal, the polishability and wear-resistance of composites increase as particle size decreases. Durability to fracture increases as the percent of inorganic loading by volume increases (percent filled). *Note: Filler loading by weight is commonly referenced, since it is the easiest to measure. Weight measurements generally are larger than volume measurements, because fillers are denser than resin matrices.*

The ideal composite would be highly filled with very small particles. Unfortunately, loading a composite with large amounts of small filler is difficult, because the large surface area causes a marked increase in viscosity. Therefore, to have reasonable

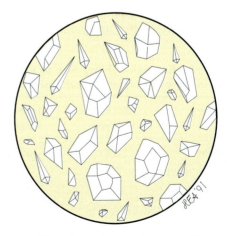

Figure 7–1. The relation between inorganic filler and resin in first-generation composites (Addent and early Adaptic).

clinical handling properties, composites with smaller particles must sacrifice some loading and strength compared with composites with larger fillers.

The relation between filler size and filler loading in the various classes of composite is shown in Table 7–1. Filler loading is critical in providing composite stiffness.

The type of filler used in a composite resin profoundly affects its clinical and handling properties. The classification system used here is based on recommended clinical uses. This classification was first presented in the first edition of this text and remains instructive.[1] It is in concordance with some of the concepts presented by Lutz and colleagues.[2]

Macrofilled composites

Macrofilled composites use relatively large inorganic quartz or glass fillers. The particles in early macrofilled composites ranged in size from 15 to 100 μm. Currently, typical composites use particles ranging in size from 1 to 10 μm (Figure 7–2). Most contain a small amount of microfill (1 to 3%) as a stabilizer to avoid particle settling. One of the major problems with glass-filled composite is the separation of the filler from the surface of the material. This results in loss of occlusal form and excessive wear, both proximal and occlusal (Figure 7–3).

The most common fillers in current macrofilled composites are ground quartz, strontium, or heavy-metal glasses containing barium. Quartz (density of 2.2 g/cm^2), the most common filler used in early composites, has excellent esthetics and durability but lacks radiopacity. Radiopaque glasses, such as strontium (density of 2.44 g/cm^2) and barium

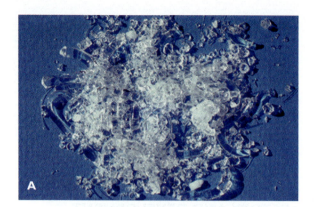

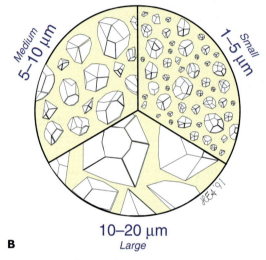

Figure 7–2. A, The raw glass material that is ground to make composite filler. B, Schematic representation of the different sizes of filler particles used in macrofilled composites. Early materials with large particles included Adaptic, Concise, Clearfil F, Smile, Simulate, and Nuva-Fil. Those with medium particles included Profile and Estilux. Those with small particles included Command and Prisma-Fil. Currently, almost all composites are hybrid composites.

Table 7–1. Relation of Filler Size to Filler Loading in Various Classes of Composite Resin

Composite Resin	Filler Particle Size (μm)	Loading by Weight (%)
Microfilled	0.04	50–60
Submicron hybrid	≤1	50–75
Micron hybrid	1–5	60–78
Heavy filled	Various sizes	80–87
Large particle	5–10+	>80

glass (density of 3.4 g/cm^2) are more brittle and more soluble than quartz. Heavy-metal glass fillers are the most commonly used because they are radiopaque and easier to grind. Composites containing quartz and zirconium fillers, because of their hardness, wear opposing enamel significantly more than composites containing microfillers or barium glass.[3] *Note: With a density of 3.4 g/cm^2, barium glass is 30 to 40% heavier than most other fillers. This greatly increases filler by weight compared with filler by volume.*

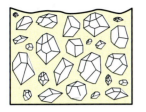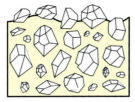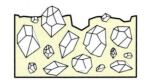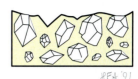

Figure 7–3. A simplified illustration of the wear process showing loss of filler in large-particle macrofilled composites.

Macrofilled composites are difficult to polish to a smooth finish because any loss of filler particles at the surface leaves a rough finish, whereas filler with a smaller particle size reduces this disadvantage (Figure 7–4).

Microfilled composites

Microfilled composites contain inorganic filler particles of pyrogenic silica (ash) averaging 0.04 μm (Figure 7–5). They were developed to achieve a more polishable restorative. The first microfilled composite introduced was Isopaste (Vivadent) in 1977. Microfill and macrofill particle size is compared in Figure 7–6.

How microfillers are made

Microfillers are made from a silicon dioxide smoke or ash, called *fumed silica* (commercially known as

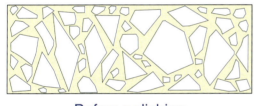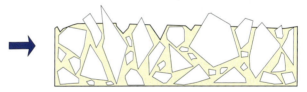

A

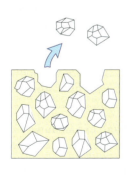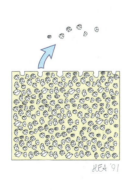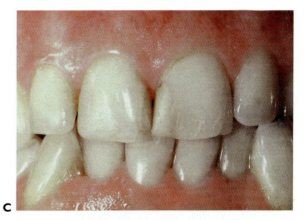

B   C

Figure 7–4. Schematic representation of, *A*, how polishing the surface of a macrofilled composite leaves a rough surface (illustration by Ralph Phillips), *B*, differences in surface roughness resulting from the loss of large and small filler particles, and *C*, typical surface of a large-particle composite after 8 years of service.

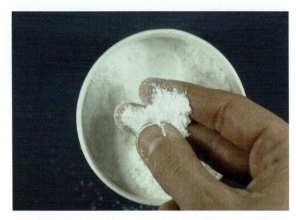

Figure 7–5. The fine silica ash used in microfilled composites. The material is called Airosil and functions as a thickening agent, owing to its small particle size; it is also used to thicken toothpastes, cosmetics, paints, and other household materials.

Airosil, Degussa Corp., Ridgefield Park, New Jersey) or by adding colloidal particles of sodium silicate to water and hydrochloric acid, which produces *colloidal silica.*

There are two types of microfilled composites, homogeneous and heterogeneous.[2] In homogeneous materials, the microfiller is loaded directly to the resin. Because of their considerable surface area, microfillers are difficult to add directly to a resin in high concentrations. An 80% filler loading by weight is impossible; therefore, microfilled composites are rarely made this way. To circumvent this problem, special methods are used to fabricate these materials; the most common is heterogeneous loading. In heterogeneous materials, the microfiller is compressed into clumps by sintering, precipitation, condensation, or silanization. The fumed silica resin is added to a heated resin at a filler loading of approximately 70% by weight, more than twice what is normally possible.

The resulting resin–filler mixture is heat-polymerized into blocks, then frozen and ground (or splintered) into filler particles from 1 to 200 μm in size. The particles average 30 to 65 μm in most microfilled composites. This process is illustrated in Figure 7–7. These filler particles, called *prepolymerized resin fillers,* are then added to a nonpolymerized resin. This resin is frequently filled with microfiller, but at only half the concentration of the cured resin filler, to avoid excessive thickening. Hence, a microfilled composite is highly loaded with precured resin particles (Figure 7–8). The final product usually contains 35 to 72% inorganic filler by weight.

In these microfilled composites, the matrix (resin) and the filler particles (resin and silica) have basically the same composition. When finished carefully, these materials can attain a smooth surface that can be maintained longer than the surface of a macrofilled composite surface (Figure 7–9).

Although surface smoothness is an advantage, there are problems associated with most types of microfilled composite.

- **Resin filler–matrix interface.** The interface between the prepolymerized resin filler and the surrounding matrix is a suspected weak link. Since the prepolymerized resin fillers are highly cured, they cannot copolymerize with the surrounding resin matrix. This inability to copolymerize can result in a loss of resin filler from the material's surface (Figure 7–10).

- **High coefficient of thermal expansion.** The lesser amount of inorganic filler in microfilled composites (vs. macrofilled) is thought to contribute to more microleakage and possibly to marginal chipping over time (Figure 7–11).

- **Low tensile strength.** In high tensile stress-bearing Class IV areas, microfill restorations fracture more frequently than macrofills.[4]

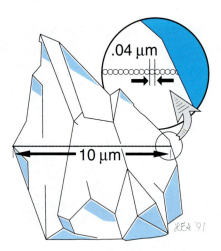

Figure 7–6. Schematic size comparison of microfiller and macrofiller particles.

Resins 115

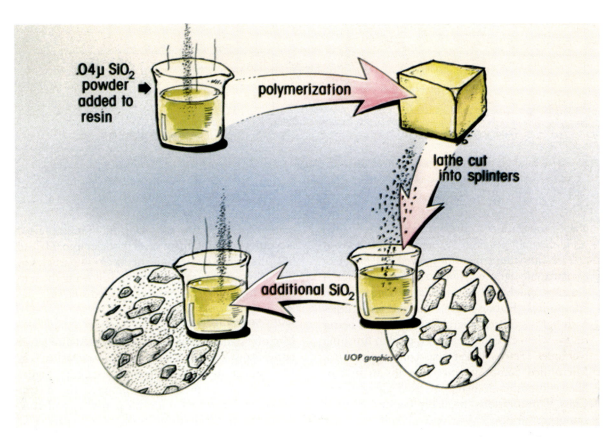

Figure 7–7. The four steps used to make a conventional microfilled composite with prepolymerized resin particles.

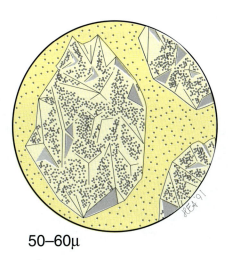

Figure 7–8. Schematic representation of the relation between filler particles and resin in conventional microfilled composites (eg, Isopast, Heliosit, Silar, Durafill, Silux, Silux Plus Filtek™ A110, and Renamel).

- **Low stiffness.** Since microfills include noninteracting particles, the resin matrix acquires little stiffness. Microfills deform easily under stress and have considerably lower fracture resistance (higher rate of crack propagation) than macrofills.[5] Therefore, most microfills are too weak to support cusps in posterior teeth.

- **High water sorption.** Owing to higher resin content, microfills generally have high water sorption, which softens the resin matrix.

- **High polymerization shrinkage.** The slightly higher volume of unset resin in microfilled composites results in slightly greater polymerization shrinkage. This shrinkage makes microfills more technique-sensitive for placement and finishing. Poor attention to placement, curing, and finishing procedures can cause damaged margins (white lines) and marginal voids.

- **More fatigue fracture.** Since the microfiller particles are less able to absorb stress, considerable

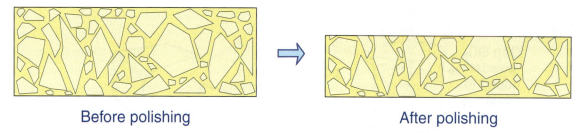

Figure 7–9. Polishing the surface of a microfilled composite leaves a smooth surface since the filler itself is polishable.

crack propagation occurs during the composite's resin phase. In posterior restorations, one study of an early autocured microfill showed a 20% rate of catastrophic failure from resin fatigue after 4 years,[6] a much higher rate than for macrofilled composites (Figure 7–12). More recent studies with light-activated microfills have shown better results when careful attention is paid to finishing techiques (Setcos J. Personal communication). Microfilled composites are superior to macrofilled composites in small, protected, Class III and Class V restorations, probably because of their smoother surface.

Agglomerated microfills

Agglomerated microfill composites, such as Visio-Dispers (ESPE), are filled with microfiller agglomerates. Agglomerates are made by combining (or agglomerating) 0.04-μm silica particles into 0.07- to 0.2-μm pellets by heating the microfill particles to just below their melting point and allowing them to clump together. This process is called *sintering*.

Condensed microfills

Microfill particles can also be condensed into larger complexes known as *condensed microfills* (eg, Heliomolar and Helioprogress, Vivadent). Figure 7–13 illustrates the relation between the microfillers, agglomerated microfill particles, and condensed microfill particles in the resin matrix.

Agglomerated and condensed microfills are considered microfills since their filler originates from 0.04-μm microfiller. Inorganic radiopaque fillers are sometimes added to make condensed microfills radiopaque. Ytterbium trifluoride, a radiopaque rare earth macrofiller, is added to some materials (eg, 25% in Heliomolar), whereas etched stron-

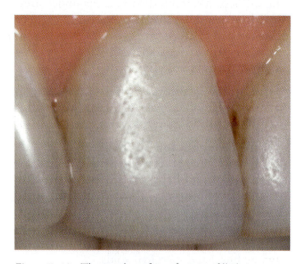

Figure 7–10. The rough surface of a microfilled composite that has lost prepolymerized particles as a result of improper placement and curing procedures.

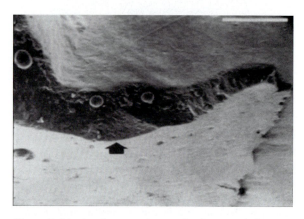

Figure 7–11. An electron micrograph of marginal chipping of a microfilled composite.

Resins

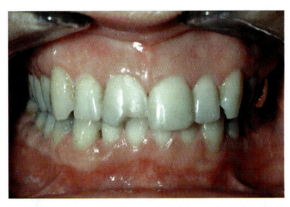

Figure 7–12. Typical catastrophic failure of a microfilled composite when placed under stress.

tium glass macrofiller is added to others (eg, 30% in Bisfil-M). Microfilled pellets and complexes can be added in large amounts to prepolymerized resin particles and to the surrounding resin matrix for additional filler loading.

Blended composites

Blended composites contain three or more types of filler: macrofiller, microfiller, and prepolymerized resin particles. If finished with dry discs, blended composites can be polished more than would be expected for their particle size, because the heat from finishing smears the resin in the prepolymerized particles on the surface. Unfortunately, this smeared resin surface wears away quickly, exposing the macrofiller particles just below the surface. These materials (eg, Valux, 3M Dental Products; Multifill, Kulzer, Wehrheim, Germany) require periodic repolishing to maintain a smooth surface.

Hybrid composites

Materials that use both macro- and microfillers in the same restorative are called *hybrids*; they show the characteristics of both microfills and macrofills. The hybrids differ from blended composites because they do not contain prepolymerized resin particles. Almost all macrofilled composites contain some microfiller (1 to 3%). Hybrids are macrofills with larger amounts (7 to 15%) of microfiller, microfiller pellets, or microfiller complexes added as a second filler to produce a material with higher loading. They vary in particle size and distribution (Figure 7–14).

Hybrids are superior to their nonhybrid counterparts because their increased filler loading (called *particulate reinforcement*) improves the stress transfer between particles in the composite. As filler loading increases with the addition of smaller-sized microfiller to the matrix, the interparticle distance decreases. This puts less stress on the resin matrix by transferring occlusal stress from one filler particle to another. This microfill–macrofill interaction becomes more significant when smaller macrofillers are used in the composite. The result is a resin that acts more like an adhesive (non–stress-bearing) and less like a matrix (stress-bearing). Since the resins used in composites are relatively weak, improved particulate reinforcement greatly increases the stress-bearing capacities of the composite and acts to toughen the material. Adding microfillers to the

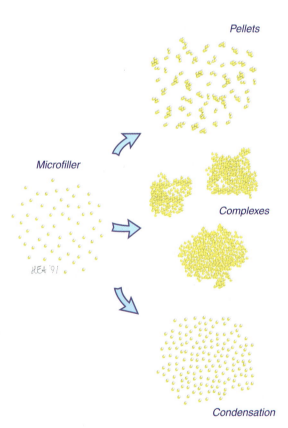

Figure 7–13. The size relation between agglomerated microfill pellets, microfiller complexes, and condensed microfillers that can be derived from 0.04-μm microfiller (eg, Answer, Nimetic Dispers, Visio-Dispers, Heliomolar RO, and Helioprogress).

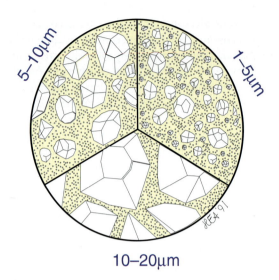

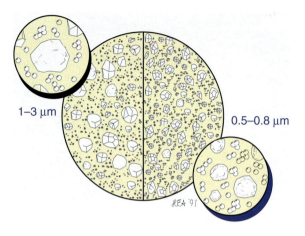

Figure 7-14. The relation between microfiller and macrofiller particles in some hybrid composites. The large particles include Miradapt (10 μm); medium particles include Pentra-Fil II and Post Com II (both 5 μm); small particles include Tetric (1.5 μm), Ful-fil and APH (both 2.5 μm), TPH and Pertac-Hybrid (2 μm), and Conquest DFC (2.5 to 3.0 μm).

Figure 7-15. *Left*, The relation between an agglomerated microfiller (smaller clumps) and submicron macrofilled particles (large glass filler) in minifilled hybrid composites. Examples include Prodigy, Herculite XRV, Herculite (all 0.6 μm), and Charisma (0.7 μm). *Right*, The relation between fillers in micron hybrids (eg, TPH and Command Ultrafine).

matrix phase of a composite also hardens the resin (called *dispersion hardening*). This increases the resin matrix cohesive strength and slows the propagation of microcracks in the matrix.

In hybrids, cracks in the matrix are initially slowed by the surrounding stress-bearing macrofillers and then stopped when the cracks encounter microparticles. The more microparticles the composite has, the more likely cracks in the resin will stop growing soon after formation. The more macrofiller present, the more slowly cracks propagate, because of stress transfer between particles. The balance between these two fillers is critical, since excess amounts of microfiller can increase brittleness.

Micron hybrids (small-particle hybrids)
A micron particle hybrid is any macrofilled composite with an average particle size of 1 to 5 μm that also contains large amounts of microfiller (7 to 15%) (Figure 7-15). These materials generally show good fracture resistance. Compared with earlier large-particle materials, these composites have improved smoothness and wear resistance because the smaller fillers leave smaller voids when they are lost from the surface (see Figure 7-4, *B*). As manufacturers make the macrofiller particles smaller, the surface area per unit volume of filler increases. More resin is required to wet the surfaces of these smaller particles. Composites with smaller macrofillers are usually less heavily loaded than those containing larger filler particles. Higher filler loading is important because composites that are more highly inorganically loaded tend to fracture less, an important consideration in restorations exposed to high stress or wear.

Quartz fillers are ideal for composites. They are highly esthetic, insoluble, form excellent bonds to resin matrices, and have performed exceptionally well clinically. The problem with quartz lies in the manufacture of filler: it is so hard it abrades the grinding equipment, resulting in impurities and 1- to 2-μm particles with jagged edges. It is also radiolucent, such that products containing quartz usually include other fillers (eg, Pertac II, ESPE) that render them radiopaque.

Submicron hybrids (minifilled hybrids)
A submicron hybrid is a macrofilled composite with a tight distribution of similar sized, more rounded particles under 1 μm, plus a relatively large amount of microfiller in the matrix. The name submicron applies because the vast majority of filler is under 1 μm and the largest particles are generally under 2 μm. The first 1-μm hybrid was

Command Ultrafine (Kerr Corp., Orange, California), introduced by Kerr in the 1970s. Kerr also introduced the first submicron hybrid, Herculite, in 1975. The second manufacturer to use this particle size was Kulzer with the introduction of Charisma in the 1980s. In the 1990s, manufacturers produced Synergy (Coltene, Altstatten, Switzerland), Vitalescence (Ultradent Products Inc., South Jordan, Utah), and others. In 1999, Kerr introduced a 0.4-μm composite, Point 4.

These hybrids are unique among composites, because they do not contain the normal distribution of larger filler particles. They are also known as *minifilled hybrids*. Minifilled hybrids are relatively highly loaded with very small inorganic filler particles. This desirable combination offers the clinician strength and surface smoothness in a single restorative.

Newer minifilled hybrid systems add microfiller or larger microfill clusters to the matrix. The advantages of using microfill clusters are (1) they displace more resin, (2) they have less surface area, and (3) they can be more heavily loaded into the macrofilled composite. These composites can be loaded up to 78% by weight (50 to 70% by volume) with an average macrofiller particle size of 0.6 to 0.8 μm. This improves particulate reinforcement and dispersion hardening.

Heavy filled hybrids

The heavy filled hybrids have more than 80% filler by weight (equal to about 60 to 70% by volume) and generally contain particles of various sizes. When compressed, this content provides a densely packed unit with few spaces. Called *gap grading*, the use of various sized particles gives a composite maximum particulate reinforcement and stiffness. These materials are called large-particle hybrids because they contain larger macrofillers, some in the 5- to 10-μm range (Figure 7–16).

The major clinical advantage of these materials is greatly improved fracture toughness. These stiffer composites also give better support to a larger restoration since they deform less when stressed, which results in less crack propagation. Most of these materials do not finish as well as smaller-particle or microfilled composites. The large filler particles in these hybrids have a rough surface, resulting in high friction that can increase

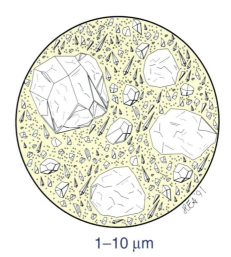

1–10 μm

Figure 7–16. The relation between resin and filler in the heavy filled composites. Note the diversity in the size of the filler particles. In these materials, the mean particle size is considerably smaller than the largest particle size. Examples of these materials (and their mean macroparticle size) include Solitaire (2 to 20 μm), Clearfill Posterior (2 to 5 μm), Z-100 (2.5 μm), P-50 (3 μm), P-30 (3.5 μm), P-10 (5 μm), Bis-Fill P (5 μm), and Occlusin (8 μm).

wear on opposing teeth. Clinically, these materials are recommended as a core or backing material.

COMPOSITE COLOR MODIFIERS AND OPAQUERS

Color modifiers are composites with more resin, more color pigment, and less filler than other composites. Color modifiers are used under or between layers of composite to characterize a restoration to suit a specific patient. They were initially used to mask opaque bases in Class V restorations, but characterization has become their main use. Opaquers are color modifiers that contain white to mask discolorations and lighten shades (increase shade value).

LONGEVITY OF DIRECT COMPOSITES

The first composites loaded with larger fillers began to fail 3 to 5 years after placement, as a result of wear and loss of form. Newer composites that are loaded with smaller fillers start to fail after 5 to 9 years, as a result of bulk fracture (Figures 7–17 and 7–18). In comparison, amalgam longevity

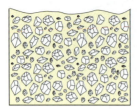 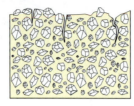 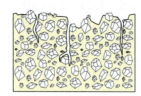 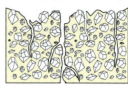

Figure 7–17. A schematic illustration of the bulk fracture process in small-particle macrofilled composites. Notice there is less wear over time but more cracks occur.

varies from 8 to 20 years and amalgam restorations are replaced because of recurrent decay rather than failure.

Heavy filled composites, which are highly loaded with filler particles of many different sizes, have both good rates of wear and good resistance to bulk fracture. They are, however, generally more opaque and offer poorer esthetics.

No single material has yet proven optimal for all restorations. Using different composites together can provide optimal success in small- to medium-size restorations. In larger stress-bearing restorations, no composite resin is as durable as metal or porcelain-fused-to-metal restorations. An enormous number of variables determine composite longevity. Nevertheless, clinicians generally agree the most critical variable is placement. Unfortunately, few practicing dentists can expect to achieve the 5-, 10-, or even 15-year longevity promised in research publications because those test restorations are placed by highly trained and skilled clinicians. In study groups run by the author, the typical life span for a small, well-placed restoration is 8 to 12 years. Larger restorations, which are subject to increased amounts of wear, breakage, and leakage, have much shorter life spans.

COMPOSITE SELECTION

A clinician must consider a number of factors in selecting a composite resin restorative material. A resin's composition in terms of filler loading and particle size determines its ability to provide any of three functions: support, form and contour, and surface finish. Some materials can be placed in more than one class of restoration and can be used for multiple purposes. An analogy to wall construction may be useful: brick and wood provide support; plaster provides form and contour; and paint or wallpaper provide the final finish (Figure 7–19).

The heavy filled hybrids, because of high loading and strength, are best for support; the minifills and small-particle composites are best for form; and the various types of microfills are best at providing a lasting, smooth finish (Figure 7–20). Figure 7–21 shows where each composite type is best used in a large restoration.

In large restorations, a heavy filled composite is used for stiffness and strength, followed by a microfilled composite for a smooth finish. The submicron hybrid and radiopaque microfilled composites are clinically acceptable for both contour and finish in small to moderate-sized restorations in areas bearing minimal stress. The submicron and microfilled hybrids mainly differ in stiffness, contour, and finish. The submicron composites are stronger and more vital, but less polishable than the microfills. The polish on a submicron composite with filler

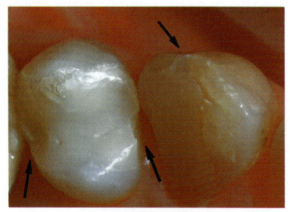

Figure 7–18. A small-particle macrofilled composite restoration that fractured after 5 years as a result of occlusal forces.

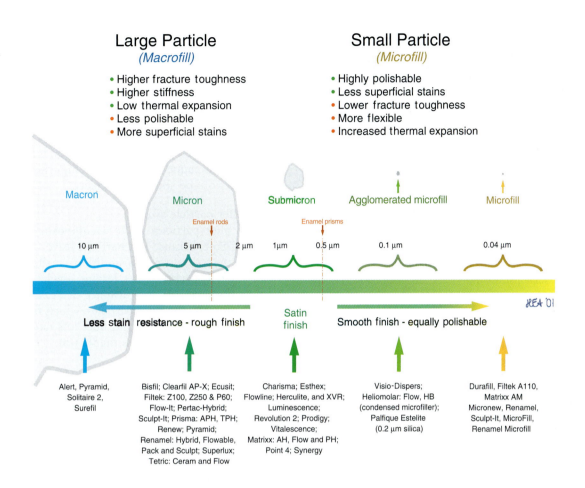

Figure 7–19. The macrofill-to-microfill balance: the relation between filler particle size and clinical properties in resin composites.

under 0.5 μm is difficult to distinguish clinically from that on an agglomerated microfill (0.1 μm). The differences in physical properties become insignificant when filler particle sizes are so similar.

Selecting an anterior composite restorative

No one material can suffice for all anterior restorations. If it is necessary to choose a single restorative for all uses, the best choice is a minifill with particles under 1 μm.

Class III restorations

Submicron composites are recommended for small preparations because they (1) are radiopaque, (2) have a good finish, (3) are durable to occlusal forces, and (4) have a favorable thermal coefficient of expansion that helps maintain a good marginal seal. Agglomerated and condensed microfills can also work well in small areas. Traditional microfills are not a good choice because they are usually radiolucent.

Class V restorations

In small restorations involving dentin, and for patients highly susceptible to caries, a modified resin glass-ionomer restorative is a good choice. In large restorations, a submicron composite is recommended. If the patient smokes or drinks a lot of coffee, placing a flowable microfill veneer over a submicron composite reduces surface staining.

In small non–stress-bearing restorations entirely in enamel, traditional microfills (eg, Durafill) have

122 Tooth-Colored Restoratives

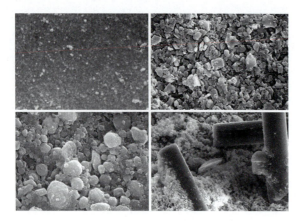

Figure 7–20. Electron micrographs showing the polished surface of (*clockwise from upper left*) a microfill, submicron hybrid, small-particle hybrid, and large-particle hybrid.

proven successful. These restorations, properly placed, show the best longevity of any material studied. Ten years postoperatively, the appearance often is indistinguishable from photographs taken at placement.

Class IV restorations
Small Class IV carious lesions are best treated with a micron or submicron hybrid. Large restorations involving an occlusal contact point are best treated with a heavy filled material. To improve esthetics, these can be coated with a micron or submicron hybrid. Where esthetics is a primary concern, coating the surface with a thin microfilled veneer is advisable. A large, complex Class IV restoration involving three materials is shown in Figure 7–21, *A*.

Selecting a posterior composite restorative
Longevity is the major concern for posterior composite restoratives. The two key unresolved issues are loss of anatomic form and bulk fracture. In addition, technique sensitivity and marginal integrity present major obstacles for most clinicians in achieving consistent clinical success. The ideal composite for a posterior restoration is a submicron, radiopaque light-cured composite with high filler volume and high viscosity.

Small filler particle size
Smaller filler particles make a composite more wear-resistant, because lost particles leave smaller voids on the resin surface. In addition, smaller particles generally pack together, leaving smaller interparticle distances. As this distance decreases, the resin is protected by filler particles, which further reduces resin matrix wear and filler loss rate. The ideal average filler size is less than 2 μm.

Radiopacity
To allow detection of overhangs and recurrent decay, radiopacity is desirable in a posterior material.

Light-cured materials
Light-cured materials are denser than their autoset counterparts. Air incorporated during mixing of autoset systems weakens these restorations. Some researchers and clinicians believe that an auto-cured resin is better suited for large posterior composites, since shrinkage might be better directed to the tooth by warmth and an active polymerizing bonding agent. This technique,

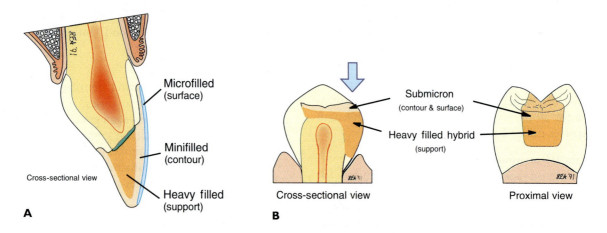

Figure 7–21. Placement of layers of different composite types in large restorations: *A*, anterior restoration; *B*, posterior restoration.

although common in buildups, is controversial for direct composite restorations.

High filler volume

Composites with more hard filler have less exposed soft resin matrix. Over 70% filler by volume (82 to 87% by weight) is desirable. Increasing the filler to these levels ensures more particle-to-particle contact, which reduces the stress on the resin matrix during function.

Putty-like composite

A high viscosity is desirable for higher filler loading. Some clinicians prefer to tightly pack putty-like composites to help improve marginal adaptation and to secure tighter proximal contacts. Owing to their lower filler volume, most microfilled composites are contraindicated for occlusal stress-bearing posterior restorations. Microfills in posterior areas may appear to be successful in the short term, by wearing exceptionally well for 3 to 5 years. However, studies on early autoset microfills show that by the fourth year up to 20% of these restorations can fracture and fail in high–stress-bearing areas. A few condensed and macrofill-reinforced microfills have been successful for 3 or more years in small conservative restorations. Some newer condensed light-cured microfills (eg, Heliomolar RO) have had better 5-year clinical results (Setcos J. Personal communication).

PACKABLE COMPOSITES

Packable composites, also referred to as high-density composites or condensable composites (a misnomer, since they cannot be condensed), are materials with a higher filler loading (eg, Solitaire, Kulzer; Surefil, LD Caulk). They also usually have larger particles. The packability of these materials makes it easier to use an amalgam condensation technique in posterior occlusal restorations. Likewise, their packability and lack of stickiness helps establish tight proximal contacts. These materials are appropriate for large posterior restorations.

Packable composites have the advantages of ease of packing, ease of establishing a good contact area, and ease of shaping occlusal anatomy.

The disadvantages of packable composites include dry spots from inadequate resin saturation, resulting in weak areas, difficult adaptation between layers since the layers do not wet each other well, and more opaque and unesthetic results for anterior restorations.

Use of extra bonding adhesive or a thin layer of flowable composite on the preparation walls can improve the adaptation and seal of a packable composite. Since many of these composites have larger filler particles, they have relatively poor wear resistance. Placing a material with smaller-sized particles on the surface improves wear. Heavy filled packable composites have good fracture resistance and can be used as the underlying support for larger composite restorations.

FLOWABLE COMPOSITES

A flowable composite is a less filled composite. Flowable composites have been available for years as cements for veneers and crowns. Many filled sealants are also flowable composites. In fact, many porcelain veneer luting agents are identical to the materials currently being sold under the name "flowable composite." These well-known materials have been repackaged (including availability in compules) and re-introduced as restoratives. The one difference is that they are offered in a full range of Vita shades for ease of use with other restoratives (whereas only a few porcelain luting agents are offered with a large shade selection).

Flowable composites are considerably easier to make than packable composites because they are lightly filled, and one of the most difficult processes in making a composite is achieving a high filler loading. Unfortunately, the problems associated with relatively low filler loading are not detectable until the composite ages. Compared with conventional composites, flowable composites shrink more upon polymerization, flex more frequently, break more frequently, fatigue more quickly, and stain more. In simple terms, flowable materials are inferior to more highly filled materials.

The main benefit of a flowable composite is the ease of adaptation to a preparation. Specifically, low filler loading makes a flowable material easier to apply to a surface as a coating material and as a thin wash that improves the adaption of the first increment of a condensable composite. However, these materials, because of their decreased strength, should not be used in large bulk additions.

Flowable composites used over glass-ionomer materials

It is common to use a flowable composite as a thin veneer over a resin-modified glass ionomer. The ionomer provides good retention, and the resin has better color stability and water resistance than most resin-modified glass ionomers. The bond between a dried resin ionomer and a flowable composite resin is good. The bond is improved if the resin-modified glass ionomer is slightly dried prior to adding the composite. These restorations can achieve good esthetics.

HANDLING COMPOSITE MATERIALS

Most direct composite restoratives have a limited shelf life. They must be stored properly to maintain maximum effectiveness.

Evaporation

All composite restoratives have volatile components. Capping tubes tightly minimizes evaporation. Materials should be dispensed onto a disposable pad immediately before use, and the tubes should be resealed as soon as possible after dispensing. *Note: Syringe-tip systems that are preloaded generally contain a more fluid composite than that found in tubes. If a tube-viscosity composite is desired, a syringe tip can be hand-filled.*

Cross-contamination

A composite should never be dispensed directly from the tube to the tooth or to a placement instrument, because tubes cannot be sterilized. If syringe tips are used, they should be discarded after use and syringe guns should be autoclaved.

Shelf life

Ideally, auto- and dual-cured composites should be stored under refrigeration when not in use and allowed to come to room temperature for at least 1 hour prior to use. Kept at room temperature, these composites have a shorter shelf life. Storing composites above normal room temperature (70°F) for extended periods may damage or prematurely age them. Most autocured composites, or the autocured component of dual-cured composites, have a shelf life of about 18 to 24 months when kept in a cool environment.

In contrast, light-cured composites are stable at room temperature if kept tightly sealed to avoid evaporation of monomer. Most viscous light-cured composites packaged in tubes have a shelf life of about 5 years when kept at room temperature. Syringe-tip systems, which are usually less viscous, have a shorter shelf life, because volatile components can evaporate more easily.

Tube labeling

On the bottom of each product box are two numbers: a batch number and a manufacturing date. Some manufacturers do not place these numbers on individual tubes or syringe tips. Since tubes and syringe tips are often removed from their boxes, it is important to transfer these dates onto the individual items. The information can be written on a piece of tape adhered to the tube. Syringe tips can be placed in small x-ray envelopes and labeled.

It is good practice to note a composite's batch number on the patient's chart. The purpose of recording the batch number is ease of patient identification if there is a bad batch of product. Noting a discard date in red aids in determining the usable life of a product. Expired composites can be used for interim or temporary restorations.

Marking calendar for reorders

It is possible to identify when a composite will expire by adding 18 months to the manufacture date, but it is difficult to remember to check every product every month or so. It is easier to anticipate product expiration by making a note on a calendar 2 to 3 months prior to expiration, and then ordering replacement material on that date. When the product is delivered, replace the old with the new.

REFERENCES

1. Albers HF. Tooth-colored restoratives. 1st ed. Santa Rosa, CA: Alto Books, 1979.

2. Lutz F, Setcos J, Phillips R, Roulet J. Dental restorative resins. Types and characteristics. Dent Clin North Am 1983;27:697–711.

3. Suzuki S, Suzuki SH, Cox CF. Evaluating the antagonistic wear of restorative materials when placed against human enamel. J Am Dent Assoc 1996;127:74–80.

4. Loeys K, Lambrechts P, Vanherle G, Davidson CL. Material development and clinical performance of composite resins. J Prosthet Dent 1982;48:664–71.

5. Papadogianis Y, Boyer DB, Lakes RS. Creep of conventional and microfilled dental composites. J Biomed Mater Res 1984;18:14–5.

6. Lambrechts P, Vuylsteke M, Vanherle G, Davidson C. Quantitative in vivo wear of posterior dental restorations: four year results [abstract]. J Dent Res 1985;64: (Spec Issue).

7. Braem M, Lambrechts, P, Van Doren V, Vanherle G. The impact of composite structure on its elastic response. J Dent Res 1986;65:648–53.

CHAPTER 8

RESIN BONDING

There are no limits to science. Each advance merely widens the sphere of exploration.
Marconi 1874–1937

The most significant development in the history of dentistry over the past 100 years is the ability to bond materials to tooth structure. This chapter provides information on this elemental aspect of direct restoration. Bonding techniques are taken for granted, but there are exceptions and limitations to standard methods. This chapter summarizes bonding methods for enamel, dentin, and pre-cemented resin. It is necessary to have a thorough understanding of the treatment methods and their critical steps, as well as knowledge of how to vary a treatment to meet the needs of a specific tooth, or restorations will fail. No one bonding system is appropriate for every mouth or for every tooth in a given mouth.

ENAMEL HISTOLOGY

The basic structural unit in enamel is the hydroxyapatite crystal. Approximately 10,000 of these long, slender crystals form a prism or rod 7 μm in diameter.[1] The enamel crystals bundled into rods start at the enamel–dentin junction and extend to the tooth surface, a distance of up to 2 mm. Most of these crystals are longer than they are wide, and behave much like fiber-optic fibers or fibers in a nylon rope. The clustering of crystals into prisms makes enamel an extremely tough and hard-wearing material; however, this strength is highly directional or "anisotropic."

The enamel prism unit is difficult to pull and break along its long axis because the crystals are oriented in the direction of surface forces. Materials bonded end-on to enamel prisms are attached in the most optimal direction. (This orientation is common in adhesive strength studies.) Attachment to the sides of prisms is much less desirable. Much weaker forces can bend and rupture a prism laterally than are required for breakage along the long axis.[2] Unfortunately, side attachment to enamel prisms occurs in the lateral walls of proximal cavities and, in combination with composite resin polymerization shrinkage, can result in a fracture and marginal leakage at the fracture.

ACID ETCHING OF ENAMEL

The first step in bonding to enamel is etching to enable micromechanical bonding. Glass ionomers stick without etching; composite resins require etching. Composite resins do not have natural affinity for tooth structure, whereas glass ionomers do. Parallel developments in composite resins and an enamel acid etch technique in recent years have made it possible to bond directly to enamel, a milestone in restorative dentistry.

History

In the 1950s, acids were used for cleaning in industry. In 1955, Buonocore described the use of acids for cleaning teeth.[3] Buonocore reported that microporosities form on enamel that has been treated with an acid and then rinsed. Self-curing acrylic resins readily attach to these microporosities via micromechanical interlock. Buonocore etched enamel with 85% phosphoric acid for 2 minutes and reported the acid (1) cleaned the surface, (2) increased the surface area, and (3) possibly made sites available for bonding through the creation of a more reactive surface. Buonocore's work went unnoticed for over 15 years. Figure 8–1 presents electron micrographs of enamel prior to and after phosphoric acid etching. Micromechanical pores develop in the etched surface as a result of removal of the enamel rods (see Figure 8–1, *B*).

In 1962, Bowen, working at the National Bureau of Standards (but funded by the American Dental Association), developed the first composite resin, Bis-GMA, which he loaded with inorganic filler. When Bis-GMA composites were made avail-

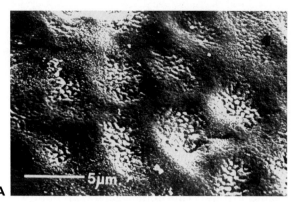 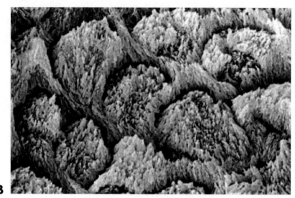

Figure 8–1. Electron micrographs. *A,* Unetched enamel. Note that the enamel rod ends are about 0.5 μm in diameter and that they are arranged in 3- to 6-μm clusters. *B,* Etched enamel. Note that the rods have been dissolved out of their 3- to 6-μm clusters and that the organic matrix remains.

able for commercial production, Lee Pharmaceuticals, 3M Dental Products, Kerr Corp, and others purchased manufacturing rights. Initially, Bis-GMA resins were sold and placed without acid etching and enamel bonding.

In 1970, Buonocore reported on a Bis-GMA activated by ultraviolet (UV) light. In 1971, LD Caulk (Milford, Delaware) introduced the UV light-activated Nuva-System™, the first to incorporate acid etching to bond composite resin to enamel. Many studies have demonstrated that a superior seal and bond between composite and enamel is achieved with this technique, regardless of preparation design (Figure 8–2).

Characteristics of etching enamel

Histologic effects of etching enamel

When enamel is treated, the acid removes about 10 μm of enamel from the surface and selectively dissolves the ends of the enamel rods in the remaining enamel. This creates porosities 25 to 75 μm deep that act as a system of channels into which an unfilled resin or resin bonding agent can flow and that increase the surface area more than 2000 times. These changes greatly strengthen the mechanical bond between the tooth and resin (Figure 8–3).

Acid strength

Buonocore used 85% phosphoric acid. Later studies have shown that etching with 20 to 50% phosphoric acid creates the deepest channels in permanent enamel.[4] Resin flowing into the etched enamel porosities is termed "resin tag formation" (Figure 8–4). Figure 8–5 shows a histologic slide illustrating resin penetrating etched enamel.

Later work by others showed that a 60-second etch with 30 to 50% nonbuffered phosphoric acid achieves the strongest bond between enamel and resin. In general, lower concentrations of acid selectively remove inorganic material from the organic matrix of the enamel surface, thereby creating faster and deeper channels. Higher concentrations are less effective since they are nonselective and are more likely to denude the surface. Gel etchants appear to be as effective as liquids, although gels need to be washed longer to remove their residue. Research suggests 37% phosphoric acid is the ideal concentration.[5]

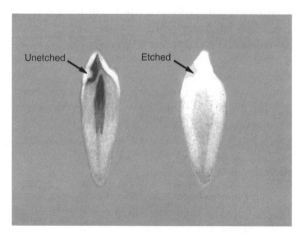

Figure 8–2. Two teeth with identical Class V preparations. *Right,* Tooth acid etched for 60 seconds with 37% phosphoric acid, rinsed, and then dried; *left,* unetched tooth. After composite placement both teeth were soaked in a dye solution and then sectioned. Note the unetched tooth shows massive leakage, whereas the acid-etched tooth is well sealed. (Image provided by Ralph Phillips.)

Resin Bonding 129

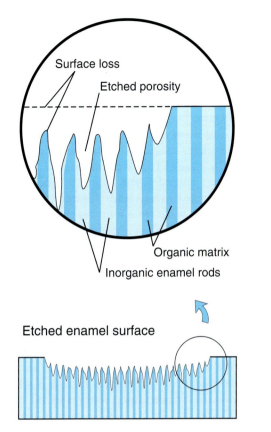

Figure 8–3. Schematic diagram depicting how acid etching produces microporosities in enamel.

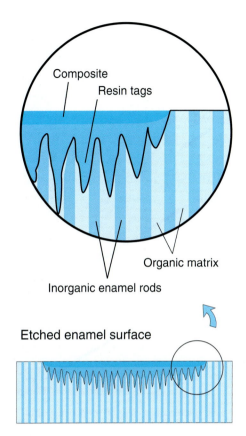

Figure 8–4. Schematic diagram depicting how resin tags penetrate the microporosities produced by acid etching of enamel.

Etching times

Etching for 15 seconds on permanent tooth enamel provides adequate microporosity for resin adhesion and sealing and bond strengths great enough to result in cohesive fracture of the enamel when separated.[6,7] On primary teeth, most research shows a 60-second etch is optimal,[8–10] but some studies show 120 seconds provides more consistent bond strengths.[11–13] This may be because primary enamel is amorphous and does not easily form the type of deep resin tags seen when etching permanent teeth. For optimum etching with a liquid etchant, the acid solution must be replenished during etching, because the acid evaporates.[14]

Variation in etching time

The endpoint of etching is an irregular surface that appears frosty white, owing to light refraction. Failure to achieve a frosty surface could result from factors such as inadequate etching or hypercalcified enamel. Etching too long (past the point of a frosted surface) can cause an insoluble reaction-product and a weak bond.

The best total etch time depends on the age of the tooth. Clinically, the most important measure of a properly etched tooth is the frosty white appearance of the surface. If the etched surface is not frosty white, it is unlikely that adequate microporosities are present for successful bonding. The average time to etch primary teeth is usually longer than for permanent teeth: the average time to etch adult permanent teeth is 20 seconds; newly erupted permanent teeth may need only 15 seconds. Clinically, it is best to etch and wash in 20-second intervals until the desired frosty look appears. Some older teeth may require over 2 minutes of etch time to achieve this endpoint.

The fluoride content of teeth affects etching time. Young teeth with mild fluorosis may need up

130 Tooth-Colored Restoratives

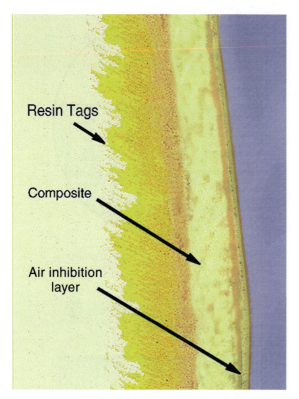

Figure 8–5. A microscopic view of resin penetration into etched enamel.

to 120 seconds.[8–10] Severely mottled teeth may require longer than 120 seconds. Freshly cut enamel etches faster than unprepared enamel.

Researchers agree that etching enamel for as long as 60 seconds is safe and reliable, but there is some disagreement about the lower limit for etching duration. Many in the field advocate etching for as little as 10 seconds. Is there a risk to shorter etch times? Almost all research on etching is done in vitro. Human teeth are not always included in the testing, and when they are, they are often third molars, which are not representative of a typical dental practice, let alone a specific patient.

The author believes that etching short of a frosty white appearance creates a significant risk of poor bonding. In most teeth, the white frosty surface appears as expected after drying. When there is no clinical evidence of an etched surface, the 20-second etch-and-dry cycle is repeated until it appears. Some highly fluoridated teeth may need the maximum published effective etch time of 2 minutes.

Washing times
Insufficient washing leaves debris that interferes with the flow of resin into the enamel channels. Acid-etched enamel must be washed for 10 seconds; gel etchants should be washed longer. Some studies have shown a 10- to 30-second wash time yields the same bond strength.[15] One study showed a 60-second wash time with a heavy water spray actually weakens the resin–enamel bond, probably because the enamel rods were crushed.[15] Current thinking has tended toward shorter wash times, often as short as 1 to 5 seconds. One consideration is that a longer wash time removes the silica used as a thickening agent in most gel etchants. It is unclear if leaving silica deposits from the etchant on the tooth has any clinical significance.

Drying
Electric hot air dryers are the best way to dry an etched enamel surface; they have been shown to improve enamel bond strengths by about 29%.[16] A high-speed vacuum, drawing warm room air past the tooth surface, is also acceptable. The least desirable way to dry an etched surface is with a three-way air syringe, since water and oil often contaminate it. Liquid drying agents do not improve bond strength.[16]

Contamination
With any bonding procedure, isolation of the working field is essential. Working with a rubber dam in place is highly recommended to avoid contaminating etched surfaces. Even a patient's breath can reduce bond strengths.

Water
The etched enamel surface must be dry. Resins are hydrophobic and do not adhere to moist tooth structure. Common sources of moisture are the patient's breath (when a rubber dam is not used) and three-way air syringes. Some of the "wet bonding" techniques start with a wet tooth and use solvents to evaporate this moisture.

Saliva and gingival fluid
The rinsed and dried etched surface must not be contaminated with saliva or intersulcular fluid or bond strength drops enormously (Figure 8–6). When contamination occurs, the enamel should be re-etched for 15 seconds, rinsed with water (usually 10 to 20 seconds), and dried again.

Oil

Oil is a barrier to both etchants and resins; it must be removed with alcohol, pumice, discs, or a water- or air-abrasion unit. Having the patient rinse with an alcohol-containing mouthwash is also effective in removing oil. The most common sources of oil are handpieces and air syringes. Oil from sterilized and recently lubricated handpieces is the major source of bond failure because the contamination is difficult to detect.

Oxygen

The surface layer of composite exposed to air does not polymerize unless the tooth is covered by a matrix or by more composite. Materials with higher filler loadings are less affected by oxygen inhibition. Special resin coatings containing highly reactive photoinhibitors are designed for surface repairs and sealing (eg, Fortify, Bisco, Schaumburg, Illinois). Alcohol weakens composites and should not be used on placement instruments. However, alcohol is a good solvent to clean composite off instruments. Eugenol inhibits polymerization. Products such as zinc oxide-eugenol (ZOE) or intermediate restorative material (IRM) (LD Caulk) should not be used as liners or bases. Likewise, copal varnish inhibits polymerization.

Etching materials

Etching liquids and etching gels

On smooth surfaces, etching liquids and gels result in similar etch patterns.[17] With deep grooves and fissures, a liquid etch is recommended, because it penetrates the irregularities of the occlusal surface. There is enormous variation in etching gels. In addition, gels can easily thicken through evaporation, making them able to wet a tooth. The ideal gel etchant is fluid enough to form a low contact angle with a tooth and viscous enough to stay where placed. When in doubt, the clinician should err on the side of a more fluid etchant.

Bonding resins

Bonding agents are low-viscosity resins that flow into the porosities of the etched enamel. These agents are polymerized to form resin tags that provide mechanical retention. No chemical bonds are formed. The filled composite (resin plus filler particles) is placed against this bonding-agent layer. A chemical bond forms between these layers. Flowable composites also can be used as bonding agents.

Remineralization

Researchers once thought that etching-induced changes in enamel were reversed upon exposure to oral fluids. Early scanning electron microscope (SEM) surveys of etched enamel appeared to show complete remineralization within 2 weeks after surface etching. Later studies revealed that organic mucoprotein from saliva filled in the etched spaces and that true mineralization could take 2 or more months to occur. Therefore, it is important to etch only those surfaces needed for bonding a restorative material (Figure 8–7).

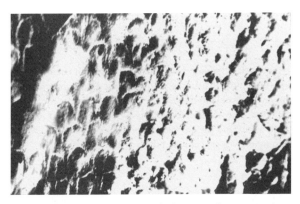

Figure 8–6. Electron micrograph showing saliva contamination of the microporosities of an etched enamel surface. Washing with water did not reopen the enamel porosities, because oral fluids bind firmly to the highly reactive etched enamel surface. To bond a resin to this surface requires re-etching the enamel.

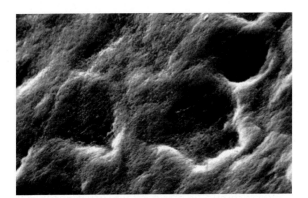

Figure 8–7. Electron micrograph of the remineralization process of etched enamel after 2 weeks. Note the complete fill-in of mucoprotein.

Adding a fluoride gel to the finished restoration before removal of the rubber dam allows the enamel to take up a significant amount of fluoride. Once saliva covers the tooth, fluoride uptake through enamel is greatly reduced.

Freshly etched enamel that remains exposed after the restoration is complete should not be subjected to coffee, tea, tobacco, or any other materials that stain. Sensitivity and staining are reduced if the patient, for a 2-week period, applies a fluoride gel or a fluoride rinse daily after brushing. This is especially helpful when extensive bonding is done on younger patients. Neither stannous fluoride nor sodium fluoride stain enamel.[18] Acidulated phosphate fluoride is not appropriate, because it dissolves some types of composite filler particles.[19]

ENAMEL MARGIN DESIGN

Bonding to enamel changes cavity preparation design because less tooth reduction is necessary.

Enamel discing

Freshly cut enamel provides a better bonding surface than nonprepared enamel.[20] The outer layer of all deciduous teeth and 70% of permanent teeth contains aprismatic enamel (ie, enamel that lacks uniform prisms) and provides less mechanical retention when etched.[21] In permanent teeth, this layer is usually 30 μm thick and is most prevalent in gingival areas. Discing off 0.1 mm of the enamel removes this layer, which improves bond strength 25 to 50%, depending on the amount of aprismatic enamel present.[20] Nonprepared enamel also often contains fluoride, which makes it acid resistant.

Preparation angles

Etching the ends of enamel rods produces the greatest benefit. Exposing cross-sectional areas of enamel allows the formation of longer tags than does exposing longitudinal sections.[22] Figure 8–8 depicts four enamel margin designs.

A 90-degree exit angle is useful when it is desirable to maintain maximum tooth structure. However, this exit angle does not expose the ends of the enamel rods and is less retentive. Natural tooth contacts should be preserved whenever possible.

A 45-degree bevel is the most commonly used finish line. This design conserves much of the

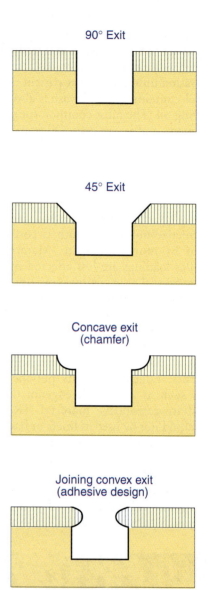

Figure 8–8. Common enamel margin designs for enamel–resin bonding. Note that in the 90-degree exit design the rod ends are not accessible to the resin. This design provides the weakest bond. The 45-degree bevel exposes more enamel rod ends at an angle, and the chamfer exposes the most rod ends. The joining convex exit provides the best seal.

original tooth structure and exposes the enamel rod ends. Compared with the 90-degree exit, the 45-degree bevel provides a superior seal for enamel, particularly at the gingival margins.[23] This is the most esthetic finish line, allowing a smooth transition and gradual shade change from composite to enamel. Bevel preparations also have less microleakage compared with preparations in which the sides of enamel rods are etched.

A concave bevel (chamfer), made by exposing the maximum surface area of enamel rod ends, is the most retentive finish line. The chamfer also allows a 90-degree angle of exit for the restoration, making it a more durable margin, particularly at occlusal contact points. However, because it is the least conservative design, the concave bevel should be used only when maximum retention from acid etching is necessary (eg, the Class IV fracture).

Some research demonstrates that a joining convex bevel (adhesive preparation) seals better than the three conventional designs.[24] This design may not always be clinically practical, but it illustrates that rounded areas of unsupported enamel provide excellent exits for bonded resins but make it more difficult to remove carious dentin from the dentin–enamel junction. The design works only with a stiff composite, because the composite must support the enamel.

After thermal cycling, adhesive designs demonstrate superior seals when examined under SEM.[24] Examinations also show that a long bevel seals better than a concave bevel (chamfer). As expected, the 90-degree exit has the poorest seal. Use of bonding agents greatly improves the seal and appearance of all margins.

Using a variety of preparation margins on the same restoration is sometimes the best approach to achieving bond retention and tooth conservation. For example, a 90-degree composite exit maintains a natural proximal contact. A 45-degree bevel on the facial provides improved esthetics. A chamfer on the lingual increases retention and reduces marginal chipping. Composite resins are softer than enamel and wear down in a crowded arch, causing considerable loss of interproximal space.

Coarse enamel surfaces
Some clinicians advocate finishing enamel margins in acid-etched preparations with a coarse diamond to provide mechanical surface retention and increase the surface area for bonding. Some research shows a 25% increase in resin–enamel bond strength (in comparison with uncut enamel) when enamel exits are cut with a carbide bur, and a 50% improvement when the exits are cut with a coarse diamond.[25] This study used unfilled resin as a bonding agent on the etched surfaces. When the surface is prepared with a diamond, numerous voids occur at the resin–enamel interface that inhibit polymerization because of air inhibition. Voids also reduce the surface area for bonding and can result in extensive marginal staining when composite wear brings voids to the surface.

Research indicates that smooth enamel margins provide maximum restoration adaptation to the tooth. Bonding research on smooth surface enamel shows that the resin–enamel bond is stronger than the cohesive strength of either composite resin or enamel. The smoothest enamel margins are achieved with straight-fissure burs with twisted flutes, and 12-fluted finish burs.[26] The finish from a diamond bur results in a more durable bond than that from a finishing bur.[25] Rough enamel can provide a 50 to 60% increase in bond strength compared with smooth enamel surfaces.[27]

A 40- to 125-µm diamond grit coarse exit is best for direct systems, because a slight roughness provides resistance form against polymerization contraction forces during curing. This reduces the incidence of bond separation caused by peel forces created at the polymerizing marginal interface. Interface peeling generally shows up after finishing, as white line margins. Although the white line may disappear in a few days because of water absorption, the resin does not reattach to the tooth and marginal staining generally increases over time.

INTERMEDIATE ENAMEL BONDING RESINS

Bonding agents are fluid, resinous materials designed to improve the bond between a viscous composite resin and the microporosities of etched enamel. Some laboratory studies show there is no difference in composite adaptation to etched enamel whether or not an intermediate bonding agent is used.[28] If the flow properties of the composite allow it to wet the surface, it may not need an enamel bonding agent. Most luting and flowable composites are fluid enough to penetrate the enamel surface without a bonding resin.

With macrofilled composites, a resin tag depth of 50 μm has been measured with and without a bonding agent.[29,30] With the more viscous microfilled composites, the absence of a bonding agent resulted in 30-μm tags, compared with 50-μm tags with a bonding agent. However, even these shorter tags tear cohesively in the resin rather than adhesively at the enamel–resin interface.[31]

Research on fractured specimens shows that use of a bonding agent reduces air-bubble formation when the composite is placed directly against enamel.[31] Clinical studies show no difference after 18 months in the performance of composites placed on enamel with or without bonding agents.[32] Laboratory studies show that using an intermediate bonding agent reduces the recurrent caries rate, compared with composites placed without a bonding agent,[33] and produces 17 to 31% less marginal staining.[34] This research suggests that it is important to use an enamel bonding agent with any condensable or stiff composite, whereas highly fluid composites (under 70% loading by weight) rarely benefit from use of a bonding agent.

The bond strength provided by flowable unfilled resins or fluid composite materials and resin cements is strong enough to result in cohesive fracture of the enamel. When used on etched enamel, the main purpose of a bonding agent is to allow more viscous composites to maximize tag formation on the resin surface. For bonding fluid composite to tooth structure, a bonding agent is required only if dentin is being bonded at the same time. Many all-purpose bonding agents contain large amounts of solvent, which if not evaporated, can severely limit bond strengths to enamel.

Bonding agents and resin compatibility

The choice of bonding agent may have implications for bond strength. A stronger bond to etched enamel may result if the resin in the bonding agent and the composite are similar.

Different manufacturers often use different monomers in their composites. Some composites are made with modified Bis-GMA resins to improve water solubility, viscosity, or durability of the resin matrix. Modifications using urethane, tricyclo, and other dimethacrylates are common. Most manufacturers provide bonding agents made of a resin similar to that in their composites and optimize their bonding agents to work with their composites. However, since almost all composite resins are dimethacrylates, almost all bonding agents work with almost all composites. Differences among the various brands of composite and bonding agents are usually not clinically significant. However, since most manufacturers supply adhesives with their composites, using them together is advisable, particularly when bonding to enamel with a viscous composite.

Which of the various types of bonding agents bond as well to themselves as to other products is not fully understood. A simple way to avoid the possibility of noncompatibility is to use bonding agents made by the composite manufacturer.

It is important to remember that some bonding agents are specifically designed to work well on dentin and do not provide good results on enamel. For example, some aqueous dentin primers can reduce etched enamel bond strengths by 15 to 30%.[35]

CLINICAL PROCEDURE FOR ACID ETCHING ENAMEL

Prior to acid etching, complete the preparation (or discing), remove all caries, and clean the tooth. Next, select an accurate shade of composite, and place a rubber dam. All enamel areas to be etched should be either prepared or disced. Use proximal finishing strips to clean the enamel in the embrasures before etching.

Step 1. Clean the tooth before placing a rubber dam and before deciding on a composite shade. Removal of debris and pellicle ensures more accurate shade selection and more effective etching. It also removes any oil deposited on the tooth by a handpiece. Clean the tooth with air or water abrasion. Discing the enamel with a disc, diamond strip, or diamond optimizes enamel bonding by providing a clean surface.

Step 2. Place a suitable liner in the very deep areas of dentin.

Step 3. Use a Mylar matrix to protect adjacent teeth from contacting the etching solution and unnecessary enamel demineralization. Failure to protect adjacent teeth could result in inadvertent bonding of surfaces.

Step 4. Place a thin layer of etching liquid or gel on the enamel with a plastic brush or sponge. (These are usually provided by the manufacturer.) Keep it wet with acid for 15 to 20 seconds.

Do not rub or apply any pressure to the enamel surface during or after the etchant is deposited since this can collapse the delicate enamel porosities that are the goal of etching. Crushing these porosities results in a weaker enamel–resin bond.

Step 5. Wash for at least 10 seconds. If a gel etchant is used, washing longer is advised, particularly if it is highly viscous.

Step 6. Dry. Use an electric air dryer, high-speed vacuum, or air syringe to dry the newly etched surface (in that order of preference). Three-way air syringes often leak oil, which can inhibit bonding.

Step 7. The enamel should look chalky white. If not, repeat steps 4, 5, and 6. If a chalky surface is not attained, disc the enamel and start over at step 3 (Figure 8–9).

HOW ENAMEL AND DENTIN BONDING DIFFER

The clinical success of enamel bonding with 37% phosphoric acid[36] led clinicians to take the same approach to dentin bonding. However, the early dentin bonding systems resulted in low bond strengths.[37]

Enamel is 95% inorganic matter (hydroxyapatite), 4% water, and 1% organic matter (a collagen substance called enamelin) by weight. Although enamel is naturally hydrophilic (readily absorbing water), hydrophobic (resistant to absorbing water) bonding resins can wet and penetrate dried, etched enamel because of the high surface energy of an etched surface.

Dentin, on the other hand, is just 70% hydroxyapatite, 18% collagen, and 12% water by weight. This collagen is normally inaccessible, owing to surrounding hydroxyapatite ($Ca_{10}(PO_4)_6(OH)_2$) crystals. The only obvious "pores" available for resin to penetrate are the dentin tubules. Because of fluid flow from the dentin tubules, dentin is more highly hydrophilic than enamel, which makes bonding a hydrophobic resin into the dentin substrate difficult.

Dentin bonding is highly technique sensitive and can be highly variable. Deep dentin exhibits far more tubules than superficial dentin, but also shows lower bond strengths, partly because the tubules are more fluid-filled near the pulp.[38] Dentin fluids can interfere with a resin–dentin bond.

Bond strengths to all dentin surfaces are consistently lower than to enamel, regardless of the material used or the presence or absence of pulpal pressure. Dentin bonding also varies from tooth to tooth in the same mouth; for example, cuspid and central incisors can have higher dentin bond strengths than molars.[39]

DENTIN HISTOLOGY

The structural unit of importance in bonding to dentin is the dentin tubule, comparable with the enamel crystal. Dentin is porous; a large number of dentin tubules run from the dentin–enamel junction to the pulp. These tubules are 1 to 2 μm in diameter and convey pulpal fluid from the pulp to the enamel (Figure 8–10).[40] The tubules maintain tooth hydration and increase the fracture toughness of the collagen matrix that holds enamel and dentin together.

The dentin tubules are surrounded by a thin coating of a highly mineralized *peritubular dentin* that is embedded in a matrix of collagen and hydroxyapatite crystals, so forming the *intertubular* dentin (Figure 8–11).[41] The peritubular dentin collar is between 1.0 and 1.5 μm in diameter. Peritubular dentin contains more mineral and less

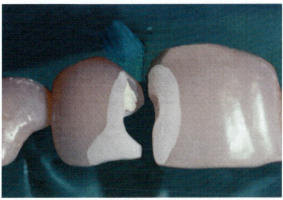

Figure 8–9. Photograph showing typical appearance after drying of an acid etched surface 2 mm past the prepared margins.

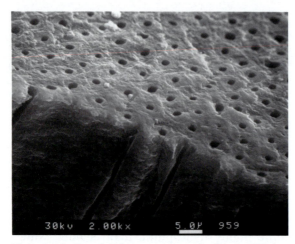

Figure 8–10. Scanning electron micrograph of a normal dentin surface. (Source: Marshall GW Jr. Dentin: microstructure and characterization. Quintessence Int 1993;24:606–17.)

collagen than intertubular dentin. As the tubules converge on the pulp chamber, the area of peritubular dentin increases and intertubular dentin decreases.

Dentin and enamel are intimately related at the dentin–enamel junction, with the enamel "protecting" the dentin from wear, and the dentin supporting the brittle enamel. Without adequate support from the dentin, the enamel shell is easily lost. Unlike enamel, dentin is neither stronger nor weaker in any particular direction; it is isotropic compared with enamel, which is anisotropic. The multiphase nature of dentin presents a number of problems for bonding, because of its water content, its resiliency, and its heterogeneity. Likewise, structural differences between superficial and deep dentin contribute to the inconsistency of dentin bonding values.

Inadequately bonded dentin–resin interfaces can exhibit microleakage that allows bacteria to migrate through the interface. Microleakage is often associated with polymerization shrinkage. Current adhesive systems, together with hydroscopic composite expansion, can compensate for microleakage. Similarly, layered application of a bonding agent, to thicken the surface layer, followed by adequate curing greatly reduces microleakage.

It has been hypothesized that a shear bond strength of 17 to 24 MPa eliminates microleakage at the dentin–resin interface.[42] These values can be achieved with most currently available bonding agents. Unfortunately, the polymerization stress of most composites can far exceed the capacity of any bonding system (Figure 8–12). Thus, the configuration of the preparation (C-factor) where the

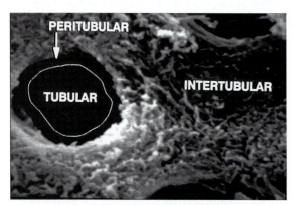

Figure 8–11. Scanning electron micrograph of a dentin surface illustrating the different components of dentin. (Image provided by Byoung Suk.)

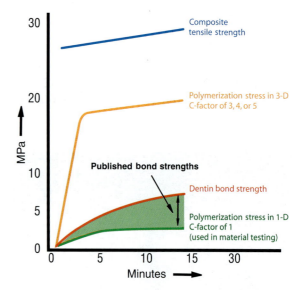

Figure 8–12. Composite polymerization strength is much greater than bond strength. In a restoration with a C-factor of 1, the composite shrinks toward the bond; this is the standard against which new bonding materials are tested. In most clinical situations, restorations have a C-factor of 3 or more, and the polyermization shrinkage competes with the bond strength.

composite is placed has the largest impact on leakage at the marginal interface.

Nanoleakage, fluid migration through a system, is also hypothesized to occur with all dentin–resin bonded interfaces. This would allow acids and other water-soluble materials to travel through these interfaces, potentially causing staining.

Smear Layer

Morphology
When a rotary or handheld instrument is used on dentin it creates a special surface texture called a smear or smear layer that closes off the dentin tubules (Figure 8–13). This layer is lightly adhered to the dentin surface and contains tooth cuttings, saliva, bacteria, and other surface debris (Figure 8–14).

Smear layer and bonding
The smear layer can reduce dentin permeability. This is helpful for hydrophobic bonding materials, since the smear layer permits a drier bonding surface with increased microporosities; however, the smear layer also has an adhesive strength of its own. This limits the potential bond strength of dentin to a fraction of the bond strength of etched enamel. For this reason, most newer dentin bonding systems remove or greatly alter the smear layer before bonding.

Smear layer removal
The smear layer is easily removed with acids, even weak ones, but cannot easily be removed mechanically with either instruments or pumice.

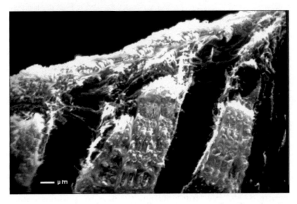

Figure 8–13. Scanning electron micrograph of a dentin smear layer. (Image provided by Byoung Suk.)

Smear layer alteration
Most primers in newer bonding systems alter, partly remove, or partly demineralize the smear layer or the peritubular area to increase micromechanical penetration and attachment into the dentin.

Effects of age on dentin histology
Dentin tubules and their contents, peritubular dentin and intertubular dentin, are the main structures of young dentin. The intertubular dentin in young teeth is well-organized "primary" dentin. With age, dentin continues to form on the pulpal surface. This "secondary" dentin, which is less organized than primary dentin, is deposited over the life of a tooth. It is formed by circular deposition of peritubular dentin and eventually closes the tubule. The rate of tubular closure increases when the gingiva recedes and dentin is exposed to the oral fluids.

A third type of dentin, "tertiary," irritational, or reparative dentin, forms in response to irritation in the oral environment, such as caries or cervical attrition. It grows along the pulpal wall adjacent to the irritation. This layer of dentin is extremely irregular and may be atubular.[43] Hence, it is also called irregular secondary dentin.

Depending on clinical conditions or lesion depth, all three types of dentin may be encountered during adhesive bonding.

Age changes in dentin
Pashley calls dentin a dynamic substrate subject to continuous change, and observes that the rate of alteration appears to be directly related to a tooth's history of insult.[44,45] Microstructural and chemical changes in the dentin relative to the caries process have been extensively investigated. The general consensus is that the dentin immediately adjacent to carious activity (transparent or sclerotic layer) has more mineral content than sound dentin. Intratubular changes observed in this zone include the obstruction of dentin tubules by large crystalline deposits that can occlude dentin tubules.[38,45–47]

Dentin sclerosis
The formation of transparent dentin, or dentin sclerosis, has been associated with abrasive lesions and is reported to result from the obstruction of dentin tubules by calcified deposits. Dentin can become transparent when the dentin tubules are obstructed with secondary dentin.[48]

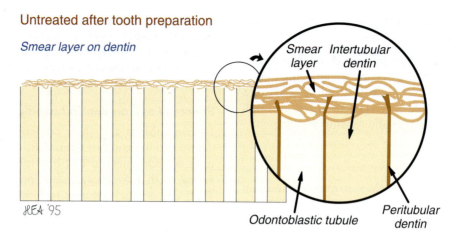

Figure 8–14. Schematic diagram showing the histology of the dentin surface with a smear layer attached.

Peritubular dentin and age

Structural changes in peritubular dentin are reported in aged and affected dentin. In newly erupted teeth, there is no peritubular dentin close to the pre-dentin near the pulp. As a result of pathologic processes and advancing age, the thickness of the peritubular dentin increases and may completely obstruct the tubular orifice.

EFFECT OF DENTIN BONDING AGENTS ON PULP

When the smear layer is removed, the resins in dentin bonding systems can penetrate the tubules toward the pulp.[49] With light-cured materials, the farther these resins penetrate, the more difficult they are to polymerize. This is because deeper resin tags are more likely to encounter dentinal fluid, which may interfere with resin polymerization. Even under ideal conditions, the conversion of monomer to polymer is only about 55 to 60%.[50] It is likely that unpolymerized monomer can leach into the surrounding dentinal fluid and toward the pulp. The long-term effect of this on pulpal irritation is not well known. Pulpal penetration of dentin bonding agents is possible in deep cavities (Figure 8–15).

Laboratory studies show the irritating properties of most dental materials are short-lived, generally lasting only 1 to 2 days.[51] In germ-free animals, most dental materials produce little pulpal inflammation.[52] Most studies have implicated oral bacteria and their by-products as the major source of pulpal irritation around leaking restorative materials.[51,53]

Dentin thickness is also important in protecting the pulp from either toxic materials or bacterial products.[54,55] Thicker dentin lowers the concentration of substances that reach the pulp, keeping these concentrations below thresholds that inflame or irritate pulpal tissues. Thin dentin is a poor barrier and does not dissipate chemicals as well. If the dentin thickness falls below 0.5 mm, there is a functional exposure because of the high permeability to the pulp. Thin dentin should be sealed.

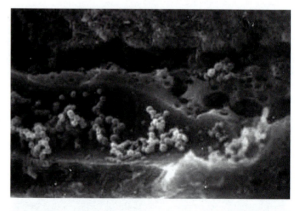

Figure 8–15. Electron micrograph of resin globules penetrating a dentin tubule.

STABILITY OF DENTIN BONDS

Dentin has a lower cohesive strength than many composites, and, unlike enamel–resin bonds, polymerization or thermocyclic stresses continue to degrade a dentin–resin bond over time. Regardless of the bonding system used, a dentin–resin bond will eventually fail cohesively below the bonding layer. A restoration that appears successfully sealed and bonded at placement will continue to degrade over time.

Currently available adhesives are thought to react with dentin surfaces micromechanically. Unfortunately, dentin tubules at the surface in such locations as Class V attrition often are obturated by peritubular dentin or by the precipitation of calcific deposits. This sclerotic dentin is less receptive to dentin bonding. In addition, aged dentin surfaces have great variability in tubular morphology. The more sclerotic the dentin, the less receptive it is to the conditioner, bonding agent, and resin composite. Clinical trials substantiate that failure of dentin–resin bonding systems occurs most in sclerotic lesions.[56]

Researchers have suggested that the extraordinary patient-to-patient variation in dentin structure and composition may account for the clinically observed variability in results with dentin adhesives.[43,56] Laboratory studies are normally conducted on ground teeth with ideal dentin, such as recently extracted third molars or bovine teeth, which do not represent the dentin restored clinically, namely, dentin affected by advancing caries or other pathologic conditions.[56]

Adhesive interactions with cervical abrasion

Micromechanics is thought to explain adhesion to unaffected primary dentin. The bond is created when monomers infiltrating demineralized dentin polymerize to form an interlocking network with the dentin matrix. Most of these systems contain an aqueous methacrylate primer (HEMA, or other water-soluble methacrylate) and an acid to remove or alter the smear layer. These primers alter the smear layer on ground, unaffected dentin, leaving clearly visible, open tubules.[57,58]

Increasing levels of sclerosis make penetration of almost all primer solutions less effective.[59] For this reason, many clinicians and researchers recommend abrading sclerotic lesions for dentin bonding. This allows dentin bonding agents better access to the organic and tubular areas of the dentin surface.

Phosphoric acid has been examined for etching heavily sclerosed dentin. However, since the intertubular dentin of sclerosed dentin is hypermineralized, etching shows less effect.[60,61]

For treating more sclerotic cervical abrasion lesions, the dentin adhesives designed to create mechanical retention in tubular orifices, or directed at specific dentin compositions, may be less successful. Successful dentin bonding depends on accurate identification of the dentin composition and matching of the adhesive system to the specific type of dentin.[54]

DENTIN–RESIN BONDING TECHNIQUES

This section classifies dentin bonding materials by their method of micromechanical attachment, which is the basis of adhesion for most dentin–resin bonding agents.[62]

Infiltrating a resin monomer into chemically conditioned dentin is the key to resin bonding. Nakabayashi and colleagues referred to this infiltration as *hybridization*.[63] It involves resin penetration into both tubular and intertubular dentin (Figure 8–16). Infiltration into the tubules accounts for about one-third of the shear bond strength of the dentin bond.[64] The remaining two-thirds is achieved through resin infiltration of the demineralized hybrid zone, and reaction and association with the underlying unaltered dentin, whose porosity and surface area contributes significantly to interfacial toughness.

Methods of attachment

Past and present dentin–resin bonding systems can be classified by their method of attachment. Currently, researchers think that many dentin bonding systems adhere by micromechanical attachment. In micromechanical attachment, wetting the dentin surface with adhesive is the key to success. This intimate relation between the primer

140   Tooth-Colored Restoratives

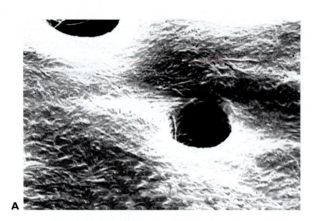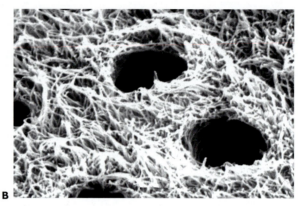

Figure 8-16. Electron micrographs. *A,* The dentin surface prior to conditioning, and *B,* the dentin surface after conditioning. The demineralized surface has voids that a primer can penetrate. (Images provided by Byoung Suk.)

and the dentin allows van der Waals forces to contribute to the attachment.

Smear layer saturation
First-generation dentin bonding materials penetrate the dentin smear layer. Some products alter this layer to improve bonding (eg, Scotchbond, XR Bond, and PUB) (Figure 8–17).

Tubular penetration
Almost all dentin–resin bonding agents that remove the smear layer allow resin to penetrate into the dentin tubules. This improves bonding by attaching to a more rigid substrate. Tubular penetration alone is marginally beneficial, although it may seal the tubules and restrict access to the pulp. Some dentin bonding agents, such as Gluma and Scotchbond II, result in maximum tubular penetration.

Tubular impregnation without smear layer
Second-generation dentin bonding agents (eg, Gluma, Scotchbond II, and Tenure) remove or alter the smear layer, demineralize the collagen, infiltrate the demineralized zone with resin, and penetrate tubular, intertubular, and peritubular dentin (Figure 8–18).

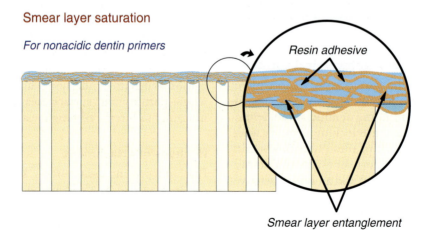

Figure 8–17. Schematic representation of attachment for first-generation dentin bonding agents (eg, Scotchbond, XR Bond, and PUB).

Resin Bonding 141

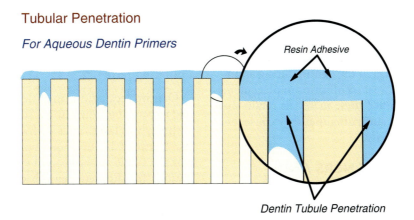

Figure 8–18. Schematic representation of attachment for second-generation dentin bonding agents (eg, Gluma, Scotchbond II, and Tenure). With smear layer removal, tubular penetration accompanies almost all dentin–resin bonding agents. The quality and quantity of this attachment varies with each dentin surface, the particular bonding materials, and the placement technique. Almost all dentin–resin bonding agents currently available involve some degree of tubular penetration.

Hybrid zone impregnation without smear layer
The third-generation bonding agents work by etching the dentin and keeping it hydrated so that a dentin bonding agent can penetrate the spaces left by removal of hydroxyapatite crystals. Products representative of this class include All-Bond, Scotchbond MP, OptiBond, and 4-META (Figure 8–19). Hydration is important to the attachment process when these materials are used; if they are used on dry dentin, the collagen layer will collapse, leaving few voids for the resin to penetrate. In the event of dentin dry out, rehydration with water for 30 seconds restores the collagen layer to permit good resin penetration.

Hybrid zone impregnation with smear layer
The fourth-generation dentin bonding agents (eg, Clearfil SE Bond, and Prompt-L-Pop) incorporate

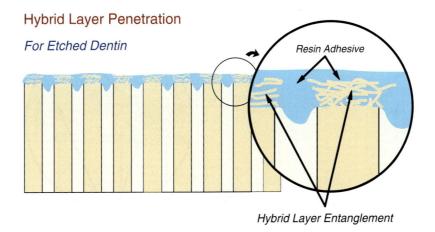

Figure 8–19. Schematic representation of the method of attachment for third-generation dentin bonding agents (eg, All-Bond, Scotchbond MP, OptiBond, 4-META materials, and almost all single-solution materials). Almost all of these dentin bonding agents also penetrate the tubules to various degrees, which is thought to account for about 20% of the overall dentin–resin bond strength.

the smear layer into the demineralized zone (Figure 8–20). These products are widely referred to as "self-etching primers." Their use eliminates the acid etching step in restoration placement. They are highly acidic and etch the dentin during application; they are not washed off prior to placement of the composite. Since these materials retain the smear layer, it is not surprising that they cause less postoperative sensitivity.

DENTIN CONDITIONERS AND ETCHANTS

Conditioners are usually mild acids that clean dentin and enhance its permeability. Most conditioners currently available are also etchants that etch enamel and dentin. Conditioners typically clean the tooth surface by removing the smear layer and demineralizing the dentin. This step is similar to etching enamel, since both processes create surface microporosities. Conditioners are almost always rinsed off. Some of the typical dentin conditioners are aqueous solutions that include one of the following as the active ingredient: 16% EDTA, 10% citric acid, 10% maleic acid, 10% pyruvic acid, 10% phosphoric acid, or 2.5% nitric acid.

Fixing agents, such as 3 to 5% ferric chloride and aluminum chloride, are sometimes combined with a dentin conditioner to stabilize collagen after etching. A solution of 10% citric acid and 3% ferric chloride (a tanning or flocculating agent) is believed to improve the stiffness and accessibility of a demineralized dentin surface to a bonding resin.

Dentin decalcification varies enormously from acid to acid and from patient to patient. The depth of the hybrid layer varies with different conditioners. Dentin has enormous buffering ability such that the single application of various acid concentrations for different periods of time results in a similar depth of demineralization. Once dentin is rinsed, the buffering capacity of the layer is removed and re-etching demineralizes a second, deeper layer. Increased depth of demineralization does not increase bond strength; it does increase postoperative sensitivity. Therefore, multiple etching cycles are contraindicated.

Following surface conditioning, a dentin primer is applied to completely penetrate the porosities in the dentin. Re-etching the dentin can make the hybrid layer deeper than the dentin primer can penetrate, particularly if the dentin has been desiccated. When the primer is unable to penetrate the deeper demineralized zones, a space is left under the bonded layer. This space can retain air when the tooth is dried, such that when the restoration is compressed, the trapped air accentuates the movement of fluid in and out of the

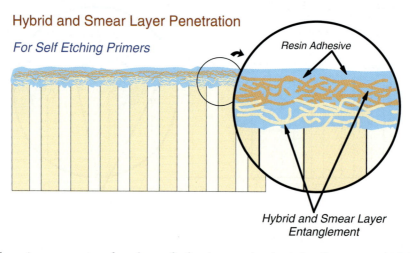

Figure 8–20. Schematic representation of attachment for fourth-generation dentin bonding agents, which incorporate the smear layer into the bonded interface. Materials using this attachment method are referred to as self-etching primers. The primer dissolves enough of the surface to allow mechanical interlocking yet limits removal of the smear layer, to reduce surface permeability.

tubules. This can cause chronic and painful sensitivity that can last up to a year. A 10-second etch time can provide good bond strengths with a lower risk of postoperative sensitivity.

DENTIN PRIMERS

Dentin primers are hydrophilic methacrylates. Full saturation of the dentin is important to ensure a sealed interface and good bond strength. This may require multiple applications of primer; it should be applied until the dentin will not absorb any more. Voids in the hybrid layer weaken the bond. The weakest spots are the top and bottom of the hybrid area, and it is at these spots that adhesive fractures occur. Each layer of primer should be gently dried to remove solvents and leave a visible, shiny layer of resin similar to the shiny, wet look achieved by licking a fingernail.

Primers aid in adhesion because they

- wet the surface (reduce the contact angle) and improve contact between the resin and the hydrophilic tooth structure;
- increase the permeability of the smear layer (if present) and allow the resin adhesive to permeate the smear layer;
- provide mechanical interlocking of the bonding agent to its surface; and
- potentially provide some chemical bonding between the resin and the altered dentin.

DENTIN ADHESIVES

The unfilled resin component, also called the bonding agent, is the intermediate layer between the primed dentin and the composite resin. This component is either a hydrophobic or a hydrophilic methacrylate resin that attaches to the resin-impregnated dentin surface, via the primer, and to the surface of the composite restorative, via copolymerization. It is the second bottle in most two-bottle systems.

Most, but not all adhesives are unfilled resins, including Bis-GMA/TEGDMA resins and Bis-GMA/HEMA resins. They are essential to dentin bonding and aid adhesion because they

- covalently bond to primer to link it to the hydrophobic resin;
- provide additional micro- and macromechanical surface retention, such that much of the bond strength comes from the adhesive wetting and interlocking in surface irregularities on the tooth surface; and
- provide an attachment mechanism for resin primers.

Some manufacturers use lightly filled resins, which may contain glass fillers, elastic-type polymers, or fluorides. Filled resins ("structural adhesives") improve the toughness of the agent. The OptiBond System (Kerr Corp.), for example, was one of the first to use such a material.

SINGLE-SOLUTION DENTIN BONDING SYSTEMS

Single-solution systems were developed to simplify application and reduce the porosities seen in most hybrid layers. They are popular because they are easy to use, but they may compromise consistent bond strength. Currently, most bonding agents sold are single-component.

One-component materials are highly volatile unfilled resins that start as thin fluids (primer mode), and become thicker (adhesive mode) through evaporation of the solvent (which is usually ethanol or acetone). Acetone-containing bonding agents include Prime&Bond, LD Caulk; One-Step, Bisco; and Tenure Quick, Den-Mat. Ethanol-containing bonding agents include Opti-Bond Solo, Kerr; and Single Bond, 3M. The problem with single-solution systems is the small window of opportunity for good bonding.

A sufficiently wet surface is crucial to successful use of single-solution systems. Loss of water and solvent from the surface when drying converts the solution from acting as a primer to acting as an adhesive. Single-solution bonding agents have the following limitations:

- High volatility
- Short shelf life
- Sensitivity to technique
- High variability in bond strength

CLINICAL PRINCIPLES OF DENTIN BONDING

The application of a dentin bonding system entails four basic steps.[65]

Step 1. An acid is used to demineralize the dentin surface. It also removes the smear layer. This creates space within the collagen network that is roughly analogous to the microporosities created by etching enamel.

Step 2. A dentin primer is placed over the demineralized surface. Dentin primers are hydrophilic solutions that have both hydrophilic and hydrophobic character (ie, they are coupling agents). These solutions penetrate the demineralized collagen to improve bonding.

Step 3. An unfilled resin (an "adhesive") is applied and penetrates the microporosities. With single-component materials, the evaporation of the volatile solvent converts the liquid from a primer to an adhesive.

Step 4. The bonding agent is polymerized.

Links in a chain

Each event in a bonding procedure is like a link in a chain; the end result depends on the weakest link. For dentin–resin bonding with direct systems, the links are conditioned dentin + dentin primer + adhesive + restorative. Links in the chain of attachment with indirect systems are: conditioned dentin + dentin primer + adhesive + composite + adhesive + porcelain or metal primer + restorative.

It is essential that each link wet (or form a low contact angle with) the following link. If at any time the contact angle exceeds 90 degrees (ie, one material forms droplets on the next), the procedure should be aborted, because there is a basic incompatibility.

Conditioners

Chemical conditioners create surface voids to which a dentin primer can attach. Conditioners are usually strong acids applied for short periods or weaker acids applied for longer times. They are always rinsed off. Because dentin decalcification varies from acid to acid and patient to patient, uniform results are hard to achieve when bonding to dentin.

When drying a conditioned dentin surface, it is important to avoid desiccation, which laboratory studies show can collapse the hybridized dentin and reduce the volume of exposed collagen by 60%, resulting in lower bond strengths (Figure 8–21).

Primers

It is generally better to prime dentin for 15 to 20% longer than it is conditioned; this helps ensure that the porosities created by the conditioner are filled by the primer (Cox C. Personal communication). When applying a primer, it is best to continually replenish the primer as it evaporates from the surface.

Adhesives

With many adhesives, layering and curing in at least two layers decreases microleakage. Most adhesives

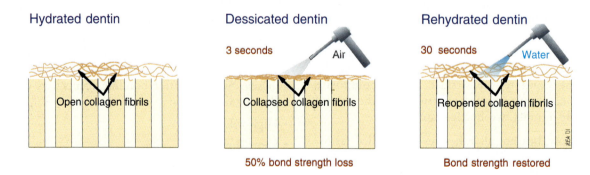

Figure 8–21. Schematic illustration of open, collapsed, and reopened collagen fibers. Open (hydrated) fibers are necessary for bond strength.

contain HEMA, and some contain water. Most are hydrophilic, which allows them to absorb water. Since water is a plasticizer (softener) of resin materials, use of dentin adhesives on etched enamel generally is not advised. When bonding to etched enamel (as with veneers), it is best to use a traditional hydrophobic, unfilled resin, because it is stronger, more color-stable, and results in less microleakage at the composite interface. Placing a hydrophobic resin over an aqueous HEMA primer on etched enamel is common practice with currently available bonding systems. Although most hydrophilic primers weaken enamel bonding slightly, the effect does not appear to be clinically significant.

Wet and dry bonding

Dentin bonding systems use three measures of dryness: wet, moist, and dry dentin.[66–70]

In dry bonding, all moisture is removed from the surface and the dentin is dehydrated. Moist bonding usually indicates that excess surface water is removed but the surface is fully hydrated. Wet bonding usually means there is a thin layer of standing water in the preparation. In wet bonding, an acetone solvent is used to remove the water and replace it with resin while, in theory, preventing the collapse of the hybrid layer.

The three types of dryness produce different results in laboratory studies of bonding with different products. Unfortunately, it can be difficult for a clinician to learn how to distinguish between different types of dryness without hands-on training. The significance of dentin dryness in terms of long-term clinical performance is unknown. With one-step materials, bond strengths are increased when they are applied to moist substrates. Using them on dry etched dentin usually reduces bond strengths by 50%, especially with the acetone-based materials. A moist surface is best achieved by removing excess water with a cotton pellet. With many two- and three-step dentin bonding materials, no differences in microleakage have been reported between wet and dry bonding techniques.

GENERIC DENTAL BONDING STEPS

For dentin bonding, the manufacturer's instructions should be followed. A clinician should vary from the instructions only if he or she understands the chemistry of the products thoroughly enough to know when a specific deviation will achieve a better clinical result.

With the exception of etchants and conditioners, mixing resin components from different bonding systems is not recommended. Mixing primers, activators, initiators, and other components that are not designed to work together can have catastrophic results.

Following is a generic set of instructions for dentin bonding. These instructions do not replace a manufacturer's instructions. They are provided to suggest how these systems work. Good technique should achieve the bonded interface shown in Figure 8–22.

Step 1. Etch only the enamel for 10 to 20 seconds with phosphoric acid.

Step 2. Condition dentin with a suitable conditioner. Condition for only 10 seconds if the etchant is phosphoric acid, longer etch times may increase sensitivity. In this way, the enamel has a total etch time of 20 to 30 seconds, and the dentin has 10 seconds. As a compromise, enamel and dentin can be treated simultaneously for 15 seconds. With self-etching primers, steps 1 and 2 are done together with a single solution. It is important not to over-etch the dentin.

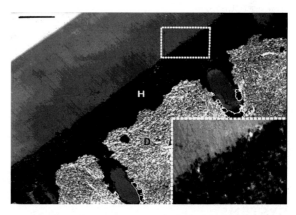

Figure 8–22. Electron micrograph showing a bonded interface. The hybrid layer (H) is saturated with a primer. This is magnified in the lower right square, which shows the mechanical nature of this attachment. The underlying dentin (D) also shows the typical intertubular penetration of the primer that accompanies almost all dentin–resin bonding agents. Bar = 1 μm. (Image provided by Franklin Tay.)

Step 3. Rinse the enamel and dentin for 5 to 15 seconds.

Step 4. Air dry with a gentle stream of air, or gently blot dry with a cotton pellet.

Step 5. Apply as many coats of primer as necessary to develop a visible resin coating (glistening appearance) on the dentin surface. Autocured bonding materials usually come in two bottles and should be used with autocured composites.

Step 6. Evaporate solvents from the enamel and dentin with a gentle stream of warm air for 3 to 5 seconds. Then dry thoroughly again to remove all residual fluid from the enamel. This will not affect the dentin since it is already sealed and will not dessicate.

Step 7. Add an adhesive (or an unfilled resin) and thin out with a dry brush or gentle stream of air. The adhesive is usually a higher viscosity resin compared with the primer. Use an autocured adhesive with an autocured composite.

Step 8. Cure the adhesive for 10 seconds.

Step 9. Add the appropriate composite resin in increments, working from the enamel walls, until the dentin wall is covered.

Step 10. After final placement and curing, wait 10 minutes to allow the dark reaction to occur. For most composites, this reaction is 90% completed in 10 minutes.

Step 11. Finish with appropriate rotary instruments cooled with a water spray. Re-etch, rinse, and dry thoroughly with a warm air dryer.

Step 12. Add glaze (which is an unfilled sealant) to seal any marginal gaps created by shrinkage and finishing. Many have extra accelerators to reduce the effects of oxygen inhibition. This is usually a higher viscosity hydrophobic resin.

COMPARING ONE- AND TWO-COMPONENT DENTIN BONDING SYSTEMS

Two-component bonding systems

Dentin bonding has traditionally involved two components, a primer and an adhesive. The primer is designed to be hydrophilic and saturate the dentin surface. The adhesive is more hydrophobic and makes a durable bond to enamel. These systems have worked well for years. A number of clinical studies have demonstrated their success.

The primer easily penetrates the dentin and quickly evaporates from the enamel. Drying the primer on the dentin surface is a critical step but is easy to do. Dried primer leaves an easily recognizable resin-rich surface. The adhesive is an unfilled resin with few solvents. Once cured, it provides good cohesive strength to retain the restorative material to the tooth.

One-component bonding systems

One-component systems, often called one-step bonding agents, combine primer and adhesive. In this case, a single solution is placed in two, three, or more layers that are dried after placement. Acetone is the common solvent in these materials because it evaporates quickly and removes moisture. One-component systems should be used on dentin that has been treated with a damp cotton pellet, since water is required for the materials to penetrate the dentin. Special bottles are required to hold these acetone-based solutions, since acetone can diffuse through most plastics.

When solvent evaporates from the solution, the remaining resin thickens. This affects bonding; the bond to dentin drops dramatically and the bond to enamel is also less effective. Preventing solvent evaporation is critical to the shelf life of single-component dentin bonding agents and to their clinical usefulness. Figure 8–23 shows the impact of solvent evaporation of a single-component dentin bonding agent: the loss of solvent changes the agent from a primer to an adhesive.

Ease of use

Although single-solution materials are considered easier to use, they give less consistent results compared with the relatively more forgiving two-component materials. The main benefit of a one-component system is that it is not possible to accidentally mistake the bottle of primer for that of adhesive, and vice versa. This may or may not be a problem in any given office.

Only a two-component system allows a clinician to apply adhesive alone, as is required when a

Resin Bonding

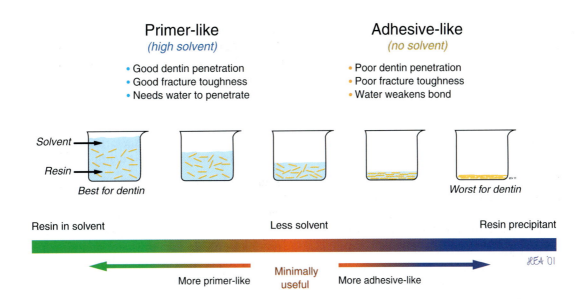

Figure 8–23. The primer-to-adhesive transition in a single-component dentin bonding agent is attributable to the evaporation of solvent.

preparation is entirely in enamel. Using just the adhesive component on an all-enamel preparation results in a consistent bond.

Dental assistants often dispense materials before use so they will be ready when the dentist needs them. This practice poses a problem with adhesives because evaporation of the solvent alters the material. With single-component bonding systems, the evaporation is so rapid the material should not be left out for even a short time. Instead, the solution should be dispensed into a clean well just before restoration placement. If a few minutes go by, the material should not be used, even if protected from ambient light. If a single-component material is dispensed and applied properly, the solvent evaporates on the tooth as it penetrates the dentin.

DENTIN BONDING FAILURE

There are a number of reasons for poor dentin–resin bonding:

- Dentin is an extremely variable substrate and changes over time.
- Dentin has varying degrees of calcification (eg, is more or less sclerotic) and changes depending on the depth and angle of the preparation.
- Structural changes in dentin closer to the pulp make it more difficult to bond in that area.
- It is difficult to avoid contaminating the dentin near the sulcus with gingival fluids.
- Polymerization contraction forces can exceed early bond strengths and result in marginal gaps and leakage.
- Dentin bonding agents can thicken, because of solvent evaporation, reducing penetration and bond strength.

Causes of Poor Bond Strength

Contamination by handpiece oil, saliva, intersulcular fluid, and hemorrhaging also result in poor bond strength.

Handpiece oil

Following lubrication, handpieces can emit significant amounts of oil for up to 30 minutes. These oils should be removed prior to bonding. Acid etching solutions do not remove oils. Alcohol, ethanol-containing mouthwash, or other organic solvent should be used to wipe down a preparation prior to bonding. An air- or water-abrasion device is another option, although generally less convenient.

Saliva contamination
The negative effects of saliva contamination are the same on resin–dentin bond strength as on resin–enamel bond strength.[71,72] The fact that dentin contamination is not as easily detected may help explain the disparity between good dentin bonding results in the laboratory and poor results or even failure clinically with the same product.

Intersulcular fluid
Intersulcular fluid contact with the bonded surfaces causes catastrophic failure. Re-etching for 15 seconds, rinsing, drying, and rebonding will recover the bond strength with most materials.

Hemorrhaging
Blood contact with the bonded surfaces causes catastrophic failure. Bleeding should be stopped with a retraction cord or an astringent (eg, ferric sulfate). The area must be cleaned to remove all signs of the bleeding. Then the procedure is to re-etch for 15 seconds, rinse, dry, and repeat the last bonding step.

STORAGE OF BONDING MATERIALS

Most dentin–resin bonding primers have a limited shelf life. They must be stored properly to maintain maximum effectiveness.

Factors to consider in storing bonding materials

Evaporation
Almost all dentin–resin bonding agents have volatile components. Containers must be capped tightly to avoid evaporation. Materials should be dispensed immediately before use and bottles resealed as soon as possible after dispensing. Unidose dispensing is highly recommended to avoid the problems caused by evaporation.

Cross-contamination
Separate brushes should always be used for primers and bonding agents. Cross-contamination can severely limit the effectiveness of these materials.

Temperature
Autocured dentin bonding primers and adhesives should be stored under refrigeration and allowed to come to room temperature just prior to use. Storage at room temperature results in a shorter shelf life for autocured systems. These materials should not be heated above normal room temperature (70°F) for extended periods.

Shelf life
When kept at room temperature, most aqueous primers have a shelf life of about 12 months (from the date of manufacture) if they are acidic solutions of HEMA (eg, self-etching primers), and about 24 months if they are neutral solutions. Alcohol- and acetone-based primers have a shelf life of 12 to 18 months at room temperature. Refrigeration extends the shelf life of most dentin bonding agents.

Labeling bottles
Two numbers are included on the label of each bonding product: a batch number and a date of manufacture. Some manufacturers place these numbers only on the boxes, not on individual bottles. In many dental offices, bottles are removed from their boxes; it is important to transfer the date of manufacture onto each bottle by attaching a piece of tape or a tag. Individual labeling is also useful in the case of a bad product batch. Noting a discard date in red simplifies determining the usability of a product.

Marking calendar for reorders
Marking the discard date on bottles provides advance notice of when new supplies will be needed. It is difficult to remember to check every product every week. An easier approach is to mark the calendar 2 to 3 weeks prior to the expiration of each product and make a replacement order on that date.

TYPES OF RESIN–RESIN BONDING

There are two types of resin–resin bonding: one type is done within 24 hours of existing resin placement, and another type is done at a later date, to repair or to modify an existing restoration. These bonds differ in bond chemistry and in the technique of placement.

In this text, the term "immediate resin–resin bonding" refers to bonding that occurs within 24 hours of original resin placement. During this period, the dark reaction of the polymerization cycle is in progress. With immediate resin–resin bonding, free, unreacted double bonds in both resins allow for copolymerization and its resulting cross-linkages between materials. Thus, immediate resin–resin bonding is chemical in nature.

The term "delayed resin–resin bonding" refers to bonding that occurs long after the original placement. In delayed resin–resin bonding there are few, if any, reactive double bonds in the old composite for bonding to the new composite. Thus, delayed resin–resin bonding depends less on chemical bonding and more on mechanical forms of attachment.

Immediate resin–resin bonding

Immediate resin–resin bonding occurs every time an uncured composite is immediately added to a composite that has just been cured. In this type of bonding, the clinician should not disturb the shiny layer on the surface of the previously cured composite. This layer is the unreacted resin resulting from the presence of oxygen on the surface. This unreacted resin is often referred to as the air-inhibited layer. This unreacted layer provides more free double bonds for attachment to the next addition of composite. This air-inhibited layer is most noticeable after the polymerization of bonding agents.

Speed produces a better chemical bond in immediate resin–resin bonding. Once a layer of composite is cured, the next layer should be added as quickly as possible. The ideal time between additions is less than 5 minutes. If more than 10 minutes pass, a thin layer of unfilled resin bonding agent should be added between the two layers of composite (Figures 8–24 and 8–25).[73] The potential for chemical bonding between composite layers continues to decrease over time.

Layering light-cured composites helps control polymerization shrinkage, improve light penetration, and create an effect that resembles the natural dentin and enamel of teeth. Composite layers should be added in thicknesses of no more than 1 to 2 mm. If contamination of the resin bonding surface cannot be avoided, use the delayed resin–resin bonding procedure and add more composite.

Ideally, the added composite has the same resin matrix as the underlying material; the filler loadings may differ. In fact, adding a microfill to small-particle material is highly recommended. The microfill and small-particle composite bond best if the microfill is added soon after the small-particle material is cured. Alternatively, the two materials can be placed together and cured at the same time. The disadvantage to this approach is that the combined layer may be too thick to completely polymerize. Curing resins in thin layers is the most desirable method.

Immediate resin–resin bonding between different products

Immediate bonding often occurs between different layers, such as bonding agents, heavy filled composites, microfilled composites, color modifiers, and surface glazes.

Generally, the strongest bonds are achieved between like materials or between materials from the same manufacturer (ie, they have the same resin). Bonds between differing resins are the weakest. The urethane resins (eg, Kulzer and Vivadent products) and the tricyclic resins (eg, ESPE products) form a weaker bond to the Bis-GMA resins. The bond strength between different resins can be greatly increased, and reach near normal limits, if a bonding agent is applied between each layer.[74]

Delayed resin–resin bonding

When a restoration has worn for a while, it may have an undesirable surface yet be sound under-

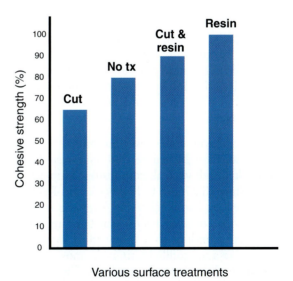

Figure 8–24. Impact of surface treatment on immediate resin–resin bond strength after 10 minutes. Cut = some of the surface was removed; resin = unfilled bonding resin was applied; tx = treatment. (Modified from Boyer DB, Chan KC, Reinhardt JW. Build-up and repair of light-cured composites: bond strength. J Dent Res 1984;63:1241–4.)

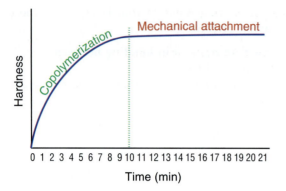

Figure 8–25. Graphic illustration of the period for transition from polymerization to mechanical attachment in immediate resin–resin bonding. The process of polymerization leaves fewer and fewer double bonds available for chemical attachment to a new composite layer. Ten minutes after curing, the conversion of free double bonds is so low that a bonding agent is required to attach a new layer.

neath. This contrast is particularly true for conventional large-particle composites, which generally undergo rapid surface deterioration. With the use of radiographs and transillumination, a clinician can determine if the remaining portion of a composite restoration is sound. When dealing with preexisting composites, many clinicians prefer to replace the entire restoration, regardless of how the restoration appears under the surface. Other clinicians may opt to veneer the existing composite via delayed resin–resin bonding. Delayed resin–resin bond strengths tend to weaken over time.[75]

Uses for delayed resin–resin bonding

It was once thought that delayed resin–resin bonding worked well with all composites. More recent studies show that it can be highly specific. Research conducted by Lambrechts and Vanherle in 1982 suggests that delayed resin–resin bonding works best when bonding to a heavy filled material.[76] Bonding to a microfilled resin is the most difficult procedure. This research concluded that delayed resin–resin bonding is a mechanical retention phenomenon in which a bonding agent interlocks with the surface irregularities of the underlying, previously cured composite. Other studies confirmed that the best results are achieved in delayed resin–resin bonding by adding to macrofilled composites. These composites have more bond strength than microfilled composites.[77]

Regardless of which types of composites are involved, for maximum bond strength, the old composite should be trimmed with a coarse disc (or diamond), etched, dried, and covered with a thin layer of unfilled resin bonding agent prior to the addition of a new composite. Many clinicians have experienced poor long-term results by bonding new resin to a smooth, previously set resin. Better clinical success is achieved by bonding new resin to a roughened surface that provides additional mechanical retention.

Bond strength values for delayed resin–resin bonding procedures are illustrated in Figure 8–26. These studies show that, at best, delayed resin–resin bonding can achieve only 50% (for microfill repairs) to 70% (for macrofilled repairs) of the original cohesive strength. Other studies show that under the best circumstances, on average, delayed resin–resin bonding provides only 36% of cohesive strength to an untreated sur-

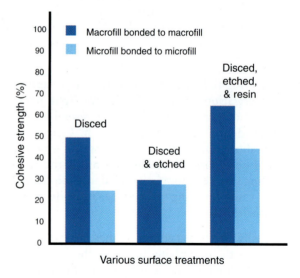

Figure 8–26. Effects of discing, etching, and adding unfilled bonding agents to macrofilled and microfilled composite surfaces in delayed resin–resin bonding. Note that the macrofill bond strengths are higher. (From Miranda F, Duncanson M, Dilts W. Interfacial bonding strengths of paired composite systems. J Prosthet Dent 1984;51:29–32.)

face.[73,78–81] This can be improved by 22%, to yield 40 to 50% cohesive strength, if an unfilled resin is used.[73,77,82,83] Some studies show even greater bond strengths if a phosphonated bonding agent is used as an intermediate layer.[84–86] This increased strength may be related to improved wetting of the resin surface. A number of resin primers are available to improve wetting (eg, Composite Repair, All Dental Prodx Prebond Primer, Bisco).

In addition to the reduced bond strengths seen with resin–resin bonding, a more serious problem is microleakage. Over time, fluids can creep between the two hydrophobic layers and cause staining. Improvements in microleakage and bond strength can be achieved if the new composite is attached on all sides to the tooth structure.

The advantages of delayed resin–resin bonding are conservation of tooth structure and elimination of a base application, since the composite acts as a liner. However, it can be difficult to distinguish resin from tooth structure when removing the outer surface of an old composite restoration. A disadvantage of delayed resin–resin bonding is that a discolored restoration cannot easily be corrected with a thin resin veneer. A clinician also must remember that placing a new radiopaque composite over an old radiolucent composite may give the appearance of recurrent caries on a radiograph. In addition, the resin–resin bond strength is less than that of a newly placed composite.

Sandblasting to increase surface area

Sandblasting greatly improves resin–resin bonding since it provides micromechanical roughening and a clean surface. Air abrasion units are well suited to this purpose. The application of a silane to the exposed glass fillers of the composite resin also increases bonding. Specialized sandblasting beads (eg, Co-Jet, ESPE) greatly increase bond strength. The beads place a thin glass layer on the resin surface; the glass layer can then be silanated and bonded to composite to yield bond strength comparable to that found when using silane on porcelain.

Caution is advised in selecting cases for delayed resin–resin bonding. The procedure is probably best suited for larger preparations, such as Class IV fractures, in which entire resin replacement could endanger the small amount of tooth structure remaining.

Etching composites to remove fillers

The solubility of glass macrofillers has been used to improve the bond strength of a resin luting agent on a pre-cured resin surface. Strong etching solutions (eg, hydrofluoric acid) have been used as a conditioner to remove soluble macrofillers from the surfaces of pre-cured indirect resin veneers. The spaces left by the glass filler particles allow formation of resin tags, creating a micromechanical bond to the composite luting agent. This bonding results in greatly improved strength for these indirect resin veneers (Figure 8–27).

This method of attachment is only effective with resin restorations in which the internal layer contains a macrofilled composite with a soluble glass filler. In addition, the etching solution used must be matched to the filler to dissolve it away effectively. This method of attachment is not advised for restorations made entirely on microfilled composite.

Delayed resin–resin bonding has become important in dentistry because of the need to bond resin indirect composites (eg, veneers, inlays, and crowns) to teeth. Unfortunately, present bond values to cured resin surfaces are low compared with other types of resin bonding. Stronger bonding would improve the viability of indirect restorations and improve the repairability of all existing resin restorations. Newer techniques and materials are being introduced to deal with these problems; however, compared with enamel bonding, delayed resin–resin bonding is the weak link in laboratory-fabricated resin restorations.

Procedure for delayed resin–resin bonding

Step 1. Remove the outer layer of resin with a coarse diamond, leaving a rough surface. If possible, extend the preparation to the natural margins of the tooth.

Step 2. Etch the resin surface for 15 seconds with phosphoric acid to dissolve any organic debris. If enamel is to be bonded in the same preparation, the enamel should be etched in the usual fashion. With glass-filled composites, sandblasting or etch-

152 Tooth-Colored Restoratives

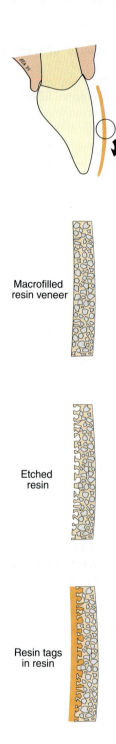

Figure 8–27. Cross-sectional view of the micromechanical bond that can exist between an etched macrofilled resin restoration and a composite luting agent. *From top to bottom:* original pre-cured macrofilled veneer, etched veneer surface (note the loss of filler particles on the surface), and a free-flowing resin bonding agent forming micromechanical tags in the spaces once occupied by filler particles.

ing with hydrofluoric acid for 5 seconds, followed by silane, may improve bonding.

Step 3. Rinse with water for 10 to 15 seconds to clean.

Step 4. Dry with an electric dryer, vacuum, or air syringe.

Step 5. Add a thin layer of silane, then dry and add a thin layer of bonding agent. Cure.

Step 6. Place and shape the composite resin. Cure and finish in the usual manner.

BONDING INDIRECT RESIN RESTORATIONS

In recent years, indirect resin restorations, such as veneers, inlays, and crowns, have become popular. Laboratory fabrication can save valuable chairtime for the clinician interested in using indirect systems. One of the major shortcomings of these systems is that they can only be bonded into place through delayed resin–resin bonding procedures. This results in bond strengths far weaker than those seen with direct restorations. In addition, these bond strengths drop over time.

A number of methods are used to place indirect resin restorations. The most popular is to roughen the lingual or internal surface of the restoration with a diamond, thereby creating mechanical grooves to which the resin can attach. This procedure is followed by the usual delayed resin–resin bonding technique. Other methods use the same procedure but add a primer to the surface prior to adding a bonding agent. An alternative treatment includes sandblasting with sand or specialized particles to expose glass filler and produce a more reactive surface.

Composite resin bonding primers

Primers are usually organic solvents that reduce the surface tension of a cured resin surface; this makes it easier for the bonding agent to penetrate surface porosities. In addition, primers are thought to cause the resin matrix to swell and to open spaces among the polymer strands. The bonding agent may penetrate some of these spaces. One drawback to the use of primers is that, since they dilute the luting agent and make it more porous, they may affect the color stability of the restoration.

Perhaps the most viable treatment for indirect veneers is the use of a micro-etched intermediate resin or glass-ionomer layer between the indirect resin restoration and the composite luting agent. These methods of attachment give the highest and most consistent delayed resin–resin bond. The mechanism of attachment involves micromechanical resin tags similar to those of enamel–resin, metal–resin, and porcelain–resin bonding.

REFERENCES

1. Boyde A. Enamel. In: Oksche A, Vollrath L, eds. Handbook of microscopic anatomy. Vol. 6. Berlin: Springer-Verlag, 1989:309–473.

2. Watson TF. Tandem-scanning microscopy of slow-speed enamel cutting interactions. J Dent Res 1991;70:44–9.

3. Buonocore MG. A simple method of increasing the adhesion of acrylic filling materials to enamel surfaces. J Dent Res 1955;34:849–53.

4. Zidan O, Hill G. Phosphoric acid concentration: enamel surface loss and bonding strength. J Prosthet Dent 1986;55:388–92.

5. Silverstone L. The current status of fissure sealants and priorities for future research. Part II. Compend Cont Educ Dent 1984;5:229–306.

6. Barkmeier WW, Shaffer SE, Gwinnett AJ. Effects of 15- vs. 60-second enamel acid conditioning on adhesion and morphology. Oper Dent 1986;11:111–6.

7. Schaffer SE, Barkmeier WW, Kelsey WP. Effects of reduced acid conditioning time on enamel microleakage. Gen Dent 1987;35:278–80.

8. Redford DA, Clarkson BH, Jensen M. The effect of different times on the sealant bond strength, etch depth, and pattern in primary teeth. Pediatr Dent 1986;8:11–5.

9. Simonsen RJ. Fissure sealants in primary molars. Retention of colored sealants with variable etch times at 12 months. J Dent Child 1979;46:382–4.

10. Simonsen RJ. Fissure sealant: deciduous molar retention of colored sealant with variable etch times. Quintessence Int 1978;9:71–7.

11. Conniff JN, Hamby GR. Preparation of primary tooth enamel for acid conditioning. J Dent Child 1976;43:177–9.

12. Silverstone LM. Fissure sealants. Dent Update 1977;4:73–83.

13. Redford DA, Clarkson BH, Jensen M. The effect of different etching times on the sealant bond strength, etch depth, and pattern in primary teeth. Pediatr Dent 1986;8:11–5.

14. Baharav H, Cardash HS, Helft M, Langsam J. The continuous brushing acid-etch technique. J Prosthet Dent 1987;57:147–9.

15. Mixson JM, Eick JD, Tira DE, Moore DL. The effect of variable wash terms and techniques on enamel-composite resin bond strength. Quintessence Int 1988;19:279–85.

16. Batchelder KF, Richter RS, Vaidyanathan TK. Clinical factors affecting the strength of composite resin to enamel bonds. J Am Dent Assoc 1987;114:203–5.

17. Asmussen E. Bonding of resins to etched enamel: Acid gel or liquid etch? Tandlaegebladet 1981;85:539–41.

18. Cooley R, Barkmeier W. Staining of composite and microfilled resin with stannous fluoride. J Prosthet Dent 1983;49:346–8.

19. Kula K, Nelson S, Kula T, Thompson V. In vitro effect of acidulated phosphate fluoride gel on the surface of composites with different filler particles. J Prosthet Dent 1986;56:161–9.

20. Schneider P, Messer L, Douglas W. The effect of enamel surface reduction in vitro on the bonding of composite to permanent human enamel. J Dent Res 1981;60:895–900.

21. Ripa L, Gwinnett A, Buonocore M. The "prismless" outer layer of deciduous and permanent enamel. Arch Oral Biol 1966;11:41–8.

22. Speiser A, Kahn M. The etched butt-joint margin. J Dent Child 1977;44:42–50.

23. Crim G, Swartz ML, Phillips R. An evaluation of cavosurface design and microleakage. Gen Dent 1984;32:56–8.

24. Porte A, Lutz F, Lund M, et al. Cavity designs for composite resins. Oper Dent 1984;9:50–6.

25. Aker DA, Aker JR, Sorensen SE. Effect of methods of tooth enamel preparation on the retentive strength of acid-etched composite resins. J Am Dent Assoc 1979;99:185–9.

26. Barkmeier W, Blankenau R, Peterson D. Enamel cavosurface bevels finished with ultraspeed instruments. J Prosthet Dent 1983;49:481–4.

27. Aksu MN, Powers JM, Lorey RE, Kolling JN. Variables affecting bond strength of resin-bonded bridge cements. Dent Mater 1987;3:26–8.

28. Jorgensen KD, Shimokobe H. Adaptation of resinous restorative materials to acid etched enamel surfaces. Scand J Dent Res 1975;83:31–6.

29. Asmussen E. Penetration of restorative resins into acid etched enamel. I. Viscosity, surface tension, and contact angle of restorative resin monomers. Acta Odont Scand 1977;35:175–82.

30. Asmussen E. Penetration of restorative resins into acid etched enamel. II. Dissolution of entrapped air in restorative resin monomers. Acta Odont Scand 1977;35:183–9.

31. Zidan O, Asmussen E, Jorgensen KD. Microscopical analysis of fractured restorative resin–etched enamel bonds. Scand J Dent Res 1982;90:286–91.

32. Smith RA, Bellezza JJ, Capilouto ML, et al. A clinical study of the composite/bonding resin–tooth interface. Dent Mater 1987;3:218–23.

33. Staninec M, Mochizuki A, Tanizaki K, et al. Effects of etching and bonding on recurrent caries in teeth restored with composite resin. J Prosthet Dent 1985;53:521–5.

34. Hansen EK, Hansen BK, Nielsen F, et al. Clinical short-term study of marginal integrity of resin restorations. Scand J Dent Res 1984;92:374–9.

35. Thoms LM, Nicholls JL, Brudvik JS, Kydd WL. The effect of dentin primer on the tensile bond strength to human enamel. Int J Prosthodont 1994;7:403–9.

36. Barkmeier WW, Gwinnett AJ, Shafter SE. Effects of reduced acid concentration and etching time on bond strength and enamel morphology. J Clin Orthod 1987;21:395–8.

37. Tao L, Pashley DH. Shear bond strengths to dentin: effects of surface treatments, depth and position. Dent Mater 1988;4:371–8.

38. Bradford EW. The dentine, a barrier to caries. Br Dent J 1960;109:387–91.

39. Pashley EL, Tao L, Matthews WG, Pashley DH. Bond strengths to superficial, intermediate and deep dentin in vivo with four dentin bonding systems. Dent Mater 1993;9:19–22.

40. Marshall GW Jr. Dentin: microstructure and characterization. Quintessence Int 1993;24:606–17.

41. Jones SJ. The pulp–dentine complex. In: Elderton RJ, ed. The dentition and dental care. Oxford: Heinemann Professional Publishing Ltd., 1990.

42. Retief DH, Mandras RS, Russell CM. Shear bond strength required to prevent microleakage at the dentin–restoration interface. Am J Dent 1994;7:43–6.

43. Mjor I. Reaction patterns of dentin. In: Thylstrup A, Leach SA, Qvjst V, eds. Dentin and dentin reactions in the oral cavity. Oxford: IRL Press, 1987:27.

44. Pashley DH. Dentin: a dynamic substrate: a review. Scanning Microsc 1989;3:161–72.

45. Pashley DH. Interactions of dental materials with dentin. Trans Acad Dent Materials 1990;3:55–73.

46. Tronstad L. Scanning electron microscopy of attrited dentinal surfaces and subadjacent dentin in human teeth. Scand J Dent Res 1973;81:112–22.

47. Kurosaki N, Kubota M, Yamamoto Y, Fusayama T. The effect of etching on the dentin of the clinical cavity floor. Quintessence Int 1990;21:87–92.

48. Lefkowitz W. The "vitality" of the calcified dental tissues. J Dent Res 1947;21:423–31.

49. Retief DH, Denys FR. Adhesion to enamel and dentin. Am J Dent 1989;2:133–44.

50. Rueggeberg FA, Margeson DH. The effect of oxygen inhibition on an unfilled/filled composite system. J Dent Res 1990;69:1652–8.

51. Cox CF. Biocompatibility of dental materials in the absence of bacterial infection. Oper Dent 1987;12:147–52.

52. Dreyfuss F, Frank RM, Gutmann B. La sclerose dentinaire. GIRS 1964;7:207–12.

53. Browne RM, Tobias RS. Microbial microleakage and pulpal inflammation: a review. Endod Dent Traumatol 1986;2:177–83.

54. Hanks CT, Craig RG, Diehl ML, Pashley DH. Cytotoxicity of dental composites and other materials in a new in vitro device. J Oral Pathol 1988;17:396–403.

55. Hanks CT, Diehl MC, Craig RG, et al. Characterization of the "in vitro pulp chamber" using the cytotoxicity of phenol. J Oral Pathol 1989;18:97–107.

56. Duke ES, Lindemuth JS. Variability of clinical dentin substrates. Am J Dent 1991;4:241–6.

57. Erickson RL. Mechanism and clinical implications of bond formation for two dentin bonding agents. Am J Dent 1989;2:117–23.

58. Wang T, Nakabayashi N. Effect of 2-(methacryloxy)ethyl phenyl hydrogen phosphate on adhesion to dentin. J Dent Res 1991;70:59–66.

59. Isokawa S, Kubota K, Kuwajima K. Scanning electron microscope study of dentin exposed by contact facets and cervical abrasions. J Dent Res 1973;52:170–81.

60. Nalbandian J, Gonzales I, Sognaes RF. Sclerotic age changes in root dentin of human teeth observed by optical, electron, and x-ray microscopy. J Dent Res 1960;39:588–607.

61. Derise NL, Ritchey SJ, Furr AK. Mineral composition of normal enamel and dentin and the relation of composition to dental caries: I. Macrominerals and comparison of methods of analyses. J Dent Res 1974;53:847–59.

62. Swift EJ, Perdigao J, Heymann HO. Bonding to enamel and dentin: a brief history and state of the art, 1995. Quintessence Int 1995;26:95–110.

63. Nakabayashi N, Kojima K, Masuhara E. The promotion of adhesion by the infiltration of monomers into tooth substrates. J Biomed Mater Res 1982;16:265–73.

64. Gwinnett AJ. Quantitative contribution of resin infiltration/hybridization to dentin bonding. Am J Dent 1993;6:7–9.

65. Erickson RL. Surface interactions of dentin adhesive materials. Oper Dent 1992;5(Suppl):81–94.

66. Kanca J. Resin bonding to wet substrate. I. Bonding to dentin. Quintessence Int 1992;23:39–41.

67. Elhabashy A, Swift EJ. Bonding to etched, physiologically hydrated dentin. Am J Dent 1994;7:50–2.

68. Vargas MA, Swift EJ. Microleakage of resin composites with wet versus dry bonding. Am J Dent 1994;7:187–9.

69. Perdigao J, Swift EJ, Cloe BC. Effects of etchants, surface moisture, and resin composite on dentin bond strengths. Am J Dent 1993;6:61–4.

70. Titley K, Chernecky R, Maric B, Smith D. Penetration of a dentin bonding agent into dentin. Am J Dent 1994;7:190–4.

71. Pashley EL, Tao L, Mackert JR, Pashley DH. Comparison of in vivo versus in vitro bonding of composite resin to the dentin of canine teeth. J Dent Res 1988;67:467–70.

72. Hansen EK, Munksgaard EC. Saliva contamination versus efficacy of dentin bonding agents. Dent Mater 1989;5:329–33.

73. Boyer DB, Chan KC, Reinhardt JW. Build-up and repair of light-cured composites: bond strength. J Dent Res 1984;63:1241–4.

74. Gordon AA, von der Lehr WN, Herrin HK. Bond strength of composite to composite and bond strength of composite to glass ionomer lining cements. Gen Dent 1986;34:290–3.

75. Walls AWG, McCabe JF, Murray JJ. The bond strength of composite laminate veneers. J Dent Res 1985;64:1261–4.

76. Lambrechts P, Vanherle G. The use of glazing materials for finishing dental composite resin surfaces. J Oral Rehabil 1982;9:107–17.

77. Miranda F, Duncanson M, Dilts W. Interfacial bonding strengths of paired composite systems. J Prosthet Dent 1984;51:29–32.

78. Forsten L, Valiaho ML. Transverse and bond strength of restorative resins. Acta Odont Scand 1971;29:527–37.

79. Reisbick MH, Brodsky JF. Strength parameters of composite resins. J Prosthet Dent 1971;26:178–85.

80. Loyd CH, Baigrie DA, Jeffery IW. The tensile strength of composite repairs. J Dent Res 1980;8:171–7.

81. Vankerckhoven H, Lambrechts P, van Beylen M, et al. Unreacted methacrylate groups on the surfaces of composite resins. J Dent Res 1982;61:791–5.

82. Boyer DB, Chan KC, Torney DL. The strength of multilayer and repaired composite resin. J Prosthet Dent 1978;39:63–8.

83. Soderholm KJ. Flexure strength of repaired dental composites [abstract]. J Dent Res 1985;64(Spec Issue):178.

84. Azarbal P, Boyer DB, Chan KC. The effect of bonding agents on the interfacial bond strength of repaired composites. Dent Mater 1986;2:153–5.

85. Chalkley Y, Jensen ME. Enamel shear bond strengths of a dentinal bonding agent [abstract]. J Dent Res 1984;63(Spec Issue):320.

86. Chan DCN, Reinhardt JW, Jensen ME. Shear bond strength of a new dentinal adhesive [abstract]. J Dent Res 1984;63(Spec Issue):320.

Chapter 9

Placement and Finishing

Perfection is not attainable, but if we chase it we can reach excellence.
Vince Lombardi

This chapter discusses the proper placement and finishing of direct composite restorative systems.

PLACEMENT

Placement is the application of a direct restorative to a prepared tooth. The selection of a shade and restorative material; tooth isolation, preparation, and etching; and restorative bonding are integral to the placement process.

Shade selection

Composite shade is selected by working with a clean, moist tooth prior to placement of a rubber dam. Once teeth are isolated by a rubber dam they dry out and get lighter in color, making accurate shade selection difficult. Since the shade guides provided by many manufacturers are not made of composite, they may not accurately represent a composite shade. Studies show custom guides made of composite are considerably more accurate than a manufacturer's mock-composite shade guide.[1] Even better accuracy is achieved if the custom shade tabs are stored in water, but problems with controlling bacterial growth make this impractical. Storing in water hydrates the tabs, maintaining conditions similar to those of the mouth. Hydrated composite shade tabs are darker than dry ones.

Once a shade is chosen for a discolored tooth, verify the masking ability of the composite by placing material on the tooth in the same thickness as will be used in the restoration and then curing. Placing a color modifier on the tooth under the composite can improve its color or masking ability. With autocured systems, if the shade of the tooth does not match one of the shade guides, different shades can be mixed to obtain a more accurate match. With light-cured systems, composites can be layered, placing darker materials underneath and lighter materials over the surface to provide intermediate shades.

Using a master shade guide system

All restoratives and chairside shade guides should be matched to a master shade guide. All materials should be tested to match this master, and restoratives should be relabeled when discrepancies occur.

Before using a new restorative product, polymermize the material and place the sample in water for 24 hours. After the sample has rested for 24 hours, match its color to the office master shade guide. Materials are often a shade or more off of the master guide. For example, shade A3 of a particular product may match the A2 master shade guide, so it should be relabeled A2. Standardizing all office restorative materials to a single shade stabilizes restoration esthetics, such that once a patient's shade is determined, all calibrated restoratives will match.

A number of shade guide systems are commercially available. By far the most common is the Vita Lumin system (Vita Zähnfabrik, Bad Sackingen, Germany), which breaks shades first into hues and then shows hues with increased chroma and decreased value. Vita's newer Vitapan system breaks shades into value (darkness), hue, and chroma (color). Value is the most important characteristic of a shade since it is not light dependent. Hence, the new Vita system differentiates shades according to their most important characteristics.

The most common shade used in indirect restorations is A2. It is so popular a shade that using it for full-mouth reconstruction pleases most patients. With older patients, this shade may appear light but is still preferred by most patients.

Polymerization lightening

Light-cured composites generally lighten in color as they cure. This is because they contain camphoroquinone initiators, the most common photoinitiators in dental resins. These yellow-brown compounds lighten during polymerization. The camphoroquinone is consumed in the setting reaction and becomes part of the polymer. The colored diketone ring changes from dark yellow to clear when it reacts with light and a tertiary amine to form a free radical (Figure 9–1). Thus, a composite cured for 15 seconds may have a darker shade than one cured for 60 seconds (Figure 9–2). Some manufacturers believe that most of the quinone in composites should react within a 60-second curing cycle. Therefore, composite cured for this length of time should not undergo much additional quinone change. Since teeth can lighten from dehydration and it takes over 24 hours for a complete composite cure, the final shade cannot be accurately determined until a subsequent appointment. The polymerization lightening effect makes it important, when making composite shade tabs or checking composite shades on a tooth, to cure the samples for at least 60 seconds. Note that some macrofilled composites are white prior to curing, owing to air refraction between the filler and resin. After curing, these composites darken and then slowly become lighter during post-polymerization curing (the dark reaction).

Brands of composite differ in their camphoroquinone content and chemistry. The mechanisms that cause the light-cured composites to change in both value and chroma after polymerization are not yet completely understood. Lighter shades of composite show more pronounced polymerization

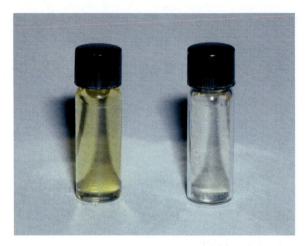

Figure 9–2. These vials show the color of a composite resin before (*left*) and after (*right*) polymerization. Note the shift from yellow to clear that results from polymerization; this color shift resolves roughly 24 hours after curing and greatly affects a restoration's final shade.

changes than darker shades. This may be because the many other pigments in darker shades mask the effect.

Color shifts can be a serious problem to practitioners. Figure 9–3 shows a composite restoration that was a perfect shade match at placement and then 2 weeks postoperatively, appeared too light. Postoperative lightening has several possible causes:

- The inherent color shift of light-cured composites owing to photoinitiation.

- Under-polymerization of the composite, often the result of inadequate energy output by the curing light. The average halogen bulb maintains the intensity necessary for curing for only 100 hours. Lights should be checked routinely to ensure adequate energy output. Under-polymerized composite absorbs water, loses pigment, and lightens. Later, it is more susceptible to staining and darkening.

- Shade selection after tooth isolation. Any isolation system, particularly a rubber dam, will desiccate a tooth. Some teeth lighten within minutes of isolation, such that matching them results in selection of a too light restorative, noticeable only after the tooth returns to its normal shade.

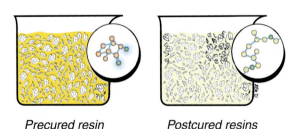

Figure 9–1. The breakdown of camphoroquione results in post-polymerization lightening of composite.

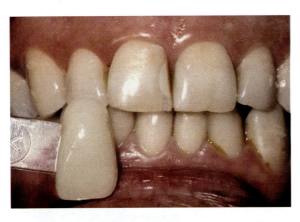

Figure 9–3. A too-light shade of composite in two Class III restorations (mesial central incisors). The shade tab shown was provided by the manufacturer to represent the composite shade.

Mixing composite resins

Composite materials should be mixed according to the manufacturer's recommendations. For an autocured system, this usually means the pastes must be mixed thoroughly into a homogeneous mass within about 30 seconds. Excessive entrapment of air should be avoided when mixing autoset and dual-cured composites by folding the material onto itself rather than beating it. The material should be mixed so that it forms a thin coating over a large area and bubbles have only a short distance to travel to the surface. If a void caused by air entrapment shows at a margin, the restoration must be repaired or redone. Light-activated materials should not be mixed because the entrapped air weakens the resin in two ways: it makes the structure less dense and it prevents setting of the resin around the air voids, since air inhibits polymerization. Voids also affect esthetics.[2]

Heavily filled autocured composites with large particles (>10 μm) should be mixed using plastic or wooden spatulas. The filler in these composites is highly abrasive to metal instruments. Metal particles abraded from the instruments can become incorporated into the resin mix and discolor the material. Plastic or metal instruments are options when mixing microfilled composites. When dispensing two-paste systems, opposite ends of the spatula should be used for each paste to prevent contamination.

Pads supplied by the manufacturer should be used for mixing composite. Pads that shed fibers that are then incorporated into the restoration are to be avoided. Many manufacturers provide plastic pads. These are especially useful for quartz-filled materials.

With light-cured systems, if a less viscous filling material is necessary, a small amount of unfilled resin can be mixed with the filled material. The resulting combination has the same potential for polishing but less durability.

Use of a composite syringe

Use of a composite syringe can reduce voids during placement. A number of studies with cylindrical preparations (C-factor of 4 or 5) have shown that composites placed with a syringe have 50 to 95% fewer voids than composites placed by hand.[2–4]

Light-cured composites can be stored in opaque syringe tips for extended periods. Many manufacturers sell composite prepackaged in syringe tips (also known as unidose systems) and label each syringe with the name, shade, and expiration date of the material. Colored syringe caps for color-coding of filled or partly filled syringe tips are also available (e.g., C.R. Black Tubes and Colored Caps, Centrix, Shelton, Connecticut). Where access is poor or a heavy-bodied material is to be used, placement with a power syringe may be considered (e.g., Omnisyringe, Centrix). These syringes have a longer reach and dispense heavy-bodied materials with much less effort. With any composite syringe system, placing a drop of bonding agent in the empty tube and blowing the excess out of the tip with an air syringe greatly reduces the amount of force required. This technique is helpful with packable materials.

Matrixing

Many composite restorations are hand sculpted and do not use a matrix or crown form for contouring. Matrices are, however, used during placement. The most common matrix is clear Mylar (Figure 9–4).

Dead-soft plastic

Sandwich bag plastic, freezer wrap, and other forms of soft plastic are ideal for protecting adjacent restored teeth from restoratives placed during the same appointment.

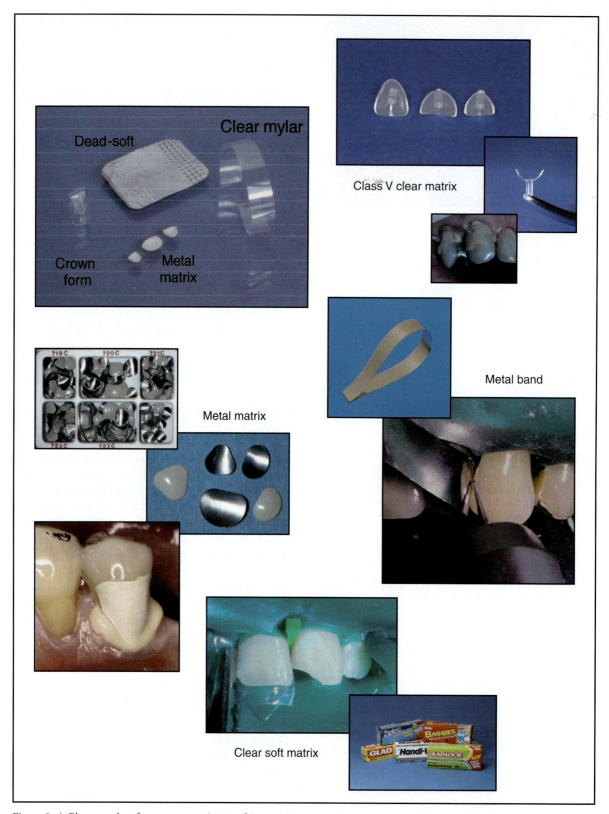

Figure 9–4. Photographs of common matrices used in anterior restorations.

Dead-soft metal matrix

A dead-soft metal matrix is a matrix that retains a new shape. In contrast, most metal matrices have "memory" and return to their original shape. There is a large gradient between dead-soft metal and matrices with memory. Dead-soft metal is helpful when contouring. It is ideal for posterior Class II composites, lingual matrixing of light-curing composites, and glass-ionomer cements. It is not desirable for Class III and Class V areas since light cannot pass through it for light curing.

Crown forms

Several crown forms are available. Some forms have the advantage of being thinner and more anatomically correct than others. When crown forms are used, their proximal surfaces are disced to thin them in this critical area.

Custom crown forms

Custom forms can be made with any polypropylene temporary splint material. They must be made on stone models that have been reproduced from a diagnostic waxup. Use of a custom form is a precise technique, but it may not be time-efficient in composite placement.

Class V matrix forms

Metal forms are ideal for glass-ionomer cements. They are easily adapted to gingival areas because they have no handle and can be more easily picked up with a piece of utility wax shaped to the tip of an amalgam condenser.

Class V cure-through matrix forms

Cure-through matrix forms are designed for light-cured composites and resin ionomers. When heated in hot water, they can be reshaped and adapted to a tooth. These forms have a small handle to aid in picking them up. A curing tip can be placed against this handle to hold the form in place during composite curing.

Placement instruments

Clinicians use a variety of instruments for placing composite, depending on personal preference and the demands of the restoration. Plastic instruments are one choice and are suited for mixing as well. When packing composite, always use a convex condenser. Concave condensers can increase voids, whereas convex condensers help pack a composite toward the cavity walls (Figure 9–5, *A*). An explorer is ideal for adapting material, because its small surface area limits the potential for composite to stick to it. A half Hollenback or interproximal carver is ideal for smoothing and contouring composite (Figure 9–5, *B*). Mylar is ideal for pulling composite proximally and shaping the proximal surface.

Fingers

Clean, gloved fingertips are well suited to shaping and smoothing composite. The composite is squeezed from the facial to the lingual to establish proximal contacts. Since gloves may contain contaminants, they should be used only when no further increments of composite are needed.

Contouring prior to polymerization

The primary goals of finishing are to obtain a restoration that has good contour, occlusion,

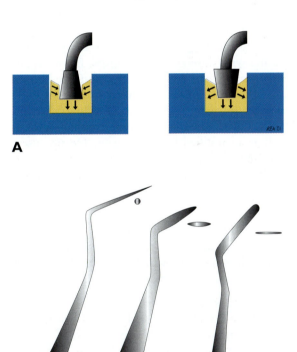

Explorer   Half Hollenback   Interproximal carver
B

Figure 9–5 *A*, Instruments used for packing. The tapered, convex condenser (*right*) is recommended, because it compacts composite toward the side walls; the concave condenser (*left*) is not recommended, because it pulls composite away from the side walls. *B*, Instruments used for sculpting and contouring, from the left: explorer, half Hollenback, and interproximal carver.

smoothness, and healthy embrasure forms. Tight margins should blend esthetically into the tooth's natural contours. Prepolymerization contouring is essential for consistently successful restorations. The amount of time required to finish a restoration is determined by how accurately the tooth was contoured before curing. A trained clinician can place an ideal restoration in 15 minutes, whereas an untrained operator can take over 60 minutes on the same restoration.

Composite layering

Visible light curing

Composite layers are cured in 1- and 2-mm increments with not more than 5 to 10 minutes elapsing between additions. When different classes of composite are added in layers (eg, a microfill to a minifill or to a heavily filled composite), an unfilled bonding agent should be placed between the layers to improve adhesion. Layering with unfilled bonding agents is even more critical when composites with different resin matrices (ie, from different manufacturers) are used. An unfilled bonding agent is a minimally filled fluid composite without solvents. A thin coat of a flowable composite, air-thinned, is an alternative that works as well as an unfilled bonding agent. Do not use a dentin bonding agent, because its components could inhibit bonding and weaken the composite.

Placing internal layers

Place the internal layers with a composite syringe or with a single-dose syringe system. Layers should be added in increments to approximately 0.5 mm below the final contours. Packing with a convex condenser is recommended.

Placing external layers

Sculpt the external layer with a hand instrument. A Mylar strip can be used proximally to distribute the composite evenly to the lingual surface to reduce voids. Most (95%) of a restoration's form, shape, and surface smoothness should be finalized before curing. The Mylar strip is removed carefully before curing, and a proximal carver is used to carefully smooth and shape areas with poor access (eg, gingival and proximal margins).

Before finishing

The resin is polymerized for 60 seconds (or as otherwise indicated) and left undisturbed for at least 10 minutes to allow the resin to more completely polymerize. This helps reduce finishing-induced surface trauma that increases wear and fracture.

FINISHING

In this text, *finishing* refers to all of the procedures associated with contouring, eliminating excess at the margins, and polishing. *Smoothness* is both the subjective appearance and the objective measurement of a polish. *Appearance* is related to texture and the nature of the material being polished. *Polish* relates to a number of other terms, such as surface smoothness, luster, or gloss. These terms imply greater light reflection from the restored surface. Polish also implies refinement or improvement of a restored surface. But finishing to improve polish is not always associated with an improved restorative surface.

There are two kinds of polish: acquired and inherent. The acquired polish is the surface placed by the operator. The inherent polish is the surface the material naturally reverts to through mastication and erosion. This surface is largely determined by the size and solubility of the dispersed phases of the material used (eg, fillers, fibers, etc).

Polishing is an inherently destructive process. The purpose of finishing and polishing should be to achieve the best possible surface with the least restorative damage and marginal leakage. There is a point of diminishing returns. Polishing high-stress-bearing surfaces to the inherent polish might provide a longer-lived restoration than extended polishing to gain an acquired polish.

For most direct dental restoratives, finishing is dependent on the hardness and polishability of the matrix and fillers that compose the material. Because autoset glass ionomers have a soft matrix and relatively large filler particles, the surface smoothness achievable through polishing is poor compared with composites that have a more durable polymerized resin matrix. Composites that contain macrofillers also have large particles, but because their matrices are more durable than that of an autocured glass ionomer, they can be finished to a higher polish immediately after placement. Resin ionomers have matrices that are stronger than those of autoset glass ionomers and have an initial polish that is better than that of an autoset glass ionomer but not as good as that of a macrofilled composite.

Placement and Finishing 163

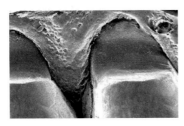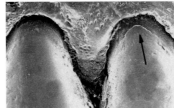

Figure 9–6. *Left*, Preoperative abfraction lesion; *Right*, postoperative composite with an open margin (arrow) resulting from the heat and friction of dry finishing. (Courtesy ESPE, Norristown, Pennsylvania).

Wet or dry finishing

Dry finishing is very harmful to most restoratives. The heat and friction generated can open dentin margins, particularly dentin–composite margins (Figure 9–6). Glass ionomers are especially susceptible to desiccation from dry finishing; however, they can rehydrate and recover if the drying is not too extensive (Figure 9–7). Dry finishing should be reserved for microfilled composite resins because they contain only resin fillers, which melt and produce an artificial smear layer of resin that enhances the surface gloss. Wet finishing, the technique used for most composites, reduces heat and friction, and thus, reduces surface damage to the body and margins of the restoration.

Acquired versus inherent polish

Inherent polish is determined by the characteristics of the restoration material. This includes the maximum particle size of nonpolishable (usually inorganic) particles and the ratio of wear between the polishable particles (those made of prepolymerized resin) and the matrix.

Heterogeneous materials such as glass ionomers and composites generally attain a smoother acquired polish than inherent polish. Heterogeneous materials revert to their inherent polish after a short time regardless of the initial finish achieved. Microfills usually attain an acquired polish that is similar to their inherent polish because there is less difference between the wear resistance of the fillers and the matrix.

Acquired:inherent polish ratio

If the acquired-to-inherent polish ratio (A:I ratio) is 1:1, the surface texture will never change. Because almost all restoratives are heterogeneous materials, they become rougher over time. Microfills have a low A:I ratio since both filler and matrix are similar. Large-particle macrofills have a large A:I ratio, because their surface becomes more rough over time: "I" becomes smaller relative to "A." The A:I ratio of submicron composites falls between that of the macrofilled and the microfilled composites. For example, if a material starts with an acquired polish equivalent to an inorganic grit size of 1000 and the surface

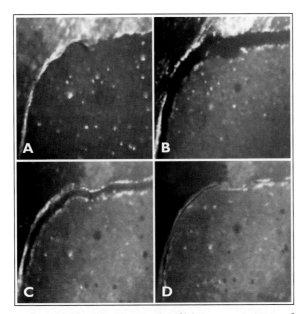

Figure 9–7. Electron micrographs of laboratory specimens of glass ionomer dehydration and rehydration: *A*, glass ionomer 10 minutes after placement, margin sealed; *B*, glass ionomer shrinkage after exposure to air for 1 hour, margin open; *C*, glass ionomer expansion after 30 minutes in water, margin closing; *D*, fully hydrated glass ionomer after 1 hour in water, margin closed. (Courtesy ESPE.)

eventually stabilizes to a grit size of 200, the A:I ratio is 1000 to 200, or 5. This means the restorative stabilizes at a roughness five times that achievable by the dentist at the time of restoration placement.

A manufacturer's claim that a composite's average particle size is 1 μm implies that the composite will provide a polish equivalent to that of other similarly sized materials. This is not necessarily true. Materials proclaimed to have the same average particle size of 1 μm may have A:I ratios from 2 to 15+ because of the difference in particle distribution. The A:I ratio takes into account the effects of adding larger particles to a restorative.

Surface transition time

The surface transition time (STT) is the time it takes a material to transition from its acquired polish to its inherent polish (Figure 9–8). Allowing for slight differences among patients, each composite has a predictable STT. The durability of the resin phase, the loading of the dispersed phase, and the bond strength and stability of the coupling interface between the filler and the matrix all profoundly affect STT. In addition, diet, occlusion, and the solubility of a restorative's components in an individual's oral environment influence STT. Bruxism and bulimia greatly shorten the STT of any material. Based on study-group experience, the typical

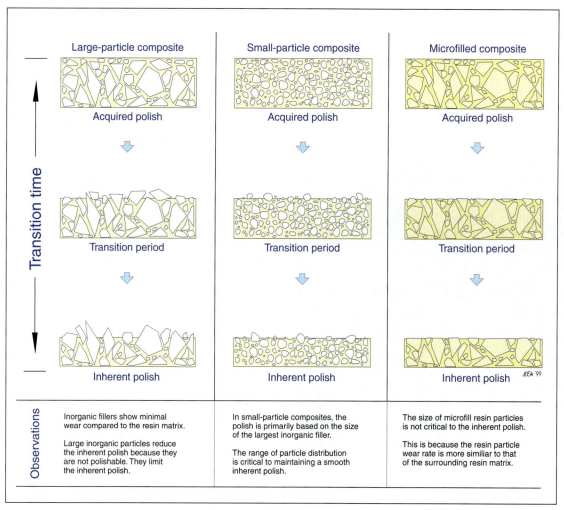

Figure 9–8. Schematic illustrations of three of the many wear patterns that composites can undergo during the transition from acquired to inherent smoothness. As the inorganic particles get larger or harder, wear on the opposing enamel increases proportionately. Submicron composites with good A:I ratios, owing to tight particle size distribution, perform well clinically.

restorative has an STT of 6 months for macrofilled composites, 1 year for microfills, and well over 2 years for ceramic materials.

Clinical significance of acquired:inherent polish ratio and surface transition time

A composite resin that achieves a high acquired polish tends to pick up fewer stains, accumulate less plaque, and show better wear. Ideally, the inherent polish should be smooth enough to be well tolerated by gingival tissue. The polish should look like enamel, and it should have an STT that allows the surface to maintain a smooth and stain-free appearance between normal cleaning visits. To maintain maximum esthetics, the STT should be greater than the time between cleaning appointments

Materials with short STT and a high A:I ratio have an inherent polish that is usually unacceptable to patients. There is wide variation in the inherent polish of composites, based on their content of particles over 2 μm in size. Generally, materials that contain only particles 0.5 μm (the size of enamel rods) or smaller retain a polish better and wear opposing structures less than materials containing larger or harder filler particles. Particles larger than 5 μm are larger than enamel rod bundles.

Predicting inherent surface smoothness

Information on the average particle size of a composite is of little value in determining its polish, because polish is dependent on the size of the largest inorganic filler particle. Many manufacturers are tempted to add large particles to their composite to increase filler loading. This improves the material's strength but is detrimental to its inherent polish.

Polish information about a composite can be ascertained from a particle size distribution graph, provided by the manufacturer, that shows the amount and size of each particle in the material. All the inorganic filler particles in an anterior composite should be less than 1 μm (submicron hybrids). Materials with particles of 1 to 5 μm are called small-particle composites and are generally more highly filled. Materials with still larger particles (>5 μm) are heavily filled hybrids and are indicated for support under high–stress-bearing restorations. Figure 9–9 shows the relative size of particles from 0.04 μm to 10 μm. Both small-particle and heavily filled hybrids can be used in posterior teeth.

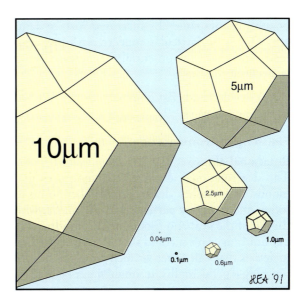

Figure 9–9. The relative size of the nonpolishable inorganic fillers used in currently available glass ionomer and composites (0.04 to 10.0 μm). Inorganic particle size is the most critical determinant of long-term surface smoothness.

In esthetically critical areas of anterior teeth, they should be covered with a microfilled composite to improve the inherent polish.

POLISHING METHODS

A composite is under stress and tension at placement. It takes 10 to 15 minutes for a composite to stabilize enough following curing to allow finishing to be accomplished without considerable damage to the restoration. A damaged composite has a higher wear rate, a tendency to fracture, and open margins (often seen as a white line at the enamel–resin interface).

After proper curing, the surface should be wet finished slowly (to reduce heat and friction) with micron diamonds, white stones, or discs. Excess material is removed in a way that allows for good tactile sense. A fine 40- to 125-μm diamond or a medium disc works well on submicron composites. More heavily filled materials may require coarser instruments. Microfills require a more delicate touch and can be trimmed interproximally with a No. 12 Bard Parker blade. Rubber points work well on microfills after contouring with discs or micron diamonds (40 μm). Polishing a material past its inherent polish should be avoided, because this results in a temporary gloss, possibly accompanied by increased surface damage. This is of particular concern with posterior teeth because of the potential for increased wear in occlusal function.

Composites and glass ionomers, can be finished in a variety of ways.[5-11]

Finishing instrumentation

Rotational abrasive, dry
The dry rotational abrasive technique uses diamonds, white stones, discs, or dry rubber points to soften and cut away particles and the matrix with the aid of the heat and friction that is produced in dry finishing. This method should only be used on materials that will soften or melt from the heat of finishing (eg, microfills). It should never be used on a glass ionomer

Rotational abrasive, wet
The wet rotational abrasive method uses diamonds or other abrasives, such as aluminum oxide discs, with water or a water-soluble lubricant. Examples are micron diamonds or white stones with water spray, or discs used wet or with a water-soluble lubricant that reduces heat and chipping.

Rotational abrasive, erosive
The erosive rotational abrasive method uses pastes to soften and erode the attachment between larger particles and the matrix. The pastes that are used with soft rubber cups generally contain submicron aluminum oxide particles. These should be prepared in a thin slurry to smooth small-particle (1–5 μm) and submicron (<1 μm) composites. Examples of these pastes are Herculite (Kerr, Orange, California) and Prisma Gloss (LD Caulk, Milford, Delaware).

Hand oscillation
Proximal strips of varying sizes and grits are available for sanding between teeth. The main concern with the strips is laceration of oral tissues. Diamond-coated stainless steel strips with polished edges and varying grits are useful with bonded porcelain restorations (eg, veneers).

Handpiece-driven oscillation
Devices such as Profin (Dentatus/Weisman Technology, New York, New York) use small oscillating diamond points (Figure 9–10). These devices are unique, have a large number of available tips, and

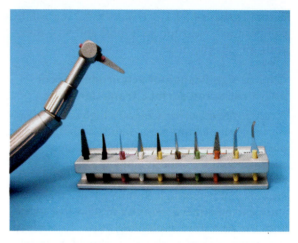

Figure 9–10. The Profin handpiece attachment device includes a variety of tips for specific clinical uses.

offer good proximal access. These devices are not recommended for routine finishing. They are best used in place of strips when more aggressive cutting is needed (eg, removal of overhangs).

Rotary instrument shapes
The two critical features of a bur are grit size and shape. Generally 100 to 150 μm is used for preparations and gross reduction; 50 to 100 μm for contouring, and less than 50 μm for polishing. The shape of a diamond cutting instrument can create or limit proper preparation design and proper fin-

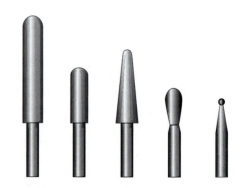

Figure 9–11. Burs for cutting internal shapes in preparations. Internal cutting shapes have rounded tips to avoid placing any sharp angles in a preparation. Rounded angles limit the stress points associated with tooth cracks and fracture.

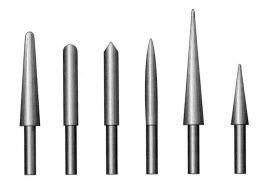

Figure 9–12. Burs for cutting external shapes in preparations. External cutting shapes are straight, beveled, or round. Beveled instruments provide good exit angles for direct composite and gold restorations.

ishing. The instrument shapes shown in Figure 9–11 are used for cutting internal shapes. Note they are all round-ended; this prevents sharp internal line angles that result in stress points and increase the incidence of tooth cracks and cusp fractures. The shapes shown in Figure 9–12 are used for cutting external margins. The shapes that are appropriate for finishing have straight or concave sides and create fewer unwanted concavities on the facial surface (Figure 9–13). A rounded instrument is used only for creating proper lingual contours.

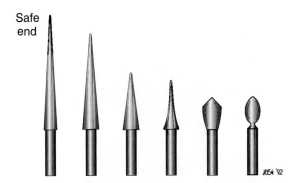

Figure 9–13. Burs appropriate for finishing composites. Finishing shapes are straight for the facial and rounded for the lingual. Convex shapes are available for proximal areas. These are useful for gross reduction but wear out much more quickly than other shapes.

SPECIFIC FINISHING MATERIALS

Burs

Six-fluted burs cut rapidly, are difficult to control, dislodge particles, and cause fissuring (Figure 9–14). They should not be used to finish composites.

Twelve-fluted burs may tear the resin matrix and actually weaken the composite near the margins. Use these burs for cutting preparations on indirect restorations. A 12-fluted bur generally provides a smoother surface than a 15-μm diamond. Thirty-fluted burs effectively finish submicron composites.[9]

Forty-fluted burs can be used to trim excess composite resin from under gingival tissues because the burs do not cut tissue and they leave a smooth burnished surface. The main disadvantage is the slow cutting, which, without copious amounts of water, can cause the fine flutes to clog. Few manufacturers make these burs.[9]

Figure 9–15 shows a representative sampling of currently available burs.

Diamonds

Coarse, medium, and fine diamonds are shown in Figure 9–16. Coarse diamonds (>125 μm) are particularly useful in resin-to-resin bonding because the roughness creates a mechanical interlock between the old and newly added composites. Fine diamonds are ideal for gross contouring.

Micron diamonds are designed for use at slow speeds and with copious amounts of water; however, most practitioners use them at near stall-out high speed. The finish is slightly less smooth than the finish achieved with flexible discs. Micron diamonds are suited for the lingual surfaces of incisors and the occlusal surfaces of posterior composites. Studies show that these diamonds do not damage the resin matrices and margins as much as do some finishing burs (Figure 9–17).

Stones

White and green stones, if used dry, can loosen fillers from the resin matrix and cause interfacial fractures in a composite, which can weaken a restoration. Since they produce large amounts of heat, they should be used with large amounts of water.

168 Tooth-Colored Restoratives

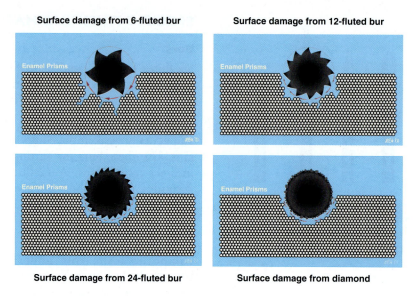

Figure 9–14. Schematic illustration of enamel surface damage associated with finishing with a 6-fluted bur, a 12-fluted bur, a 24-fluted bur, or a fine diamond. Note the decreased fracturing as the number of flutes increases.

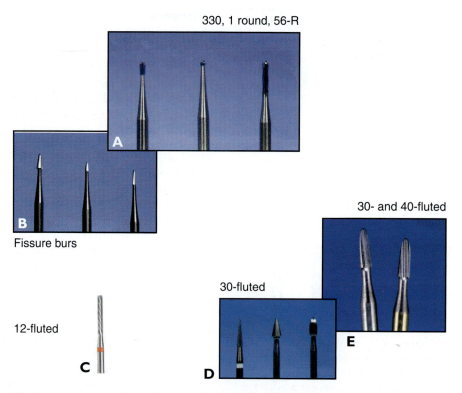

Figure 9–15. *A*, The three most commonly used burs; from left to right: 330, No. 1 round, and 56-R. *B*, Fissure burs. *C*, Twelve-fluted finishing bur. *D*, Three 30-fluted finishing burs. *E*, Thirty-fluted and 40-fluted finishing burs.

Placement and Finishing 169

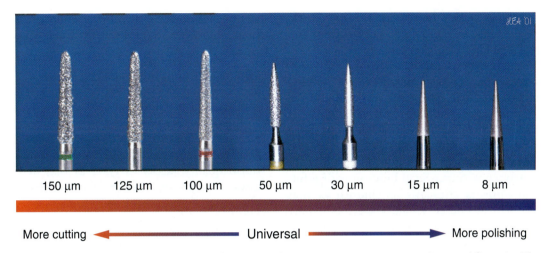

Figure 9–16. Diamonds are available in a range of micron particle sizes, representing coarse, medium, and fine grits. The more coarse diamonds are used in resin-to-resin bonding, whereas the finer diamonds are used for finishing.

Finishing Discs

Discs and strips, unlike diamonds, are typically measured by grit rather than by micron particle size (Table 9–1). Grit is determined by mesh size during manufacture; a disc with a grit of 200 would include a mixture of particles, all measuring 74 μm or less. Figure 9–18 shows a representative sampling of currently available disks. The major types are described below.

Sof-Lex Discs (3M Dental Products, St. Paul, Minnesota) are popular flexible composite finishing discs. The abrasive is aluminum oxide. A soft backing allows these discs to curve to the tooth. The discs provide a smooth, even finish by selectively removing the raised projections from the resin surface. Using all four grits in sequence provides the best finish. They are available for either Moore's standard mandrels (E.C. Moore Co., Inc., Dearborn, Michigan) (16-mm diameter) or "Pop-On" mandrels. The Pop-On mandrel has a smaller circular head and uses smaller discs (13- and 9.5-mm diameters).

Micro-Fill Composite Finishing Discs (E.C. Moore Co., Inc.) rapidly and grossly reduce any composite, but because the discs are rigid, they cannot give the best final polish on most composite resins.

Flexidiscs (Cosmedent, Chicago, Illinois) are available in four grits. These discs are 16 mm in diameter and fit a standard Moore's mandrel. They are thin, making them ideal for proximal areas, but are less flexible than Sof-Lex Discs. Flexidiscs cause more surface scratching on microfills and small-particle hybrids than do Sof-Lex Discs.

Table 9–1. The Relationship of Grit Size to Microns and Inches for Grits Commonly Used in Dental Instruments

Use	Grit Size	Microns	Inches
Finishing	1250	10	0.0004
	625	20	0.0008
	550	25	0.0010
Contouring	400	36	0.0014
	325	44	0.0017
	270	53	0.0021
	200	74	0.0029
	140	100	0.041
Cutting	120	125	0.0049
	100	149	0.0059
	80	177	0.0070
	70	210	0.0083
	60	250	0.0117

Super-Snap Discs (Shofu Dental Corp., Menlo Park, California) are more rigid than Sof-Lex Discs and not as rigid as Moore's discs. Super-Snap Discs are thin and easy to use in interproximal areas. Because the mandrel is mounted behind the disc, there is no metal hub. This gives excellent access in hard-to-reach areas and reduces the possibility of the mandrel damaging the restoration. Super-Snap Discs were introduced in 1983 and come in two diameters: 8 mm and 12.5 mm. When used in proper sequence, Super-Snap Discs provide a finish that appears clinically as smooth as that achieved with any other system. The grit is on only one side of the disc, so two discs are needed to change the grit from the face to the back.

Sof-Lex XT Discs (3M) are among the thinnest and most rigid of the composite finishing discs. The abrasive is aluminum oxide. The relatively stiff backing allows access to tight proximal areas. When all four grits are used in sequence, these discs give a finish close to that achieved with the original Sof-Lex Discs. Sof-Lex XT Discs are available in the standard 3M Pop-On mandrels. These discs come in 13-mm and 9.5-mm diameters and work nicely in finishing composites as well as porcelain–enamel and metal–enamel margins.

Vivadent Polishing Discs come in three grits with a 16-mm diameter and are used with Moore's snap-on mandrels. They are relatively rigid. The fine grit disc is coated with tin oxide; the coarse discs use conventional aluminum oxide and zirconium silicate.

The proper methodology for using a disc on anterior teeth is illustrated in Figure 9–19.

Rubber wheels, cups, and points

Figure 9–20 shows a representative sampling of currently available rubber wheels, cups, and points.

Soft rubber

Burlew wheels have an intermediate grit that is good for initial contouring and smoothing.

Medium rubber

Centrix polishing cups come in two grits and are suitable for gross and final finishing. LD Caulk's "Enhance" polishing cups and points are useful for a combination of gross and final finishing, especially in posterior and occlusal areas. Shofu polishing cups and wheels provide smoother finishes than microfine diamonds and burs. Cups and wheels are popular in many study groups.

Vivadent polishing cups and wheels are excellent for characterizing microfilled resins. The cups and wheels cut rapidly yet leave a smooth surface. The gray wheels are used for gross reduction, whereas the green wheels are used for final finishing. Studies show that wheels and discs produce a finish quality nearly as good as that of flexible discs. They are available in a range of shapes.

Hard rubber

Ceramic discs (Shofu) have abrasive points for gross reduction and rubber points for final finishing. They are available in a number of different shapes.

Proximal finishing strips

Figure 9–21 shows a representative sampling of currently available proximal finishing strips. Proximal finishing strips are ideal for enamel discing before cutting a preparation, and for finishing a restoration after final contouring.

Metal strips

Metal strips cut almost all tooth and restorative materials evenly. They are superior to plastic strips in almost every respect. They are excellent for gross

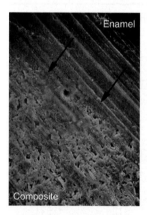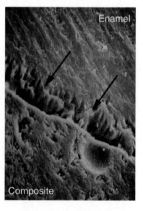

Figure 9–17. These scanning electron micrographs show the difference between finishing a composite–enamel margin with a micron diamond or a bur. *Left*, Minimal damage caused by a micron diamond; *right*, the marginal chipping commonly associated with burs. (From Lutz F, Setcos J, Phillips R. New finishing instruments for composite resins. J Am Dent Assoc 1983;107:575–80, with permission.)

Placement and Finishing 171

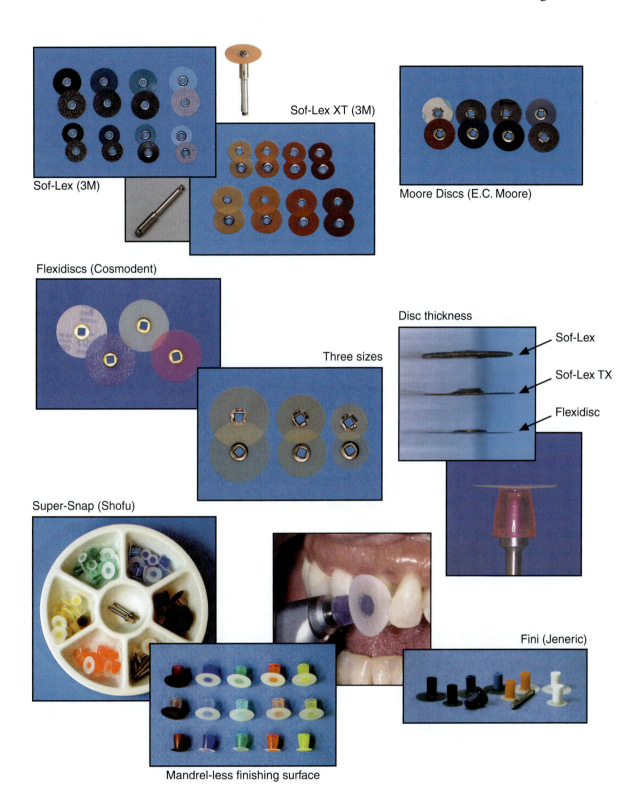

Figure 9–18. Some of the more commonly used finishing discs: Sof-Lex Discs, Flexidiscs, Super-Snap Discs, Fini Finishing and Polishing Disks (Jeneric/Pentron, Wallingford, Connecticut), and Micro-Fill Composite Finishing Disks (E.C. Moore Co., Inc.).

172 Tooth-Colored Restoratives

Use the edge of a small, thin, stiff disc to establish gross proximal contouring. This should be done by gently rotating the disc from 90 degrees toward the facial at a very slow speed.

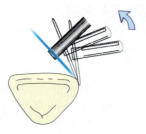

Use the face of a flexible disc for gross contouring. Use it at three distinct planes that are gently blended together. To avoid flat spots, keep the disc moving in gentle circular motions.

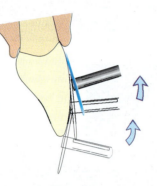

Use the outermost 1 mm of a disc at 90 degrees to the surface to place developmental grooves. Use a gentle sliding motion along the groove length. A more textured look is achieved by intermittantly touching the surface.

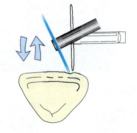

Use the edge of a very thin disc to adjust incisal edges. Adjust out any interferences that could contribute to wear or loss of the restoration.

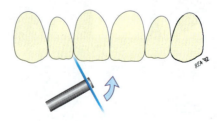

Figure 9–19. Discs play different roles in contouring and finishing anterior teeth. They are used for removing excess composite, shaping composite, and placing anatomy.

Placement and Finishing

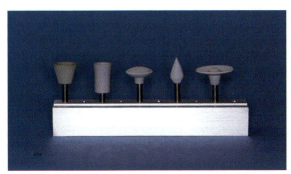

Figure 9–20. Polishing cups and wheels yield smooth finishes. They come in a variety of shapes, sizes, and grits.

interproximal reduction, particularly as a first step in interproximal finishing. They must be used carefully, because they easily remove tooth structure as well as composite. The major disadvantage of metal strips is cost. However, they are autoclavable and can be reused.

Diamond Strips (Brasseler, Savannah, Georgia) are thin metal strips (0.13–0.08 mm) with a safe spot (no grit) in the middle. They are available in three grits: medium (45 μm), fine (30 μm), and extra-fine (15 μm) in 2.5-mm and 3.75-mm widths.

Compo-strips (Premier, King of Prussia, Pennsylvania) are thin metal strips with a safe spot (no grit) in the middle. Compo also offers a matching set of handheld discs for opening embrasures.

GC International Metal Strips (GC, Tokyo, Japan) were the first of the high-quality diamond strips with polished sides. Current improved versions are still the standard to which others are compared. The strips are available in an extensive array of grits (eg, 200, 300, 600, and 1200). The 300-grit is an intermediate grit for initial finishing, whereas the 600 and 1200 are ideal for smoother finishes. These strips are more durable than many others on the market.

Moyco Metal Strips (Moyco Technologies, York, Pennsylvania) are used for gross reduction. Moyco also makes a narrow strip for proximal access. They are not as highly refined as many other strips on the market.

The Teledyne Proflex Scaler (Teledyne, Fort Collins, Colorado) is a unique cutting system that involves many perforations in a soft metal strip.

The strip is thin and easily enters tight proximal spaces. Because it cuts slowly, it is ideal for final composite polishing or to remove proximal stains. It is a special item and should not be compared with the other metal strips mentioned.

Plastic strips

Flexistrips (Cosmedent) are available in two grits, one for finishing and one for polishing. The strips provide a smooth surface on microfilled composites and are tear resistant.

Moyco Plastic Strips are thick, color-coded strips. They cut more slowly and are less useful for gross reduction.

Sof-Lex Strips (3M) are excellent for final finishing of proximal areas and are understandably popular among dentists. They have an uncoated area in the center of the strip for easy initial placement. They come in two widths and two pairs of grits, one for finishing and one for polishing. Use both strips for optimal results.

Vivadent Strips are available in coarse and medium aluminum oxide. They are similar to those manufactured by 3M. Vivadent's fine strip is coated with tin oxide and is excellent for polishing when no reduction is desired.

Hand instruments

Hand instruments include Bard Parker blades and tungsten carbide carvers (Figure 9–22). A standard No. 12 or No. 15 Bard Parker blade can remove excess restorative material interproximally. Because the blades dull quickly, it sometimes takes several to trim a single restoration.

Carbide composite carvers, such as those sold by Brasseler and GC America, are available in several shapes, trim a microfilled composite with ease, and hold their edge well. Instruments numbered 150.17 to 150.20 are bladed instruments that are excellent for chipping away excess veneer cement. Instruments numbered 150.18 and 150.19 are curved to the shape of a tooth and can be used subgingivally to remove small amounts of composite flash. Some clinicians find the discoid-shape carver the most useful because it effectively removes flash from the lingual of central incisors. Although they are expensive, these carvers are more effective in cutting composite than Bard Parker blades.

174 Tooth-Colored Restoratives

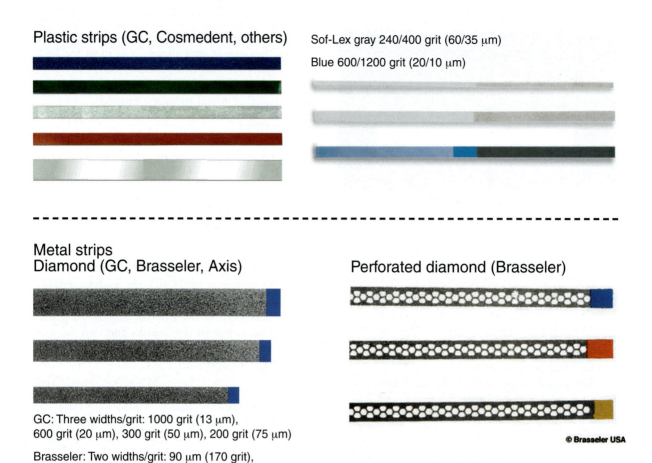

Plastic strips (GC, Cosmedent, others)

Sof-Lex gray 240/400 grit (60/35 μm)

Blue 600/1200 grit (20/10 μm)

Metal strips
Diamond (GC, Brasseler, Axis)

GC: Three widths/grit: 1000 grit (13 μm), 600 grit (20 μm), 300 grit (50 μm), 200 grit (75 μm)

Brasseler: Two widths/grit: 90 μm (170 grit), 45 μm (300 grit), 30 μm (500 grit), 15 μm (600 grit)

Perforated diamond (Brasseler)

© Brasseler USA

Proper Use

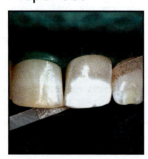

Handheld separator

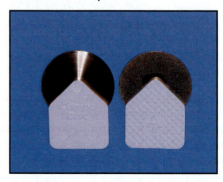

Figure 9–21. Plastic and metal finishing strips are available in various thicknesses. Metal strips are easier than plastic strips to place through tight contacts. Some plastic strips (eg, Sof-Lex) have a grit-free area in the center, which aids interproximal placement.

Placement and Finishing 175

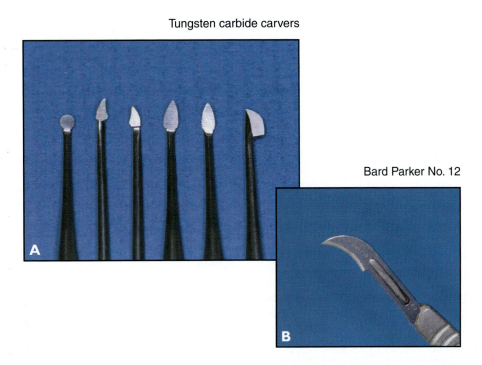

Figure 9–22. *A*, Tungsten carbide carvers are used to remove marginal excess on facial and lingual surfaces. *B*, Bard Parker blades are used to remove interproximal excess.

Polishing pastes

Aluminum oxide
A thin mixture of aluminum oxide powder can be used on microfilled composites and some small-particle hybrids. In conventional macrofilled composites, pastes may induce plucking by preferentially removing resin from around the macrofiller particles.

Luster Paste (Kerr) is a 0.3-µm paste that gives a higher polish than pastes with larger particles. The grit in the polishing material should be smaller than the inorganic filler size of the composite. Prisma Gloss (LD Caulk) gives a polish similar to Luster Paste on submicron composites, and improves the polish achieved with extra-fine discs.

Creating texture
Creating a textured surface requires polishing to the ideal contour and leaving a slight extra thickness over the area to be textured. Then, with a micron diamond or small disc, indentations of the desired texture are carefully and slowly cut. The tip of the instrument is in constant motion. Generally, horizontal indentations that are straight or broken are made in the gingival third (ie, lift the instrument on and off of the surface), and vertical indentations are made in the incisal two-thirds (Figure 9–23). A polishing paste in a prophy cup or the edge of a polishing disc may be used, with a light tapping motion, to bring out areas of luster.

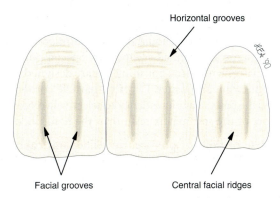

Figure 9–23. Schematic representation of the placement of horizontal and vertical contours to match the natural anatomy of a typical central incisor.

FINISHING TECHNIQUES

Diamonds and burs

Micron diamonds (40 to 60 μm) are used for bulk reduction on surfaces unreachable with discs. Micron diamonds used at slow or stall-out speeds with copious amounts of water provide a smooth surface with minimal resin damage. Diamonds are generally better than discs for placing surface texture. Medium or coarse diamonds leave a rough surface that could extend finishing and polishing times.

Stones should not be used, because the heat and vibration they generate can loosen the composite filler particles and increase surface porosity. The effect of using finishing stones on submicron and small-particle hybrid composites has not been studied.

Burs cut the composite surface, which increases the likelihood of resin fatigue fracture. The greatest roughness occurs when large-particle composites are finished with a 12-fluted bur. The proper use of a rotary instrument is shown in Figure 9–24.

Flexible discs

Flexible discs and strips (eg, Sof-Lex, 3M) give an excellent finish. The coarse discs are used with water and with a very light touch. Because heat and friction weaken the composite and enamel–resin interface, discs should be moved constantly to prevent heat and flat spots.

Flexible discs cut composite more rapidly than enamel and can easily ditch composite. Discs with more rigid backing are used to polish the margins of materials with different cutting rates (Figure 9–25). Special discs are made for this purpose (eg, XT, 3M; and several by Cosmedent).

Polishing pastes should be used on micron and submicron macrofilled composites. Special polishing pastes with a fine polishing grit are designed for submicron composites. On large-particle composites, the pastes have a tendency to selectively remove more of the soft matrix resin than the hard filler.

Use of flour of pumice, tin oxide, and rubber wheels should be avoided because they increase the roughness of large-particle composites.

Incorporating surface texture

It is easier to create a textured surface with micron diamonds and polishing pastes than with discs. Discs are used for the final polish when a very smooth surface is desired. The edge of a disc is used to place conservative developmental grooves.

Metal hand instruments

Metal instruments effectively trim microfilled composites because resin filler is not abrasive to metal. In areas that are difficult to reach, micron diamonds are also effective. Scalpels, blades (No. 12 and No. 15), or gold knives also remove flash from microfilled composites. Their use is particularly helpful in proximal areas with limited access. Micron diamonds used at slow speed and with copious amounts of water provide good margins.

Discs

When discing a microfilled composite, a final superfine disc is used dry (ie, without water spray). The heat from dry discing produces a highly cured smear layer of resin over the microfilled surface. This creates a smooth and durable finish.[5] Coarser discs for gross reduction should be used wet. Heat and friction can result in white line formation during finishing. This occurs when microfill polymerization shrinkage creates tension on opposing margins, particularly during the first 15 minutes after light initiation. Later, water absorption expands the matrix and relieves this tension to some extent.

Rubber cups

A number of manufacturers make rubber cups for finishing areas a disc cannot reach. They are effective with microfill composites because of the homogeneous nature of these materials. Some cups (eg, Enhance, LD Caulk) are designed as a single-use instrument for contouring and polishing.

Small-particle hybrids

The small-particle hybrids (fillers <1 μm) should be finished with water spray and 20-μm diamonds or flexible finishing discs. However, unlike microfilled composites, a polishing paste of very fine particle size (eg, Luster Paste, Kerr; Prisma Gloss, LD Caulk) must be used in the final finishing step. A 60-second polish with a wet slurry on a soft rubber cup gives the best finish to submicron composites.

SURFACE COATINGS

Placing unfilled resin on a composite margin increases sealing and reduces marginal leakage

Placement and Finishing   177

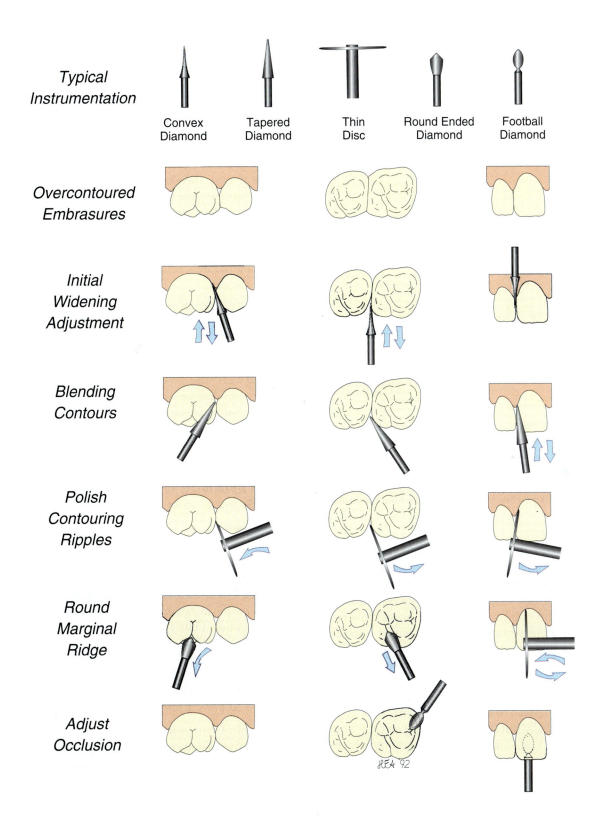

Figure 9–24. Schematic representation of the proper use of rotary instruments during finishing.

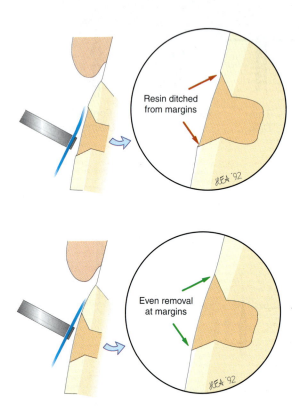

Figure 9–25. A flexible disc is not recommended for finishing a composite restoration at its enamel margins. A flexible disc bends under pressure, which tends to result in a flat or concave surface because the disc removes more of the softer restorative. Stiff discs are easier to use when placing convex contours or finishing the margins between two or more materials of dissimilar hardness.

from contraction gaps (Figure 9–26). Composite shrinks immediately upon setting, but usually expands as it absorbs water. Sealing, although not strong, will last long enough for the composite to expand and stabilize the margins. Some clinicians apply a fluid surface coating of resin to create a smooth surface on a roughly finished restorative surface. Although quick and easy, the result usually is a large amount of air inhibition in the outer surface, preventing a complete cure. Materials added through delayed resin–resin bonding have weak bonds; usually just 30 to 50% of the original bond strength. These fluid surface resins wear rapidly and then expose the underlying rough surface. Surface resins traditionally have a short surface transition time, and because they are so short-lived, the final polished surface is often poor when compared with the inherent finish of the restoration.

Surface glazes

Surface glazes can help reseal margins and repair surface defects after finishing.[12] This glaze is more critical if the post-cure rest time is inadequate (ie, is less than 10 min) prior to the start of finishing.

Indirect restorations

Surface glazes have been used on both temporary and provisional composite restorations to reduce processing time. Because these units are polymerized in a vacuum, the surface glaze is nearly completely polymerized. These glazes are successful as provisional restorations and can maintain a polish for a year.

Specialized glazing products

Some materials are specially made for surface repairs. Most of the glazes are thin resins with highly reactive accelerators that compete more successfully with oxygen to reduce air inhibition. Surface sealers (eg, Fortify, Bisco, Schaumburg, Illinois, and other fluid resins) can repair surface defects that occur during finishing. Studies show this sealing improves the initial wear rates of posterior composites and can decrease microleakage around Class V restorations. In study group experience, these sealers are useful over posterior composites and on restorations that involve dentin cavosurface margins, where they help close any immediate contraction gaps.

MAINTENANCE OF COMPOSITE RESINS

Types of wear

Abrasion

Heavily filled macrofilled composites with large particles often have an inherent polish that is abrasive to enamel. These restorations need special attention at recall prophylaxis appointments to regain their acquired polish. (The type of composite used in a restoration should be clearly marked in a patient's record.) Mechanical cleaning devices, such as a Prophy-Jet or Cavitron (LD Caulk) destroy the surface finish and pit the restoration. Coarse prophy pastes can dull a composite restoration.

Many clinicians agree that one of the best polishers for microfilled composite and small-particle restorations is a slurry of very fine aluminum oxide. The finish can be maintained by periodic polishing with a thin mixture of aluminum oxides on a soft rubber cup (chemical grade aluminum oxide powder works effectively). With small-particle

Placement and Finishing 179

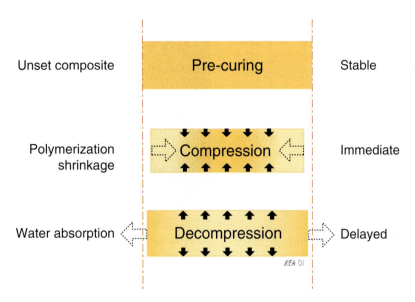

Figure 9–26. Schematic representation of changes in restoration size that occur as a result of polymerization shrinkage and subsequent water absorption.

hybrid composites, there is some clinical evidence that polishing pastes with very small particles give superior results (eg, Kerr's Luster Paste).

Erosion
Composites are susceptible to chemical erosion. All resin systems have some susceptibility to hydrolysis. Acidulated phosphate fluoride (APF) can dissolve the fillers and pit the surface of many macrofilled composites. Laboratory studies show that composites filled with strontium glass and, to a lesser extent, those filled with quartz are dissolved during normal applications of APF gels. Microfilled resins are the least affected by APF. It is therefore prudent to use non-APF fluorides on patients with macrofilled composite restorations.

Problems on recall visits

White line margins
If a composite restoration has any thin, knife-edge margins, a white line at this margin may be noticeable at placement. Microfills generally produce more white lines at the margins than do more heavily filled materials. White lines seen immediately after placement are thought to be related to finishing techniques that cause the enamel tags to tear as a result of the tension of polymerization shrinkage. Finishing burs cause the most white line margins, whereas micron diamonds and flexible discs cause the least (Figure 9–27).

The exact cause of white lines is not established. Research suggests that these margins stain. Because of the large disparity in the coefficient of thermal expansion between the tooth and the restoration, staining at an unsealed edge is a long-lasting problem.

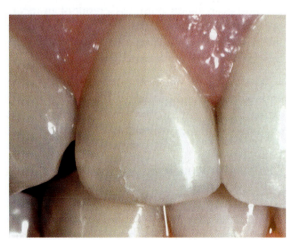

Figure 9–27. Postoperative view of a restorative margin lifting off a tooth because of polymerization tension and trauma from finishing. The result is a white line margin.

The simplest way to treat a white line margin on the end of a thin flash of microfilled resin is to trim it with a sharp instrument (Bard Parker blade, gold foil knife, or carbide hand instrument) and then polish the restoration with flexible discs in the usual fashion. This approach is appropriate only for restorations with sufficient bulk for additional finishing. Restorations with no excess bulk should be removed with a diamond, and resin should be added by the delayed resin–resin bonding technique.

White line margins at 90 degrees and chamfer margins must be removed with a bur. The preparation should then be filled with new composite, using delayed resin–resin bonding. Finishing burs are not recommended for removal of white line margins. They cause microtears of the resin matrix and ditching of resin–enamel margins.

Pits

Pits are caused by porosity or air incorporation. They are sometimes hard to detect during placement but become readily apparent at recall, because they stain easily. Aging is another factor in pit formation. When composites get old, they sometimes dry out. This can result in pitting throughout a restoration.

Light-cured materials are the least porous. In fact, some products have virtually no voids. Poor placement is the major cause of pitting in these materials. In general, highly viscous materials are more likely to have voids during placement, owing to poorer adaptation during layering and injection. Viscous autoset composites are highly porous as a result of air incorporation during mixing. Powder-liquid systems are the most porous of the composite types; it is difficult to achieve a consistently mixed paste.

The treatment of a pit begins with enlarging it with a small round bur into a box-shaped preparation. Next, composite is added using the delayed resin–resin bonding technique.

Chipping

Chipping is common with larger composites, such as veneers (Figure 9–28). In general, microfills chip in large pieces when stressed, which can cause a shear failure. More heavily filled materials tend to chip in small increments that are easier to repair. The most frequent cause of chipping is excessive occlusion. Ideally, all composite restoratives should

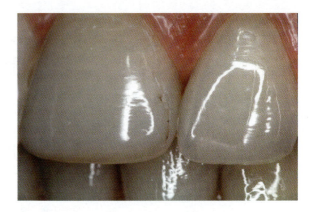

Figure 9–28. Three-year postoperative view of chipping owing to the long-term effects of composite contraction and expansion on thin restorative margins.

be cleared of any occlusal forces, including protrusive and parafunctional movements.

Marginal chipping is treated by removal of the chipped portion of the composite with a coarse diamond and the addition of new composite, using the delayed resin–resin bonding technique.

Cohesive fracture

Cohesive fracture is more common with microfills than macrofills (Figure 9–29). Heavily filled composites are the least likely to fracture and should be considered as replacements for more lightly filled materials.

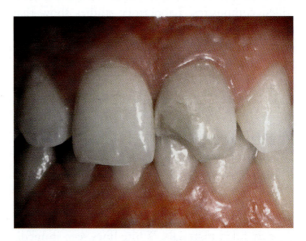

Figure 9–29. A cohesive fracture resulting from composite fatigue; these fractures are more common when composites with low filler loading are placed under occlusal stress. Case selection is critical to the longevity of stress-bearing restorations.

A cohesive fracture is treated by completely removing the restoration or, in less severe cases, with delayed resin–resin bonding. If there is no obvious occlusal interference or other placement error, the restoration is replaced with a more highly filled composite.

Color change

Light-cured composite resins are generally color-stable. Most color discrepancies are attributable to incorrect shade selection. There are three common explanations for a color that appears too light: (1) the tooth was allowed to dehydrate before final shade selection, (2) there was a disparity between the shade guide and the composite restoration, and (3) the composite was not completely cured.

Composites lighten during curing because of color transformation of the camphoroquinones that are activated during polymerization. Therefore, determining shade color based on a partly cured composite is likely to yield a shade that is too light when the restoration is fully polymerized. If the final restoration color is too dark, there was likely a problem in shade selection. A common cause is clinician "color saturation" from looking at a tooth too long, which tends to lead to selection of a too dark color.

REFERENCES

1. Pink FE. Use of custom composite shade guide for shade determination [abstract]. J Dent Res 1989;68(Spec Issue):302.

2. Fischel HF, Tay WM. Effect of manipulative techniques on porosity in composite resins [abstract]. J Dent Res 1977;56(Spec Issue).

3. Medlock J, Zinck J, Norling B, Sisca U. Composite porosity comparisons with hand and syringe placement [abstract]. J Dent Res 1983;62(Spec Issue):219.

4. Gjerdet NR, Hegdahl T. Porosity of resin filling materials. Acta Odontol Scand 1978;36:303.

5. Davidson CL, Duysters PP, De Lange C, Bausch JR. Structural changes in composite surface material after dry polishing. J Oral Rehabil 1981;8:431–9.

6. Dennison JD, Craig RG. Physical properties and finishing surface texture of composite restorative resins. J Am Dent Assoc 1972;85:101–8.

7. O'Brien WJ, Johnson WM, Fanian F, Lambert S. The surface roughness and gloss of composites. J Dent Res 1984;63:685–8.

8. Herrgott AL, Ziemiecki TL, Dennison JB. An evaluation of different composite resin systems finished with various abrasives. J Am Dent Assoc 1989;119:729–32.

9. Boghosian AA, Randolph RG, Jekkals VJ. Rotary instrument finishing of microfilled and small-particle hybrid composite resins. J Am Dent Assoc 1987;115:299–301.

10. Quiroz L, Lentz DL. The effect of polishing procedures on light-cured composite restorations. Compend Cont Educ Dent 1985;6:437–9.

11. Chen RCS, Chan DCN, Chan KC. A quantitative study of finishing and polishing techniques for a composite. J Prosthet Dent 1988;59:292–7.

12. Lambrechts P, Vanherle G. The use of glazing materials for finishing dental composite resin surfaces. J Oral Rehabil 1982;9:107–17.

CHAPTER 10

ANTERIOR RESTORATIONS

Choose a job you love and you will never have to work a day in your life.
Confucius

This chapter discusses the restorative treatment of Class III, Class IV, and Class V lesions with light-cured composite. For each class, it outlines preparation design, restoration placement, and finishing. The procedures described minimize the problems of voids and open margins often associated with polymerization shrinkage.

The following armamentarium applies to all three classes of lesion. Additional materials are identified in the restorative treatment for each class of lesion. The standard setup includes operator items, such as a gown, gloves, mask, and face shield. Isolation materials include retraction cord, rubber dam, interproximal wedges, and Mylar strips with a Mylar retention clip. Standard supplies include anesthetic, a caries indicator, and placement supplies, such as cotton forceps and placement brush. Instruments that are standard include an explorer, mouth mirror, periodontal probe, small spoon excavator, and handpiece with assorted cutting instruments. Standard equipment includes a curing light, radiometer, tooth dryer, air and water syringes, suction mechanism, and color-corrected light source.

Anterior restoration materials include:

- Suitable liner
- Appropriate conditioning or etching liquids or gels
- Appropriate enamel and dentin primers with bonding agents
- Pulp-capping material

Anterior restoration equipment includes:

- Quarter- and half-round burs
- Round-ended preparation diamonds
- Regular tapered and pointed 40-µm straight-sided diamonds

- Safe-ended 40-µm straight-sided diamonds (eg, Brasseler Finishing Safe-Ended Flame 8859 GKEF [fine]; Safe-Ended Flame 859 GKEF [extra fine], Brasseler Inc., Savannah, Georgia)
- Wood, plastic, or Cure-Thru wedge (Premier, King of Prussia, Pennsylvania)
- Small ball-ended applicator
- Interproximal carver and condenser
- Finishing discs (eg, Sof-Lex, 3M Dental Products, St. Paul, Minnesota)
- Finishing cups (eg, One Gloss, Shofu Dental Corp., Menlo Park, California)
- Diamond metal strips (eg, GC Metal Strips 300 and 600 grit (GC America Inc., Chicago, Illinois) or Premier Compo-strips)
- Bard Parker No. 12 blade and handle

CLASS III RESTORATIONS

When Class III preparations are surrounded by enamel, they are usually restored with a composite resin. In deeper restorations, a resin–ionomer liner can be used to replace the dentin portions of the tooth. In shallower restorations, a dentin–resin bonding agent is generally preferred to replace the dentin.

The rationale for using an internally placed glass ionomer is long-term sealing for reduced incidence of caries or pulp death. With larger direct resin restorations, a perfect seal is difficult to achieve and often impossible to maintain, providing access for caries development.

In restorations involving dentin margins, which are frequent in mature patients, a glass ionomer is often recommended for the entire restoration. Some clinicians coat this restoration with a composite resin immediately after placement to improve its durability.

Class III restorative treatment

Class III restoration requires the following materials in addition to the armamentarium prescribed at the beginning of the chapter:

- A radiopaque, agglomerated microfilled, submicron, or small-particle composite in compules, or a material that can be loaded into a syringe. In some clinical situations, an autoset composite or resin-modified glass-ionomer restorative is best. It would be ideal to place these materials with a syringe.

- No. 1 and No. 2 round-end diamonds (medium to fine grit)

Restoring enamel-only lesions

The goal of composite resin dentistry is the conservation of tooth structure. Since bonding allows composite restorative retention without mechanical undercuts, more conservative restorations are possible. If caries in a tooth can be removed without entering the dentin, no additional tooth reduction is necessary. This type of preparation and restoration is illustrated in Figure 10–1.

Preparation of dentin-involved lesions

Prior to rubber dam placement, clean the tooth and select the appropriate shade of composite.

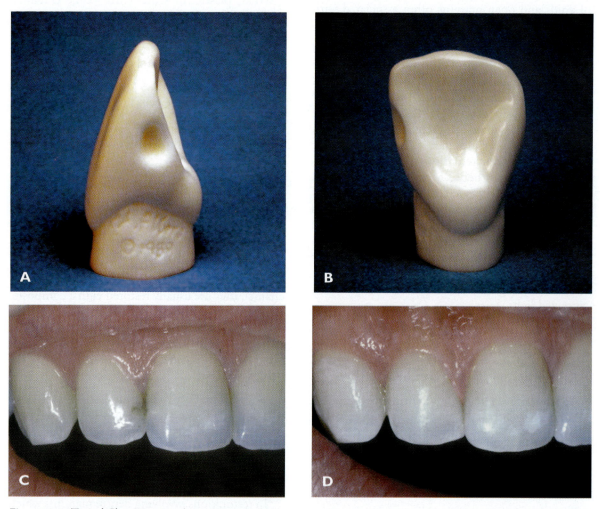

Figure 10–1. Typical Class III carious lesions treated with intra-enamel preparations: *A*, proximal view; *B*, lingual view; *C*, preoperative view; *D*, immediate postoperative view.

Outline. Make the initial entry with a small diamond or new round bur. If the lesion is equidistant between the facial and the lingual surfaces, using a lingual approach conserves labial tooth structure and is generally more esthetic (Figure 10–2). If the caries is mainly on the facial, a facial entry conserves tooth structure.

The outline form is dictated by the extent of caries and is roughly defined with a rotary instrument. If possible, maintain all or part of the proximal contact point. Since there is no "extension for prevention" in composite preparations, caries in dentin is removed with a spoon excavator or a slow-speed bur. Using a caries indicator is highly recommended.

Use a flame-shaped finishing diamond (or fine flame bur) to smooth the enamel walls and to round any unsupported enamel rods. Wherever possible, bevel the cavosurface margins to a 45 degree angle and a width of 0.5 mm or more on the lingual surface (Figure 10–3).

Retention. Acid-etching the enamel provides adequate retention for most restorations. In areas where there is little or no exposed enamel for bonding, use a trough undercut, usually at a depth of a quarter-round bur, 0.5 mm inside the cementoenamel junction. The undercut should not be placed at the expense of the axial wall. Retention is evaluated by seeing the tip of the explorer disappear into these retention areas. If a trough develops during excavation of caries, the resulting undercut may provide sufficient retention.

Enamel etching. Clean the preparation of all debris, making sure the enamel cavosurfaces are free of debris and base or liner. Place Mylar strips and wedges to protect adjacent teeth from the etching solutions. Isolate teeth and etch the enamel.

Placement of composite

Place a Mylar matrix and wedge. The Mylar strip contains the material, restores the proximal contact, and reduces flash. The wedge seals the gingival margin, separates teeth to ensure proximal contact, pushes the proximal dam and tissue gingivally, and opens the gingival embrasure.

Etch, rinse, and dry the enamel in the usual fashion. Place a bonding agent. Wet the cavosurface margins by brushing on a bonding agent as thinly and evenly as possible. Apply a stream of air to spread the bonding agent in a thin layer, and remove the excess. Polymerize.

Step 1. Place the composite with a composite syringe and wedge it between the preparation and a piece of Mylar (Figure 10–4).

Step 2. Pack the composite into the preparation with a condenser; score the edges with a carver.

Step 3. Pull the Mylar strip slowly through the contact to adapt the composite to the facial wall of the preparation.

Step 4. Remove the Mylar swiftly, with a quick snap. If the composite comes out with the Mylar, the composite either was too soft or had more surface area on the Mylar than on the tooth.

Step 5. Using an interproximal carver, remove any excess composite, and cure (40 seconds at 400 mW/cm^2 if EOP = 16 joules).

Step 6. Place another Mylar strip and inject composite from a syringe tip to fill the remaining

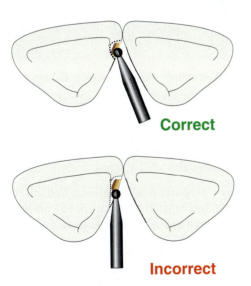

Figure 10–2. Schematic representation of the correct angled approach of the cutting instrument when making a Class III preparation. Angling preserves lingual tooth structure. The straight approach weakens the tooth and places more composite in function.

186 Tooth-Colored Restoratives

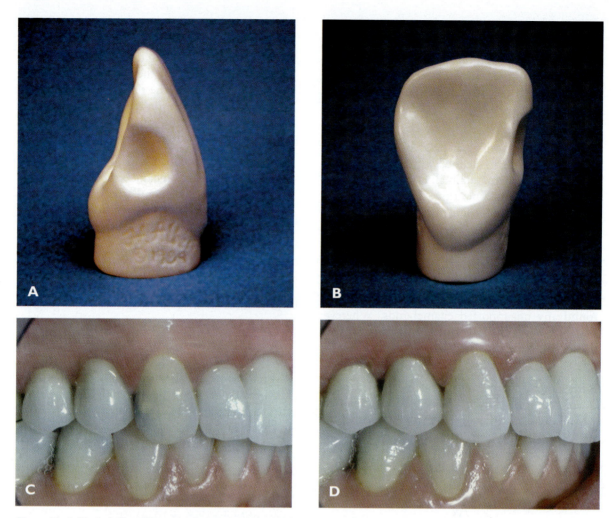

Figure 10–3. Typical Class III carious lesions treated with dentin–enamel preparations: *A*, proximal view; *B*, lingual view; *C*, preoperative view; *D*, immediate postoperative view.

area of the preparation. (Preparations with dentin involvement should be filled in at least two light-cured layers, as described here.)

Step 7. Pack the composite into the preparation with an interproximal carver.

Step 8. Pull the Mylar strip slowly through the contact to adapt the composite to the facial wall of the preparation.

Step 9. Remove the Mylar swiftly, with a quick snap.

Step 10. Remove any excess composite and completely contour the composite. Care should be taken to remove excess in difficult-to-reach areas, such as interproximal spaces. The contact area can be tightened by pressing the composite from buccal and lingual.

Large preparations involving dentin require multiple (more than two) layers of composite to control polymerization shrinkage (Figure 10–5).

Finishing and polishing

Step 1. Remove proximal flash with a sharp hand instrument or a No. 12 or No. 15 Bard Parker blade.

Step 2. Use fine diamonds for gross reduction. Also use a lubricant to reduce heat and friction. Overzealous gross reduction of composite can result

Anterior Restorations 187

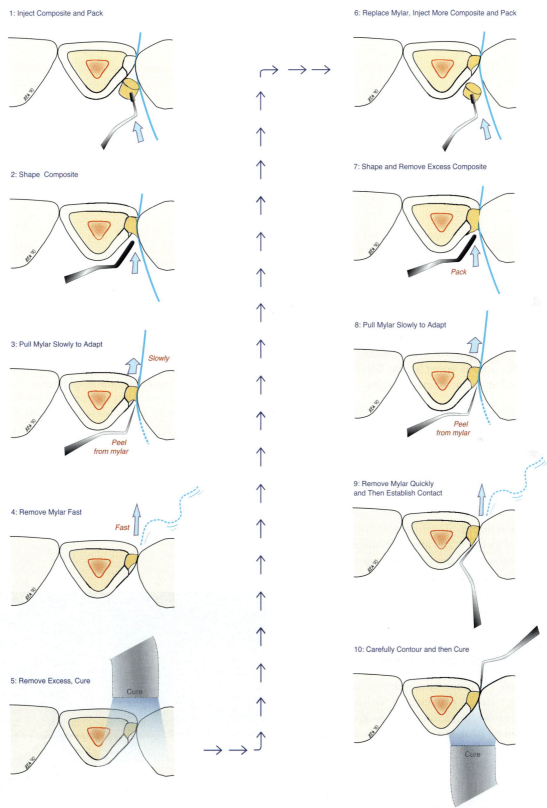

Figure 10–4. The procedure for treatment of a medium-size Class III preparation involving dentin. Two increments of light-cured composite are layered and contoured to create the restoration.

188 Tooth-Colored Restoratives

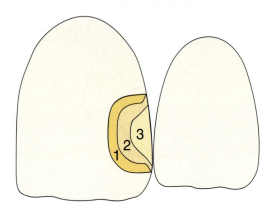

Figure 10–5. Treatment of a large Class III lesion requires at least three layers of composite to minimize polymerization shrinkage.

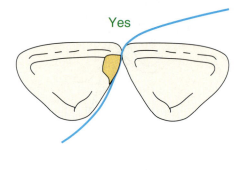

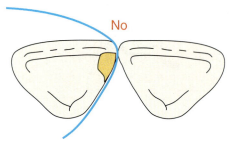

Figure 10–6. Correct use of a proximal strip to finish a Class III restoration involves pulling the strip through in an S-shaped pattern to maintain the contact point (top). Pulling the strip from the same side tends to open the proximal contact point (bottom).

in interfacial composite fractures and white line margins. These can weaken the restoration.

Step 3. When approaching the margins, use only micron diamonds, white stones, or flexible discs, with copious water spray. Finishing strips may be used at the proximal margins.

Step 4. Finish with a proximal strip (Figure 10–6).

It is common practice to remove all unsupported enamel in dental preparations. By bonding composite, however, unsupported enamel can be retained (Figure 10–7). The procedure involves bonding a stiff composite to the lingual surface of the enamel to support it as the dentin once did. The incisal edge is minimally affected. Once the restoration is completed, care must be taken to avoid occlusal contact over the composite supporting the enamel, since composite flexure can cause cracks in the enamel. A great amount of enamel can be preserved with this technique, which also results in better esthetics and longevity (Figure 10–8).

CLASS IV RESTORATIONS

When Class IV preparations are surrounded by enamel, they are usually restored with a composite resin. In deeper restorations, a resin–ionomer liner can be used to protect the dentin portions of the tooth. In shallower restorations, a dentin–resin bonding agent is generally preferred to replace the dentin.

When treating larger Class IV restorations with direct resin restoratives, it is often preferable to use two composite resins: a stiff internal material for support (such as a heavily filled hybrid) to increase stiffness and reduce fracture from cyclic fatigue, and a small-particle material (such as a microfilled or submicron composite) to provide the outer contour and finish.

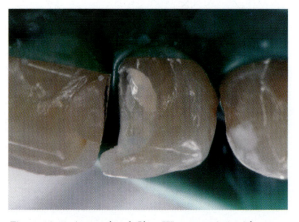

Figure 10–7. A completed Class III preparation with extensive caries removal and intact facial enamel.

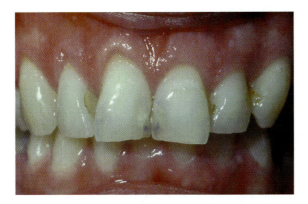 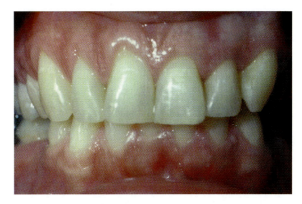

Figure 10–8. *A*, Preoperative view of multiple large Class III lesions with extensive dentin involvement. *B*, Immediate postoperative view. Note the high esthetics possible by retaining facial enamel.

A bonded porcelain restoration should be considered for restorations that are large and have no remaining enamel in the incisal edge or contact areas.

Class IV restorative treatment

The standard setup and supplies required are listed at the beginning of the chapter. Specific additional materials needed for Class IV restorations include:

- A light-cured submicron or small-particle composite in a tube, or a material that can be shaped without slumping. In some clinical situations, a heavily filled composite is used as a core. Some operators prefer to use a microfilled composite as the final surface material for these restorations.

- A bullet-shaped chamfer diamond

Preparations

Decide on the tooth shade prior to rubber dam placement. Anesthesia is often unnecessary for small fractures where the preparation is limited to enamel. Larger fractures with exposed dentin may be sensitive to air, cold water, and bur vibration and often require anesthesia. Determine the tooth shade, then place a rubber dam and clean the tooth with pumice and water.

Outline. These preparations are appropriate for fractures that run one-third to two-thirds of the incisal edge, which often expose dentin. Typical Class IV fractures are illustrated in Figure 10–9, *A*.

Most anterior teeth have horizontal and vertical grooves that can be used to hide the margins and increase the color-match and esthetic outcome (Figure 10–10).

Chamfer design. Prepare a chamfer 1-mm long (or half the length of the fracture) to half the depth of the enamel on the labial and lingual surface. This type of preparation results in the most durable restorative margins (Figures 10–9, *B*, and 10–11). It is important that the chamfer is cut only halfway through the enamel surface (Figure 10–12). Horizontal and vertical lines are easily hidden in anatomy, whereas oblique lines conflict with natural anatomy and surface texture and are, therefore, more visible. Stair-stepping the labial enamel with a good chamfer cavosurface margin into the tooth anatomy helps achieve a good esthetic result (Figure 10–13).

Beveled margins. An alternative to a stair-step chamfer design is to prepare a 2- to 3-mm bevel in place of a chamfer (Figures 10–9, *C*, 10–14, and 10–15). This bevel creates a gradual change of color from the tooth to the restoration. Although the beveled margin is not as durable as a chamfer, beveled preparations usually provide more consistent esthetic results. Scalloping the labial enamel with a beveled cavosurface margin is less important in achieving an esthetic result. It is best to finish these bevels in a curve, going from horizontal to facial (Figure 10–16). The major problem encountered at recall with beveled margins is chipping.

Enamel conditioning. Clean the preparation of all debris. Make sure the enamel cavosurfaces are clean of any dentin lining materials. After protecting the

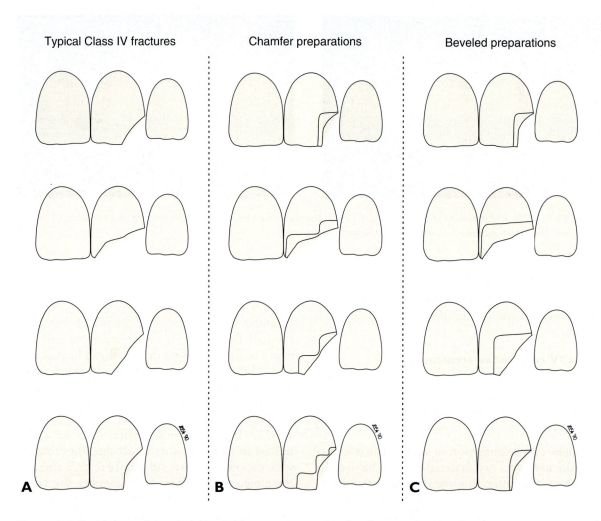

Figure 10–9. Facial views of *A*, typical Class IV fractures, *B*, typical outline forms used in chamfer Class IV preparations, and *C*, typical outline forms used in beveled Class IV preparations.

adjacent teeth with a Mylar strip, etch with acid using an enamel–resin bonding technique. This technique usually involves a 20-second etch of the enamel and a 10-second (or less) etch of the dentin, rinsing for a minimum of 5 seconds, then drying according to the manufacturer's recommendation for the specific bonding agent.

Composite placement

Prepare, etch, and dry the tooth; add bonding agent, and cure. Place a Mylar strip. Place and form the composite in a minimum of three increments, each 1- to 2-mm thick (Figure 10–17). For the first layer, the composite core, use a heavily filled ma-

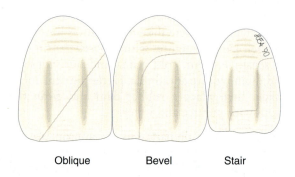

Figure 10–10. A facial view of the horizontal and vertical grooves that can be used to hide Class IV preparation margins and increase color-match and esthetic outcome.

Anterior Restorations 191

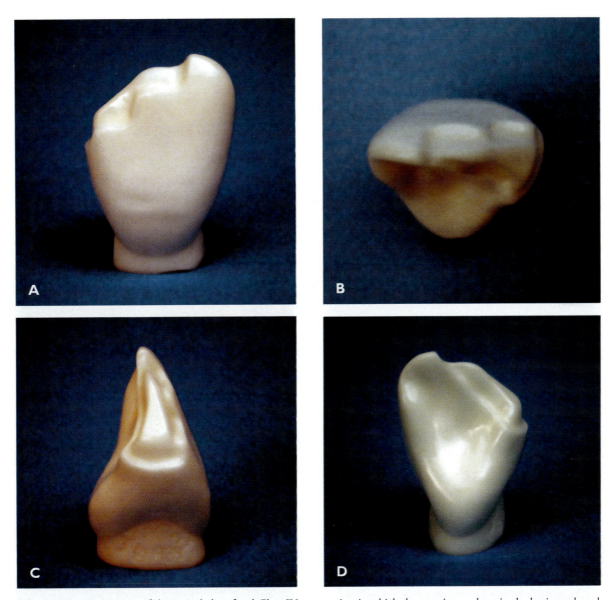

Figure 10–11. Four views of the typical chamfered Class IV preparation in which the margins are kept in the horizontal, and the vertical anatomic forms of the tooth are used to help hide the margins.

terial. Form it to the proper contour with Mylar, an interproximal carver, and an explorer. Remove the excess material from the gingival and proximal areas with an explorer. Polymerize for a minimum of 40 seconds on each side. For darker shades, polymerize for 60 seconds on each side (for materials with an EOP of 16 joules.)

Step 1. Place the composite core, using a heavily fill material. Wedge the composite between the Mylar strip and tooth fracture.

Step 2. Shape the composite core by slowly pulling the Mylar through to wrap the composite to the lingual, which draws the composite around the tooth.

Step 3. Polymerize the composite core.

Step 4. Place the contouring layer, using a submicron material.

Step 5. Slowly pull the Mylar strip through to wrap composite to the lingual.

192 Tooth-Colored Restoratives

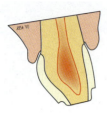

Figure 10–12. A facial-lingual cross-sectional view of a completed chamfered Class IV restoration.

Step 6. Separate the composite from the Mylar strip, and contour. Remove the strip quickly.

Step 7. Polymerize for a minimum of 40 seconds on each side (60 seconds for darker shades).

Step 8. Replace the Mylar strip. Add a final layer of composite, and contour. Slowly pull the Mylar strip through to wrap composite to the lingual. Pull the Mylar strip through rapidly to separate the strip from the composite. Remove the strip.

Step 9. Remove excess composite and carefully contour.

Step 10. Polymerize for a minimum of 40 seconds on each side (60 seconds for darker shades).

Step 11. When set, check for voids and excess material. Repair any voids.

Step 12. Wait 10 minutes after the last addition of composite before contouring the restoration.

Most composites do not cure thoroughly if built to a thickness greater than 2 mm. If the thickness of the fracture is in excess of 4 mm across the center of the restoration (from labial to lingual), the central area will be more than 2 mm from the surface. In this situation, multiple placement steps are necessary. Without the crown form in place, add and cure a central core of composite within 2 mm of the final surface of the restoration. After this addition, a crown form can be used for composite final placement. If a crown form is not being used, add the composite in layers with a plastic instrument. Make sure each layer is less than 2 mm thick, and cure after each addition. The final layer should be contoured and shaped until it closely resembles the desired shape of the tooth, and then polymerized.

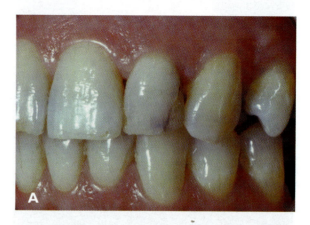

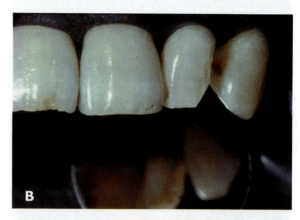

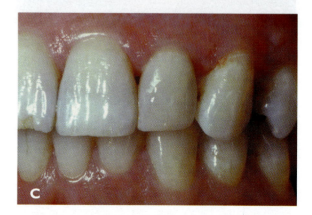

Figure 10–13. Chamfer design: *A*, Preoperative view; *B*, completed preparation; note stair-stepping; and *C*, immediate postoperative view.

Anterior Restorations 193

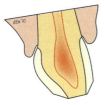

Figure 10–14. A facial-lingual cross-sectional view of a completed beveled Class IV restoration.

Finishing
Step 1. Remove flash with a sharp hand instrument or a No. 15 Bard Parker blade.

Step 2. Use fine diamonds for gross reduction. Also use a lubricant to reduce heat and friction.

Step 3. When approaching the margins, use only micron diamonds or flexible discs. A finishing strip is a good alternative at the proximal margins.

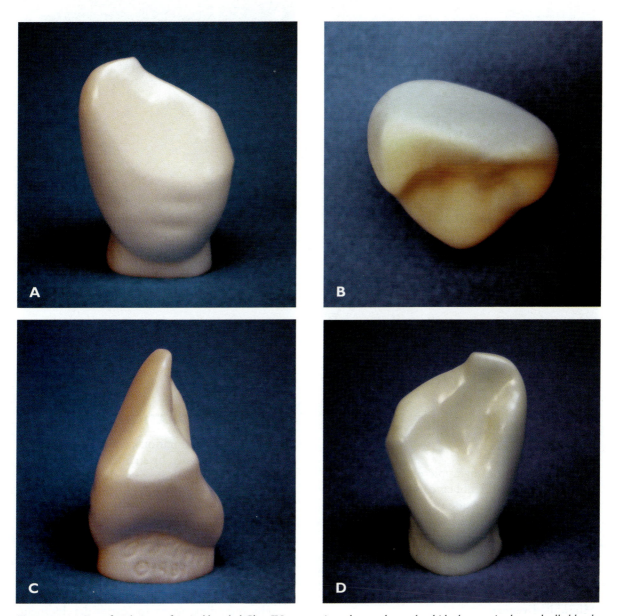

Figure 10–15. Four facial views of typical beveled Class IV preparations that can be used to hide the margins by gradually blending into the tooth surface.

194 Tooth-Colored Restoratives

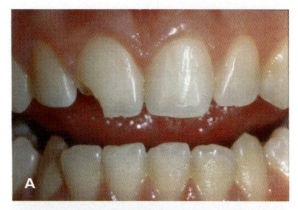
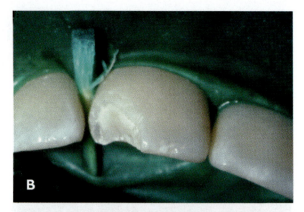
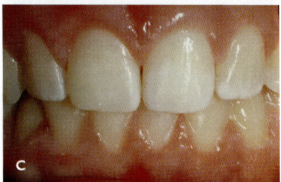
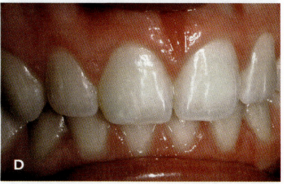
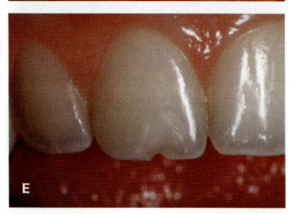

Figure 10–16. Bevel design: *A*, preoperative view; *B*, completed preparation; *C*, immediate postoperative view; *D*, six-month postoperative view; and *E*, fracture at 2 1/2 years postoperative, owing to fatigue and occlusal trauma.

Step 4. When using a microfill or submicron particle composite, rubber composite finishing cups and aluminum oxide pastes may be used to place the final finish. Occlusion plays an important role in the longevity of a restoration. The restoration should be in light occlusion (especially protrusive), since composites expand slightly over time.

Microfilled veneer
When it proves difficult to match a composite to the tooth, one solution is to veneer the restoration surface with a microfilled resin. If a full veneer is required, finish the resin away from tissue. In any case, finish it proximally just short of the contact (Figure 10–18).

CLASS V RESTORATIONS

As with Class IV restorations, when Class V preparations are surrounded by enamel, they are usually restored with a composite resin. In deeper restorations, a resin–ionomer liner is recommended to replace the dentin portion of the tooth. In shallower restorations, a dentin–resin bonding agent is generally preferred to replace the dentin.

Again, a glass ionomer is recommended with larger restorations because an adequate seal is difficult to achieve and often impossible to maintain, thereby providing access for caries development. The glass ionomer provides long-term sealing and reduction in caries or pulp death. In restorations

Anterior Restorations 195

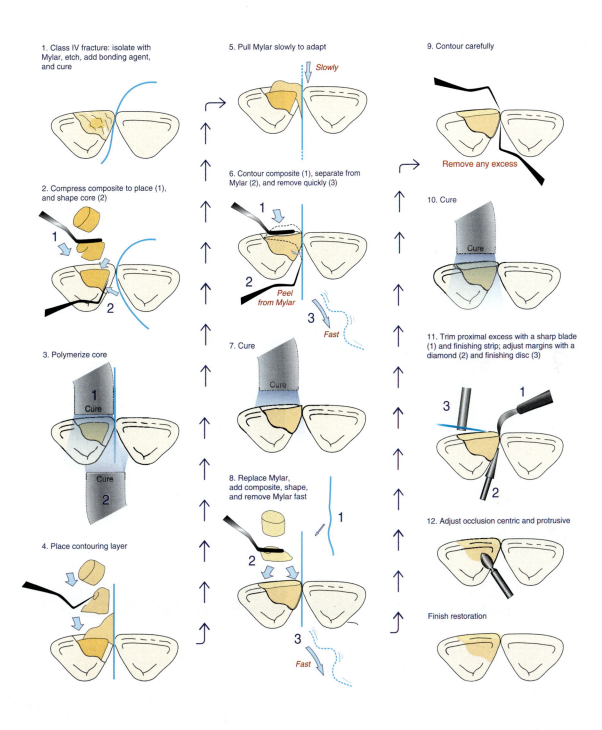

Figure 10–17. The procedure for treatment of a Class IV preparation involving dentin. Three increments of light-cured composite are layered and contoured to create the restoration.

196 Tooth-Colored Restoratives

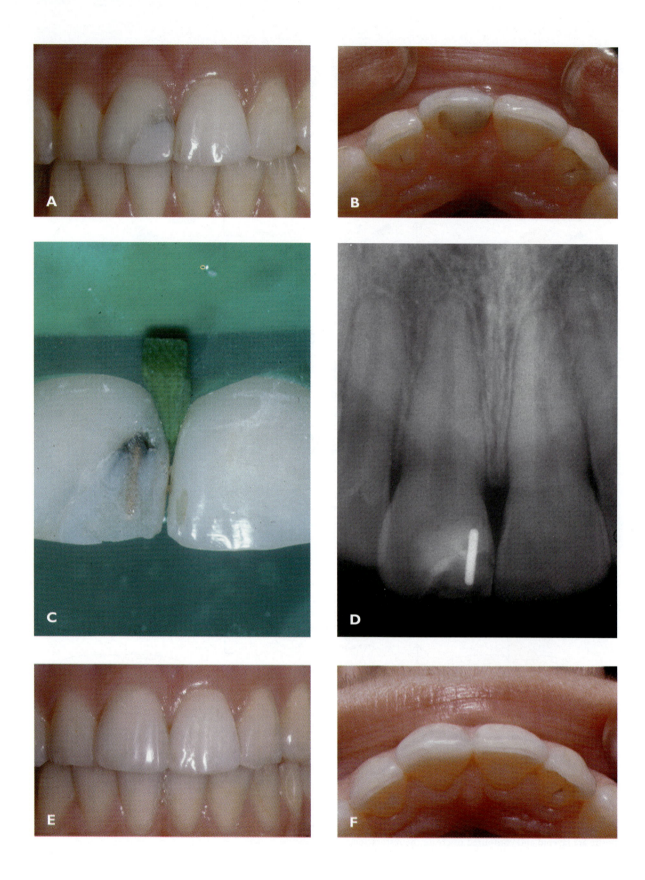

Anterior Restorations 197

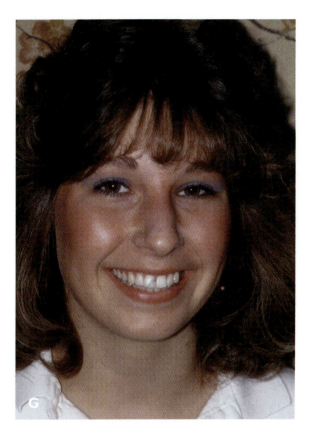
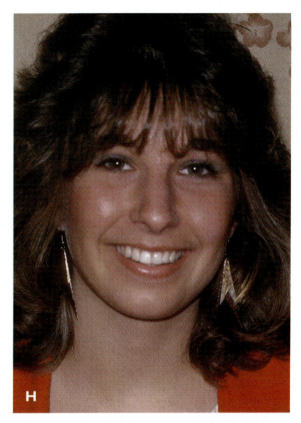

Figure 10–18. Large Class IV with discoloration owing to previous restoration with a metal pin. *A*, Preoperative facial view. *B*, Preoperative incisal view. *C*, Facial portion of restoration, prepared. Note severe discoloration from metal pin. *D*, Radiograph showing pin position. *E*, Postoperative facial view. *F*, Postoperative incisal view. *G*, Preoperative facial view. *H*, Postoperative facial view.

involving dentin margins, common with Class V lesions, a glass ionomer is often recommended for the entire restoration. Some clinicians coat the restoration with a resin glaze to improve the seal.

Class V restorative treatment

Specific materials needed for Class V restorations, in addition to the standard setup and materials identified at the beginning of the chapter, include:

- A restorative, such as a light-cured glass ionomer or a composite with dentin bonding
- No. 1 and No. 2 round-end diamonds (medium to fine grit)
- Cure-Thru cervical matrix

Caries in enamel only

The goal of composite resin dentistry is conservation of tooth structure. Bonding composite allows retention without mechanical undercuts. If it is possible to totally remove caries without entering the dentin, no additional tooth reduction is necessary; the composite is bonded to the remaining enamel. This type of preparation is illustrated in Figure 10–19.

Preparation for dentin-involved caries

Prior to rubber dam placement, pumice the tooth and select the appropriate shade of composite. Anesthetize for sensitive or deep lesions.

Outline. Make the initial entry with a medium-grit, small, round diamond. Keep the diamond perpendicular to the enamel surface. The ideal depth is the minimum depth to remove caries. The outline is determined by the caries present. Remove only carious tooth structure. The ideal preparation, viewed from the facial, should have rounded line angles (Figure 10–20).

198 Tooth-Colored Restoratives

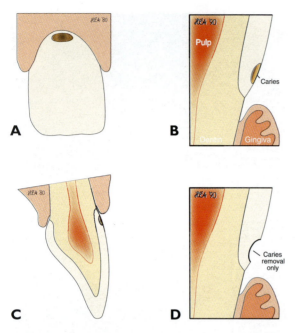

Figure 10–19. A typical Class V carious lesion in enamel only: *A*, frontal view, *B*, cross-section, *C*, close-up view and *D*, a typical intra-enamel preparation for this lesion.

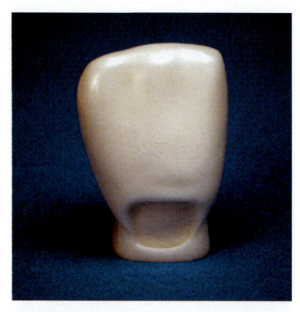

Figure 10–20. Typical Class V preparation.

Use a flame-shaped finishing bur or diamond to bevel the enamel cavosurface margins to achieve a 45-degree exit angle for the composite in the final restoration. A width of 0.5 mm is usually adequate. If the gingival margin is in dentin, leave a 90-degree exit.

Retention. Figure 10–21 illustrates a typical dentin–enamel preparation in the cervical area of an incisor. The portion of the preparation that is in dentin needs additional retention. Make a 0.5-mm groove inside the cementodentin junction with a quarter-round bur (Figure 10–22); place it 0.5 mm deep (or to 100% of the cutting flutes of the bur). It should not be placed at the expense of the axial wall. Figure 10–23 shows a typical clinical application of a Class V restoration with a gingival groove.

Pulpal protection. In deeper restorations, a glass-ionomer liner is usually placed on the axial wall over the dentin that leads to the pulp. In deep preparations that extend within 0.5 mm of the pulp, place a thin liner of calcium hydroxide (eg, Life, Kerr, Romulus, Michigan or Dycal, LD Caulk/Dentsply, Milford, Delaware) just over the exposure or near the exposure and then cover it with a glass-ionomer liner.

In the event of pulp exposure, dry and apply a calcium hydroxide liner over the exposed pulp. Cover this with a glass-ionomer liner.

Dentin bonding agents. If dentin bonding agents are to be used, limit the base to the deep areas of the exposed dentin. A base is unneccessary for maximum dentin bonding in shallow preparations.

Enamel conditioning. Acid etch the enamel with a gel etchant. Rinse with water and dry thoroughly with air.

Polymerization shrinkage considerations
Composite shrinkage upon polymerization is a problem in larger preparations, especially when a preparation has both enamel and dentin margins.

One-phase addition. In small preparations that have margins entirely in enamel, the restorative contracts away from the axial wall (Figure 10–24). This is called a contraction gap. Larger restorations may show white lines (or open margins) and should be filled in two steps to minimize the contraction gap.

When dentin margins are involved, the one-step placement technique often results in an open dentin margin (Figure 10–25). The opening of the dentin margin is reduced but not eliminated with the use of dentin bonding agents. Because the enamel–resin

Anterior Restorations

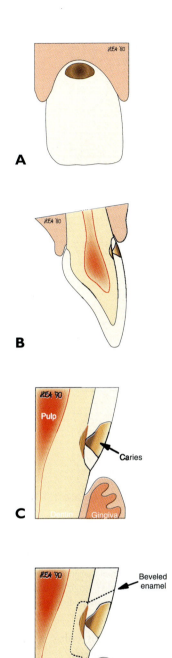

Figure 10–21. A typical carious lesion, *A*, front view, *B*, cross-section, *C*, close-up view; and *D*, the preparation outline for a Class V restoration involving enamel and dentin.

bond is usually greater than the dentin–resin bond, the dentin margin fails first as the composite shrinks.

Multiphase additions. Because composite resins shrink, filling preparations in multiple steps or

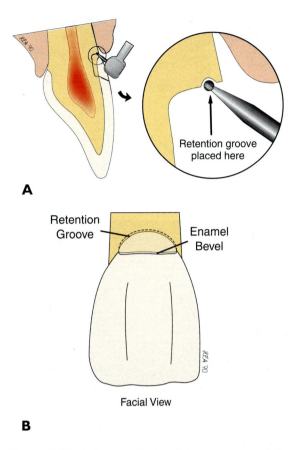

Figure 10–22. *A,* Cross-sectional and close-up views and, *B,* facial view of placement of a retention groove just inside the cavosurface margin of a Class V preparation for dentin bonding of composite.

layers is recommended to minimize opening of the dentin margin. The multilayer technique for a moderate size Class V preparation is illustrated in Figure 10–26.

Step 1. Place composite in the upper half of the preparation and contour with an interproximal carver. Cure.

Step 2. Add a second layer of composite to cover from the first layer to just short of the retention groove. Cure.

Step 3. Add a third layer of composite to fill in the retention groove and add the surface layer. Cure.

Step 4. Finish the margins with a safe-end diamond.

200 Tooth-Colored Restoratives

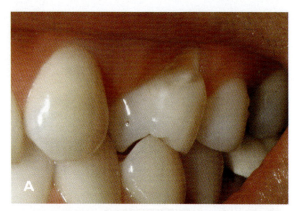
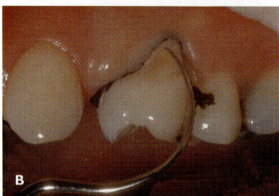
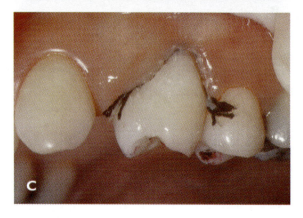

Figure 10–23. *A*, Preoperative view. *B*, Completed preparation of a Class V restoration with a gingival groove. *C*, Composite buildup, done in three layers.

Step 5. Smooth and polish the surface with rubber cups.

Note how the multiphase placement technique effectively reduces the impact of polymerization shrinkage (contraction gap) on the dentin margin. To improve esthetics, use a darker shade for the dentin addition and a lighter shade for the enamel

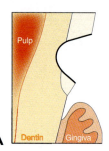
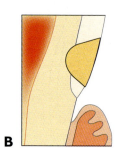
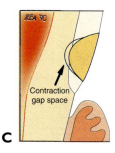

Figure 10–24. A facial-lingual cross-sectional view showing the contraction gap resulting from one-phase technique in a Class V restoration with all-enamel margins: *A*, finished preparation; *B*, single layer pre-cure; and *C*, single layer post-cure. This type of contraction gap is not desirable but is acceptable.

addition. This change of color is natural in the gingival third of many teeth.

Composite placement

The following technique is for preparations completely surrounded by etched enamel.

Step 1. Control moisture with retraction cord, suction, or a rubber dam.

Step 2. Wet the etched enamel margins with a bonding agent as thinly and evenly as possible. With an air syringe, apply a stream of air to the preparation to spread the bonding agent in a thin layer; remove excess, and polymerize.

Anterior Restorations   201

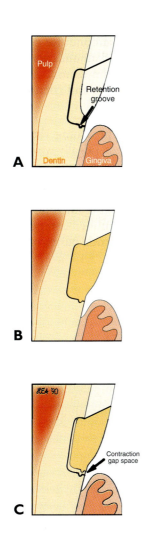

Figure 10–25. A facial-lingual cross-sectional view showing the contraction gap resulting from one-phase technique in a Class V restoration with dentin–enamel margins: *A*, finished preparation; *B*, single layer pre-cure; and *C*, single layer post-cure. This type of contraction gap is not acceptable.

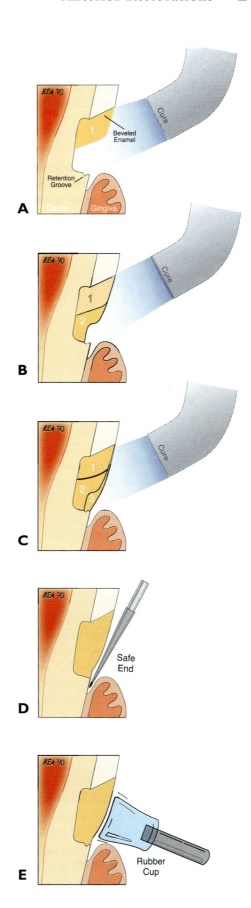

Figure 10–26. The recommended multiphase procedure for treatment of a Class V lesion with enamel and dentin margins: *A*, first layer cured; *B*, second layer cured; *C*, third layer cured; *D*, finishing; and *E*, polishing. A contraction gap is less likely to occur with multilayer placement of composite. Composite is always placed and cured on the enamel first.

Step 3. Place the composite, using a plastic instrument or a composite syringe. For restorations more than 1-mm thick, add composite in 1-mm increments and cure each increment for the appropriate time.

Pre-polymerization contouring

Pre-polymerization contouring is an alternative to the Class V matrix. To use this option, shape and sculpt the composite with a fine explorer. Completely remove the excess on the margins and shape to ideal contour and smoothness prior to curing.

Finishing and Polishing

Step 1. Remove flash with a sharp hand instrument or a No. 12 or No. 15 Bard Parker blade.

Step 2. Use fine diamonds for gross reduction. Special straight-sided diamonds with safe-cut tips help avoid ditching the dentin. Use water as a lubricant to reduce heat and friction when gross reduction is needed.

Step 3. When approaching the margins, use only micron diamonds (ideally with safe-cut tips) or flexible discs. Finishing strips may be used at the proximal margins.

Step 4. When using a microfill or submicron particle composite, rubber composite finishing cups and aluminum oxide pastes may be used to place the final finish.

CHAPTER 11

DIRECT POSTERIOR COMPOSITES

Change is the law of life. And those who look only to the past or the present are certain to miss the future.

John F. Kennedy

The major benefit of a posterior composite is that it allows the practitioner to place a conservative initial restoration, one that preserves considerably more tooth structure than an amalgam restoration. The typical amalgam restoration occupies 25% of the occlusal surface, whereas the typical composite restoration occupies 5%.[1] Composite can be placed in an existing amalgam preparation, but this type of restoration does not provide the durability of an initial composite restoration.[2]

Posterior composites generally are indicated for initial carious lesions in low–stress-bearing areas. They have advantages, such as more conservative preparations and better adhesiveness, and disadvantages, such as softness and high wear rate. Specifically, composite resins can support weak cusps and provide an excellent bond. But because the stiffness, wear rate, and fracture resistance of even the best composite is less than that of other restorative materials, a large composite that holds cusps together should be considered only a temporary measure.

CONSIDERATIONS WITH POSTERIOR COMPOSITE RESTORATIONS

Many clinicians have used amalgam preparations for posterior composites. This results in a restoration that does not take advantage of the benefits of composite preparation design. For example, resin restorations are often prepared with beveled cavosurface margins to increase the surface area of enamel rods for bonding, and extensions for caries prevention are unnecessary. Uninvolved grooves are sealed, not prepared and restored, and effort is made to retain the proximal contacts. Unlike amalgam, no bulk is required for durability, such that there is no minimum thickness or width for strength except to accommodate the size of the syringe tip and condenser used for placement.

These differences in preparation design result in restorations that are considerably more conservative than their amalgam counterparts, often 1 mm or less when placed over enamel.

A caveat on size: if a composite is to be placed in a large conventional amalgam preparation with occlusal holding contacts or no proximal enamel holding stops, or if over 50% of the intercuspal area is to be replaced, it should be considered an interim restoration only. The preferred treatment is an indirect restoration.

Advantages

Posterior composites can perform well in highly esthetic and conservative preparations. They bond to enamel with an excellent seal and can hold weakened cusps together. They can be placed in stress-bearing restorations, which makes them ideal for lengthening cusp tips; however, adequate resistance-form is critical to protect the restoration from shear forces. They have low thermal conductivity, no galvanism, and eliminate the possibility of mercury toxicity. Their cost is not affected by fluctuations in precious metal prices. In terms of placement, composites have a shorter setting time, can be polished during the placement appointment, and are easily repaired.

Disadvantages

Posterior composites are susceptible to wear or breakage, especially in large stress-bearing restorations. They have no caries inhibiting properties (whereas glass-ionomer materials do), a poor coefficient of thermal expansion, less stiffness than other restoratives, and a greater tendency to fracture than amalgam. Placement is technique-sensitive and requires hands-on training. Restoring with composite also takes longer than restoring with amalgam. Owing to leakage and flexure, composite restorations show increased potential for pulpal irritation, especially when used by a clinician who does not understand each component of the materials.

Small, well-protected areas are the best locations for these restorations. Extreme care must be used to ensure marginal integrity, since microorganisms are the major cause of recurrent caries and pulpal sensitivity. A void at the margin could result in postoperative sensitivity, recurrent caries, and rapid failure of the restoration. Even with careful placement, inherent polymerization shrinkage makes it difficult to maintain a tight seal in preparations with opposing margins (eg, margins on the mesial and distal boxes).

Polymerization shrinkage

Polymerization shrinkage is of critical concern with posterior restorations because of the potential for gaps. Composites shrink 1.2 to 4.5% by volume and 0.2 to 1.9% by linear measure. Polymerization forces are generally 2.8 to 7.3 MPa,[3] which is considerably less than the tensile strength of enamel (20 to 40 MPa).[4] Enamel bonding procedures help compensate for this shrinkage by directing it away from the margins; but polymerization shrinkage generally results in marginal gaps in posterior composites.[5,6]

Almost all Class II composites leak at the gingival margin.[7] These spaces are called contraction gaps and usually occur at the gingival cavosurface margins, where the enamel is thin. Polymerization shrinkage averages 1.5 to 2.5% in most posterior composites. This corresponds to a gap of 2 to 10 μm in the typical proximal box. Bacteria are only a fraction of this size and easily enter this space. The typical contraction gap of a posterior restoration is illustrated in Figure 11–1. If there is no enamel at the gingival floor, these gaps can spread greatly. Layering composite in many individually cured increments can compensate for this polymerization shrinkage, since each addition shrinks less.

Sensitivity

Postoperative sensitivity is of particular concern with posterior composite restorations. There is evidence that patients are more likely to experience postoperative sensitivity to biting with composite restorations (19%) compared with amalgams

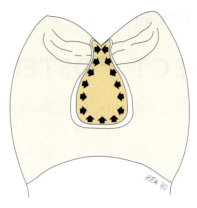

Figure 11–1. Schematic representation of the proximal view of the contraction gap that results from polymerization shrinkage in a composite resin.

(3%).[8] Although a variety of factors can cause or contribute to sensitivity in these restorations, tooth movement and stress under function increase the likelihood of problems.

Cuspal strain results from the constant movement of weakened cusps under function and can result in pain during chewing as well as enamel crazing near the gingiva. This problem is less severe with smaller composite restorations. Inadequate stiffness is of particular concern with large composites. Few composites are able to stabilize weakened cusps. Although large composite restorations show improved fracture resistance, they do not prevent cuspal movement (Figure 11–2).

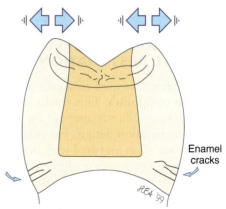

Figure 11–2. Polymerization shrinkage of large restorations can pull cusps together and cause facial and lingual cracks in enamel. In addition, the lack of stiffness in composites allows cusp movement during function, which can cause or increase buccal and lingual enamel fractures.

Polymerization shrinkage can cause intercuspal tension (experienced as sensitivity) between bonded cusps, especially with large autocured resin restorations. Layering the composite in increments so that just a few walls are involved in each polymerization reduces this tension and the overall stress on the bonded interface and the opposing cusps.

Hyperocclusion is also common with composite restorations, since, unlike amalgam, they do not go through a soft stage that deforms under stress. After curing, high spots are more obvious to a patient. In addition, most composites enlarge slightly as they absorb moisture.

Other sources of sensitivity include contamination and loss of seal at the margins, and inadequate polymerization of the resin components in bonded systems. Incomplete polymerization can cause voids when unset monomers leach out. In this case, the tooth sensitivity is attributable to bacterial invasion.

Perhaps the most common cause of sensitivity is open odontoblastic tubules, the result of the clinician's failure to adequately close the tubules after acid etching. Open tubules are more permeable to chemicals and bacteria. Patients can experience sensitivity during flossing and increased sensitivity to air owing to dentin permeability.

Longevity

An average amalgam and a properly placed composite last between 5 and 10 years.[9] Small non–stress-bearing posterior composites last considerably longer. These are typically used in conjunction with occlusal sealants. The sealant portion of the restoration may require small repairs over time.

The 5-year failure rate of all posterior composites is 9.2%, according to one study.[10] The causes were wear (0.4%), caries (3.2%), fractures (2.8%), and other (2.8%). Some studies show the wear rate of posterior composites decreases over time.[11]

One clinical study placed amalgams on one side of the mouth and composites on the other.[12] All preparations followed conventional amalgam preparation technique. After three years, 80% of the amalgams were clinically acceptable, whereas only 46% of the composites were clinically acceptable. The major difference in the composite restorations was occlusal wear.[12] Composites do not perform as well when used as a replacement for amalgam in large preparations. Composites should be used in conservative preparations and mainly kept out of occlusion.[13] These recommendations are based on the best existing research, most of which was conducted over a decade ago. Materials have since been improved and perform well under more clinically demanding applications; however, few clinical studies over the past 10 years have evaluated the longevity of posterior composites, and the studies completed have looked at only 2- to 3-year results.

POSTERIOR PIT AND FISSURE SEALANTS

Among the most conservative and successful of the posterior resin restorations are the occlusal sealants.[14–16] Applied before known caries invasion, sealants are a great preventive: an unsealed first molar is 22 times more likely to become carious than a sealed tooth.[17] In adolescents, 65% of molar sealants last 7 years. In this same age group, the average life span of an amalgam is 4 to 8 years.[18]

Many studies show a high degree of caries prevention after a single application of sealant. In one long-term clinical study, 10 years after a single sealant application, sealant was totally retained on 57% of the teeth treated, and partially retained on 21%.[19] In addition, 84% of teeth sealed only once remained sound after 10 years. Sealants in primary teeth have a retention rate similar to that noted in permanent teeth.[20] Premolars are more retentive than molars.[21] Sealants in maxillary molars have only 60% of the retention rate of mandibular molars.[22]

Sealants are also quicker to place than amalgam, taking less than half the time, and since their average cost is half that of an amalgam, they are highly cost-effective.[23] One 10-year study reported that the cost of a nonsealed tooth was 1.64 times higher than that of a sealed tooth. For every two surfaces sealed, the patient benefited by needing one less surface restoration because of caries.[19]

Patients lose more sealant in the first 6 to 12 months after placement than during later recall periods. The call for retreatment is greatest at 6 months, when typically 17% of placed sealants need enhancement or replacement. The average success rate for a sealant varies between 50% and

90% for first-time placements. Apparently, once a satisfactory seal is obtained, it is maintained until lost through abrasion.

What if decay is left under a sealant?

There is strong evidence that sealants without microleakage arrest any carious activity under them. Micik,[24] Handelman and colleagues,[25,26] Going and co-workers,[27] and Mertz-Fairhurst and co-workers[28] reported a reversal of carious activity when pits or fissures were sealed (100%, 100%, 100%, and 83%, respectively). Other 2-year retrospective studies have confirmed a lack of carious activity under restorations that remained sealed.[29,30] The researchers in the follow-up studies noted that these results held only for sealants that remained intact. Thus, recall visits are important to monitor sealant integrity.

Despite such clinical evidence, a patient is realistically much better off when all the caries is removed. All sealants eventually fail, and when they do on teeth with previously arrested caries, the result is rapid and extensive recurrent caries. Complete removal of decay also increases retention.

Preparation and placement

Isolation

Tooth isolation is key to achieving a well-sealed restoration. Fortunately, isolation of occlusal areas is relatively easy. Figure 11–3 shows a photograph of a slit or sleeve dam. The dam provides good isolation of the occlusal surfaces, avoids patient aspiration of objects, and aids in evaluation. When this technique fails, cotton rolls and suction or retraction devices are proven alternatives.

Sealant preparations

Studies show that acid etching solutions are unable to penetrate the deeper recesses of pits and fissures, and that debris also remains in these areas (Figure 11–4). Thus, cleaning these areas with a bur or air abrasion and making small preparations is essential to sealant retention. Clinical studies show that appropriate preparations can improve the overall 6-year retention rate of sealant from 65% to 85% and can double the 6-year retention rate for upper molars from 47% to 87%.[22]

Etchants

There has been some concern about whether liquid etchants and gels are equally effective. Gener-

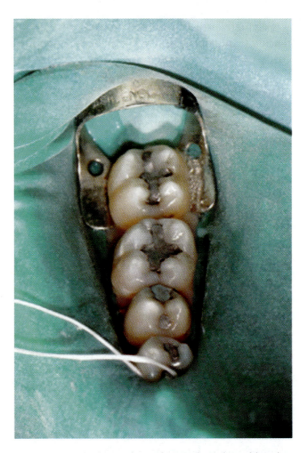

Figure 11–3. A slit or sleeve dam with molar rubber dam clamp in place. The dam is made by cutting a slit through two holes, usually at the first molar and first premolar. The dam is then stretched over the clamp and into the proximal space distal to the cuspid.

ally speaking, gels are as effective as liquid etchants,[31] providing the gel has access. In deep pits and fissures, a clinician must carefully verify the completeness of an etch.

Sealant repairs

Repairing sealants that have become worn improves their integrity. If a portion of sealant is lost, the tooth can be rebonded. In some studies, reapplication has twice the success rate of first-time placement. In cases where the sealant is lost and not repaired, in vitro research shows that enamel areas adjacent to the remaining sealant are more resistant to decay than areas not initially sealed.[32] This is thought to occur because of the remaining resin tags in the enamel. One 7-year clinical study showed that partial loss of a sealant leads to a caries incidence on that surface similar to the caries

Direct Posterior Composites 207

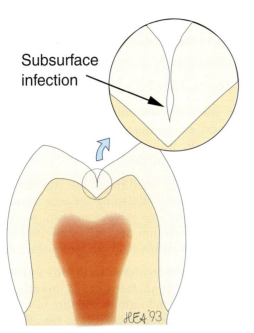

Figure 11–4. Cross-section diagram of a typical pit and fissure.

incidence on an untreated control surface.[18] No studies have reported an increased rate of caries when sealants are totally lost. Most clinical evidence concludes that sealant efficacy is associated with complete sealant retention. With proper recall evaluation and maintenance, intact sealants are nearly 100% effective in controlling occlusal decay.

Types of materials available

Both autocured and light-cured sealants are available. The light-cured sealants give a clinician more time for placement and cure more rapidly. In addition, when multiple teeth are being sealed, the total time required for light-curing may be greater than if an autocured system were used. Laboratory studies have shown that the bond strength and abrasion resistance of autocured and light-cured sealants is the same.[33] Some clinical studies have shown no difference in their retention rates on 2-year follow-up examination.[21,34] In other research, autocured sealants demonstrated a slightly better retention rate than light-cured sealants after 1 year.[35]

Sealants are usually made of filled or unfilled resins. In the past, unfilled resins were used for occlusal sealants, and success rates varied from 65% to 100%.[16] Case selection and placement methods had a role in the longevity of these restorations. Long-term studies on filled sealants have been favorable, showing that the wear rate of a sealant is directly proportional to its filler content: the higher the filler content, the better the wear.[33,35] A highly filled sealant placed with a bonding agent is significantly better at preventing occlusal caries.[36] One 10-year study showed complete retention of filled sealants in 72% of treated teeth after 5 years, and in 37% of treated teeth after 10 years.[37] Filled sealants also yielded better results than unfilled sealants in a 5-year clinical study.[38]

Adding filler increases a sealant's durability and reduces its polymerization shrinkage and coefficient of thermal expansion, thereby reducing the potential for microleakage and chipping (Figure 11–5). Filled sealants are commercially available or can be made by mixing a composite with an unfilled resin.

A disadvantage of filled sealants is that the more viscous they become, the more they require a bonding agent. The optimum amount of loading for a filled sealant is not known, although materials of 30 to 50% filler (by weight) have been clinically successful. Occlusion must be checked after placing a filled sealant, because if it is high, the patient will not be able to chew it into place as is common with unfilled sealants.

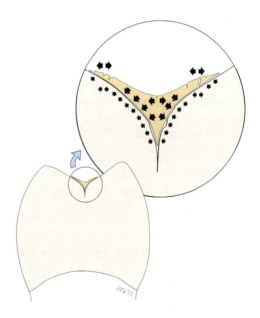

Figure 11–5. The insert depicts how changes in the coefficient of thermal expansion can cause a sealant to loosen—the result of long-term thermal contraction and expansion of the resin matrix.

A sealant material must have enough flow to penetrate pits and fissures and enough fracture toughness to resist chipping from occlusal forces and resistance wear. Generally, filler rates between 30% and 65% by weight can be used for this purpose. Composites with this filler range are available under a variety of product names: composite resin cement, porcelain veneer luting cement, flowable composite, and occlusal sealant. These materials vary in viscosity, color, and mode of initiation, and any of them can be used successfully as a sealant. Since these low-fill flowable materials have multiple uses, a dentist can select one for multipurpose application. An untinted or universal shade of fluid composite can be used effectively as a sealant, veneer luting agent, and repair material. Such a material, if it were dual-cured, could also be used to cement crowns, conventional bridges, and bonded bridges.

Altering the viscosity of a composite

A composite's viscosity can be altered in three ways: temperature (the higher the temperature, the higher the viscosity), vibration (vibration increases flow or viscosity), and mixing with a lower-viscosity resin, such as an unfilled bonding resin (not a water-soluble dentin-bonding primer or adhesive). Thus a dentist can manipulate viscosity to meet the needs of a particular clinical situation.

A filled sealant can be made by mixing about two drops of resin to a 4-mm length of composite (this varies depending on the viscosity of the composite). The result should be a creamy but flowable mix. Beware that mixing incorporates air, which weakens the resin. Commercially filled sealants are mixed in a vacuum and do not have this problem.

When a filled sealant is used, the unfilled resin (ie, bonding agent) is placed and spread into a thin, even layer with air. Then the composite-sealant mixture is added with a brush, plastic instrument, or composite syringe.

Restorative treatment: light-cured sealants

Clinical studies show that when light-cured sealants are cured for only 20 seconds (which is half the advisable time but is recommended by many manufacturers), their retention rate is lower than that of autocured sealants. In one clinical study of the 20-second cure method, the retention rate for 1 year was 86% for light-cured sealants and 94% for autocured sealants.[39]

Procedure for placement of sealant

Step 1. Place a rubber dam or slit dam to isolate the teeth to be treated.

Step 2. Teeth with heavy debris and plaque should be cleaned with a particle blasting device, either water abrasion or air abrasion. Relatively clean teeth can be treated with 3% hydrogen peroxide on a bristle brush. Do not use pumice, since it can plug pits and fissures.

Step 3. Use a small round bur (eg, fissure bur or 1/4-round) or sandblasting device to remove any organic stain in deep grooves and fissures. A drop of disclosing solution can be used to determine if all the organic debris has been removed.

Step 4. Etch deciduous teeth for 15 to 30 seconds, primary teeth for up to 2 minutes (until frosty) in the usual fashion. Be sure to carry the etchant 2 mm up the cusp inclines. Liquid etchant is preferred because it penetrates pits and fissures better than gels.

Step 5. Trace grooves with an explorer to ensure air bubbles are not preventing the etchant from reaching the deepest grooved areas. Wipe the etching solution off the explorer immediately after use to prevent corrosion.

Step 6. Wash for at least 15 seconds. If the pits and fissures are unusually deep, rinse longer (30 s).

Step 7. Dry using a warm air dryer, high-speed vacuum, or an air syringe (in that order of preference) for a minimum of 15 seconds. If disclosing solution was used, none should remain in the pit or fissure. Repeat steps 3, 4, 5, and 6 if the enamel does not appear uniformly chalky white. A second etch may be applied for 30 seconds if only a slight additional etch is required.

Step 8. Place unfilled sealants using a manufacturer's applicator, brush, explorer, or ball burnisher. For filled sealants, apply and cure the bonding agent before placing the sealant. *Note: Do not shake the sealant bottle as this incorporates air bubbles into the material. If the coloring agent settles in the bottle, use a brand of sealant that will not do this.*

Step 9. Trace the sealant through the grooves with an explorer to remove entrapped air bubbles.

Step 10. For unfilled sealants, remove the excess with a dry cotton pellet. For filled sealants, remove excess material with a dry plastic brush. In either case, a thin line of sealant should remain in the deepest part of the grooves.

Step 11. Cure light-activated sealants for at least 40 seconds. If the occlusal surface is wider than the diameter of the curing tip, repeat the cure, overlapping the cure areas.

Step 12. Check the occlusion. Adjustments are usually necessary when using a filled sealant. Micron diamonds are the instruments of choice for this purpose.

Figure 11–6 shows the clinical sequence for placement of a conservative sealant.

PREVENTIVE RESIN RESTORATIONS, CLASS I

A Class I posterior composite preparation should be conservative and affect only enamel whenever possible. Tooth structure is removed only to gain access to and eliminate decay. There is no extension for prevention: any preventive procedure should be done with an occlusal sealant and should not involve removal of sound tooth structure. This restoration is called a preventive resin restoration (Figure 11–7).[40–42]

The preparation should affect dentin only when caries is present. When deep caries is removed, a durable base or liner should be placed (eg, a glass-ionomer liner) prior to placement of composite. Teeth with larger caries, involving extensive removal of enamel, should be restored with a heavily filled composite resin (ie, a Class I composite resin).

Restorative treatment, Class I

The occlusal outline of a posterior composite restoration does not have the form of an amalgam preparation. There are major differences in depth, width, and exits. Only carious enamel and dentin are removed in composite preparations. Figure 11–8 illustrates a typical conservative composite preparation.

A posterior composite preparation should extend into dentin only when required for caries removal. To clean tight grooves, cut a preparation half the thickness of enamel. To remove caries in enamel, cut the preparation to the width of a composite syringe tip or condenser tip so the preparation can be easily filled. If no caries is present, remove no enamel. Protect noncarious developmental grooves with a sealant.

There are a number of acceptable occlusal exits for composite restorations. The most common in smaller preparations is a 90-degree cavosurface margin that is beveled to expose the enamel rod ends. Such exposure improves bonding and ensures an optimal seal. The horizontal component of this design helps maintain the seal that may be lost during composite polymerization. Some clinicians believe that bevels are unnecessary since conservative 90-degree exits in central pits already expose many enamel rod ends (Figure 11–9); however, studies show preparations with a bevel have a bet-

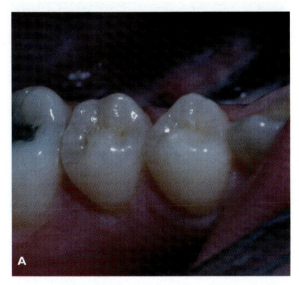
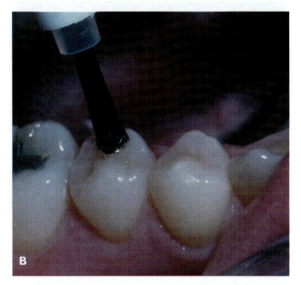

Figure 11–6. Placement of a conservative sealant. *A*, Preoperative view of the molars to be sealed. *B*, Application of etchant.

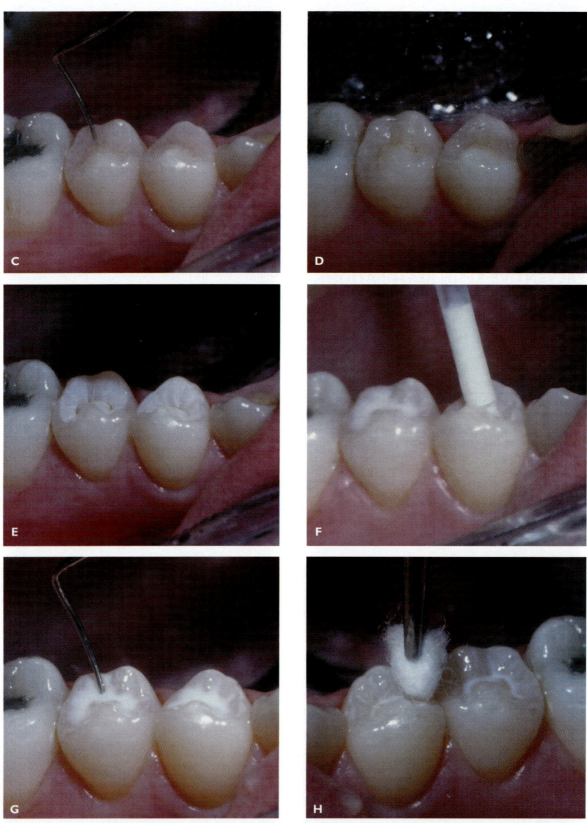

Figure 11–6. *C*, An explorer is used to release air bubbles and ensure that etchant reaches the bottom of the fissure. *D*, Gentle rinsing with water. *E*, After thorough drying with air, the site is inspected for uniform etch. *F*, Sealant is applied. *G*, An explorer is used to trace the fissure, removing bubbles and ensuring that sealant reaches the bottom of the fissure. *H*, Excess sealant is removed with a cotton pellet to reduce occlusal interference.

Direct Posterior Composites 211

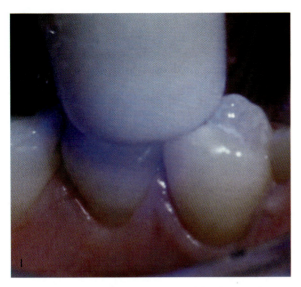
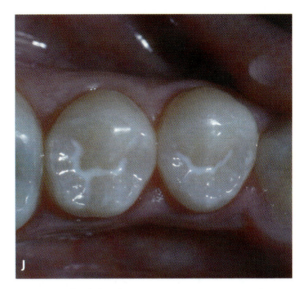

Figure 11–6. *I*, The sealant is light-cured for 40 seconds. *J*, Postoperative view of sealed molars.

ter seal than those without one.[43] Large restorations on worn teeth do not expose many rod ends, so a beveled preparation is recommended.

With larger preparations, the use of an adhesive enamel exit conserves unsupported enamel by rounding the tooth and etching three sides (Figure

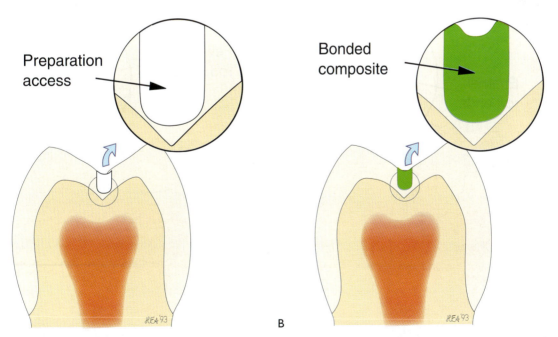

Figure 11–7. Cross-section diagram of Class I composite restoration: *A*, area of caries removal in enamel; *B*, composite placed in enamel defect.

212 Tooth-Colored Restoratives

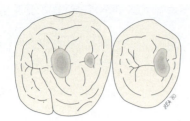

Figure 11–8. Diagram showing occlusal view of a typical conservative Class I composite preparation.

11–10). When using this design, a clinician should be careful to remove any decay that might remain under the unsupported enamel. Studies show that this design provides the best seal.[43]

Procedure for preventive resin restoration

Figure 11–11 demonstrates the procedure for preventive resin restoration.

Step 1. Place a rubber dam or slit dam to isolate the teeth that will be treated.

Step 2. Apply caries indicator (see Figure 11–11, *A*). Rinse with water for 10 seconds. Reexamine tooth to detect decay (see Figure 11–11, *B*).

Step 3. Use a small spoon to remove any stained (decayed) areas (see Figure 11–11, *C*).

Step 4. Restain, wash, and re-check tooth to ensure all decay has been removed (see Figure 11–11, *D*). Use a spoon or slow-speed round bur to remove additional stain, as necessary.

Step 5. Acid etch the tooth for 30 seconds, rinse with water for 10 seconds, dry thoroughly with an air syringe, and examine (see Figure 11–11, *E* and *F*).

Step 6. Apply bonding agent according to manufacturer's directions (see Figure 11–11, *G*).

Step 7. Place composite. Light-cure for 40 seconds (see Figure 11–11, *H*).

Step 8. Apply sealant to cover the restored surface (see Figure 11–11, *I*). Light-cure for 40 seconds.

Step 9. Remove rubber dam (or slit dam). Check occlusion with articulating paper (see Figure 11–11, *J*). Adjust occlusion as necessary with a fine diamond or white stone.

Composite and sealant

A preventive resin restoration using a resin in conjunction with a sealant minimizes extensions (for prevention) and preserves tooth structure.[44,45] Placement of a free-flowing sealant over an occlusal

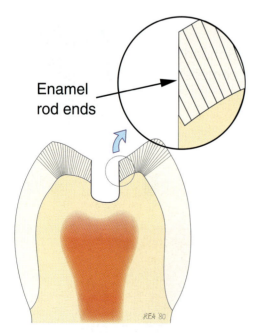
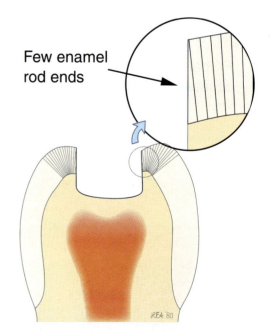

Figure 11–9. *A*, Diagram of proximal view of a Class I composite restoration preparation using a standard amalgam-type 90-degree exit. This preparation is appropriate when only small lesions extend into dentin. Note that enamel rod ends are exposed owing to the angle of the cusps. *B*, Diagram of a larger Class I restoration on a worn tooth. Note that few rod ends are exposed.

Direct Posterior Composites 213

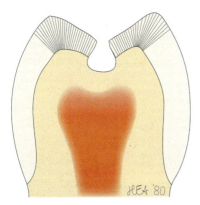

Figure 11–10. Diagram of proximal view of a Class I composite restoration preparation using an adhesive enamel exit. This preparation is used with larger lesions that extend into dentin that is under thick areas of enamel.

composite yields a six times reduction in microleakage around the restoration.[46]

A glass ionomer can be used to fill the entire Class I cavity prior to placing a sealant over the occlusal surface.[47] This procedure can be used for short-term filling in deep carious lesions while pulp health is monitored. It is not recommended as a final restoration because glass ionomers are subject to fracture.

In vitro research has shown that a preventive resin restoration provides greater caries resistance than an occlusal amalgam restoration.[48] The combined effect of conservation of tooth structure and more effective caries prevention makes a sealant restoration the treatment of choice for initial caries treatment of occlusal surfaces.

PROXIMAL SLOT AND TUNNEL RESTORATIONS

It is sometimes possible to restore a posterior proximal lesion from either the facial or the lingual surface without involving the occlusal surface. Proximal slot restoration means using facial access to remove interproximal decay in a posterior tooth. Proximal slot preparations are the right choice when carious lesions are below the contact point and the caries is clinically visible and accessible.[49] These direct access preparations preserve the occlusal surface and marginal ridge rather than remove them, as would be the case with a conventional preparation (Figures 11–12, 11–13, and 11–14).[50,51] The marginal ridge is a critical portion of tooth structure, and its removal often results in loss of contour and weakened cusps.

A tunnel preparation removes proximal caries through an occlusal access while leaving the marginal ridge intact. Like the proximal slot, this preparation conserves and maintains both the marginal ridge and the contact. When a glass ionomer is used, unsupported enamel need not be removed and mechanical retention is not required; however, because an autocured glass ionomer is recommended, placement time is limited.

Tunnel preparations

Jinks suggested that adjacent proximal surfaces of primary teeth could be "inoculated" with fluoride ions from a fluoride-containing cement, such as a silicate cement, via a "tunnel" from the occlusal surface.[52] He showed that primary teeth can be successfully treated with internal preparations. His suggestions led to one of the most conservative and esthetic proximal restorations, the tunnel preparation. This preparation has been refined and is commonly employed by replacing the carious dentin with a glass ionomer and the occlusal enamel portion with a composite.[53,54]

A tunnel preparation reduces the strength of a marginal ridge to 61% of a sound ridge.[51] Placement of glass ionomer to support the ridge can restore ridge strength to 92% of the original.[51] If amalgam is placed, no additional support is needed, but proper condensation is difficult and there is no cariostatic ingredient.

Although the tunnel concept is simple, the preparation is difficult because it is so conservative. Access and visibility are limited, and anatomic landmarks are unclear (eg, knowing where the lesion is buccolingually or occlusogingivally while trying to preserve the marginal ridge), and there is risk of pulpal or periodontal ligament exposure. Additional radiographs may be required to check for excess material after restoration placement.

Tunnel preparations are also difficult to fill and finish.[55] To fill, syringe or inject a glass ionomer to replace the dentin. It is important to have a fluoride-releasing material at the proximal opening. Restore the outer stress-bearing enamel portion of the access opening with a wear-resistant composite.[56,57]

Studies show microleakage may occur when a glass ionomer is the only material used in a tunnel

214 Tooth-Colored Restoratives

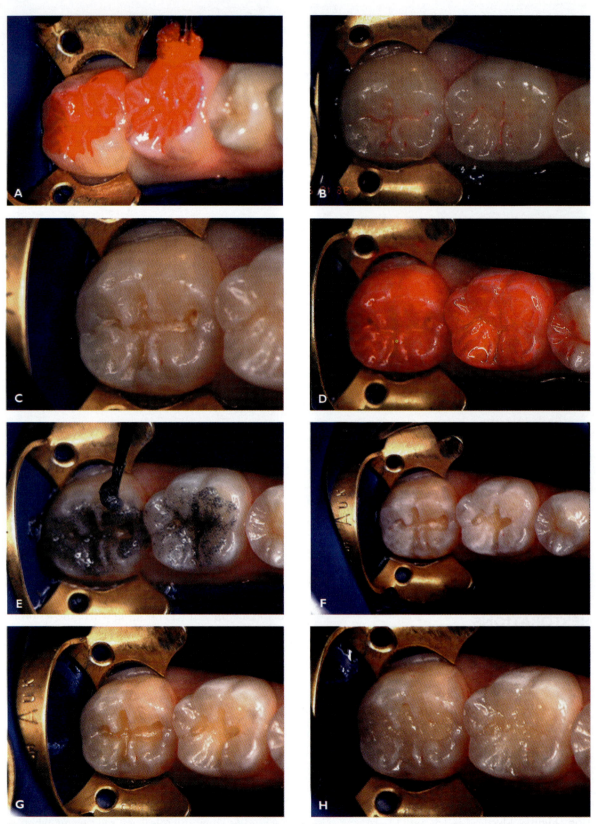

Figure 11–11. The procedure for preventive resin restoration. *A*, Caries indicator is applied. *B*, After 10-second rinse carious defects can be seen. *C*, Stained areas are removed with a spoon. *D*, The tooth is restained, rinsed, and checked again for decay. *E*, The tooth is acid etched, *F*, rinsed, dried, and examined. *G*, Bonding agent is applied. *H*, Composite is placed and light-cured.

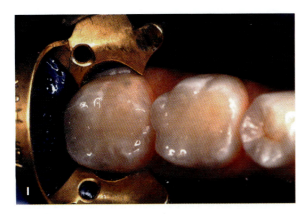 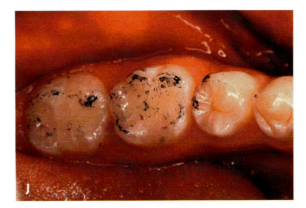

Figure 11–11. *I*, Sealant is applied to cover restored surface. *J*, Occlusion is checked with articulating paper.

preparation.[58] The author's experience is that the remaining proximal enamel is more likely to fracture when a glass ionomer is used to replace the enamel portion of the access preparation. Restoration of the enamel portion with composite is a better approach. Using an incremental fill and cure technique helps minimize marginal gaps resulting from polymerization shrinkage.[6,59]

Indications
Incipient proximal lesions on premolar or molar teeth are candidates for tunnel restorations. This preparation is contraindicated where the marginal ridge is undermined with decay.

Examine the bite-wing radiograph to be sure there are no pulp horns in the proposed access area. It is helpful to take a depth measurement with a periodontal probe from the occlusal surface to the top and bottom of the incipient lesion under treatment. Remember that radiographs show only 40% of a lesion. When caries is radiographically detected, it is likely that the lesion has penetrated the dentin.[50]

Transillumination and magnification are useful in detection, but a caries detector is required. Staining with a disclosing solution, such as 1% acid red in an ethylene glycol base differentiates

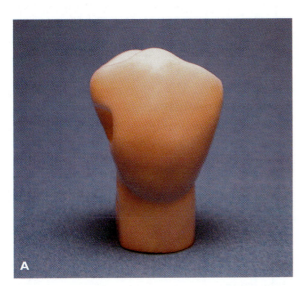 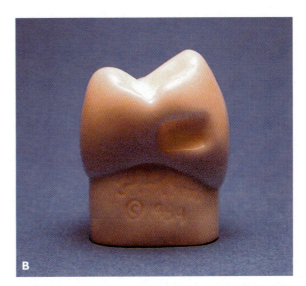

Figure 11–12. A proximal slot preparation: *A*, facial view; *B*, proximal view.

216 Tooth-Colored Restoratives

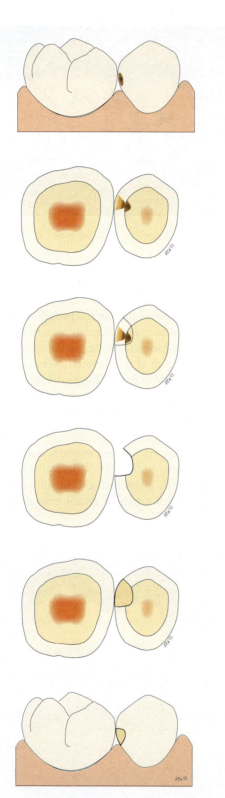

Figure 11–13. Schematic illustration of stages in the restoration of a posterior proximal lesion.

infected carious dentin that should be removed (ie, infected dentin that is completely denatured and bacterially invaded) from affected carious dentin. Affected dentin should be left since the protein matrix remains intact and remineralization from the ionomer is near certain.[60] A good caries detector only stains infected dentin.

Armamentarium

The basic setup includes operator items (gown, gloves, mask, face shield, etc), isolation materials (retraction cord, rubber dam materials, and Mylar strips with retention clips), supplies (anesthetic, a caries indicator), instruments (explorer, mouth mirror, periodontal probe, small spoon excavators to remove caries, handpiece with assorted burs and micron diamonds, small ball-ended applicator, interproximal carvers, condensers), and placement supplies (cotton forceps, placement brushes).

The basic equipment required includes a curing light, radiometer, tooth dryer, air and water syringes, suction device, and color-corrected light source.

The specific materials needed include the following:

- Radiopaque, capsule-injectable glass ionomer (autocured)

- Light-cured minifilled or small-particle composite in compules, or a material that can be loaded into a syringe

- Bard Parker No. 12 blade and handle

- Transillumination light

Restorative treatment

Use a bite-wing radiograph to determine the location and extent of caries. With an explorer, determine whether the carious defect can be reached from the facial or lingual surface. If one or the other is possible, use a facial or lingual proximal slot access and preserve the occlusal surface. If a tunnel preparation is indicated, use a periodontal probe to measure the depth of the lesion on a bitewing radiograph (Figure 11–15). In the patient's chart, record both the occlusal and gingival extent of the lesion.

Direct Posterior Composites 217

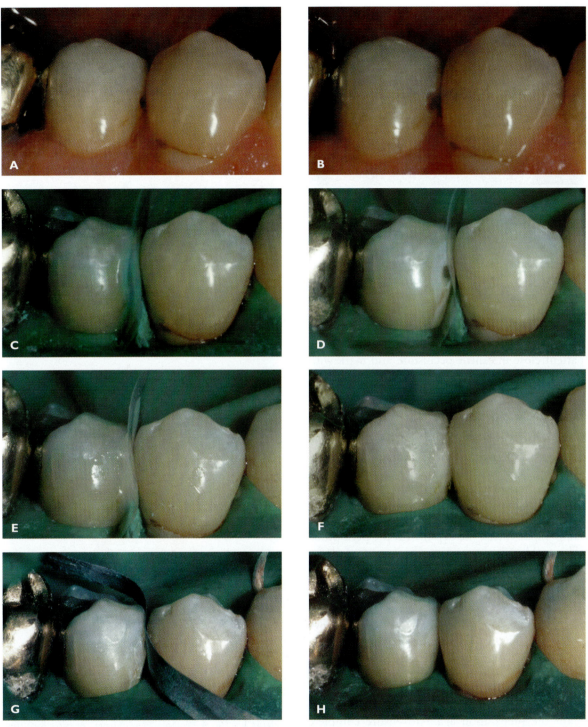

Figure 11–14. Restorative procedure involving a proximal slot preparation to treat proximal caries. *A*, Preoperative view. *B*, A thick metal matrix is placed between the tooth to be restored and the adjacent tooth for protection from nicks during preparation. The interproximal lesion is removed with a quarter-round bur to complete the direct access preparation. The preparation is limited to removal of carious tooth structure. *C*, The protective metal matrix is removed, a wedge and a Mylar matrix are placed, and etchant is applied. *D*, The preparation is rinsed and dried and inspected for uniform etch. *E*, After bonding agent is applied and cured, composite is injected into the preparation and against the Mylar matrix. *F*, The wedge is removed and the strip is pulled slowly to the lingual to remove excess composite. Any proximal excess is removed with an interproximal carver. Composite is cured. *G*, Margins are finished with a Bard Parker blade (No. 12) and a 300- or 600-grit metal diamond strip. A fine finishing disc is used for final polishing. *H*, Postoperative view.

218   Tooth-Colored Restoratives

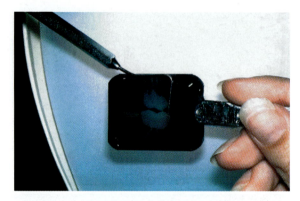

Figure 11–15. Use of a periodontal probe to measure the distance from the marginal ridge to the bottom of a carious lesion.

The ideal type of lesion for these preparations is illustrated in Figure 11–16. Either premolars or molars can be treated.

Procedure for tunnel preparation

Step 1. Dry the tooth to be restored. Have the patient close in centric occlusion, and mark with articulating paper.

Step 2. Place a wooden wedge below the proximal surface to be restored.

Step 3. With a No. 2 round diamond, prepare an access through the enamel 2 mm inside the marginal ridge. Avoid removing any centric holding contacts marked with the articulating paper. Once through enamel, use a slow-speed round bur or a spoon excavator to the depth measured on the radiograph. Check the depth with the perioprobe (Figure 11–17). Determine the extent of decay using a caries indicator and an explorer. Transillumination helps visualize the lesion.

Step 4. Stain the caries and remove it completely by cutting into the proximal wedge. Remove the wedge and view the restoration from the proximal to determine the extent of the preparation. Small preparations may not be visible when the gingiva completely fills the proximal space. A typical preparation path is shown in Figure 11–16, C. Stain the preparation again to ensure complete caries removal.

Step 5. Take another bite-wing radiograph if necessary to ensure the preparation includes the carious lesion. Treat any portions of the preparation near the pulp with a thin lining of calcium hydroxide.

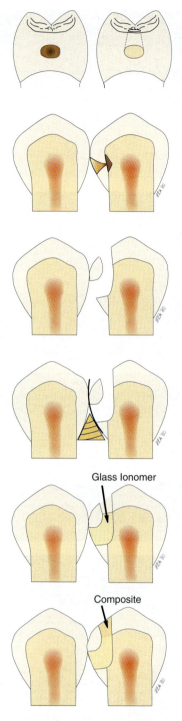

Figure 11–16. A, Proximal view of a path of entry for a tunnel preparation. Schematic mesial-distal cross-sections: B, an ideal lesion for treatment with a tunnel preparation; C, a tunnel preparation for caries removal; D, matrix and wedge placement prior to filling of a tunnel preparation; E, an ionomer placed as a base for composite resin in a tunnel preparation; F, completed tunnel restoration filled with an ionomer base and a composite resin.

Direct Posterior Composites

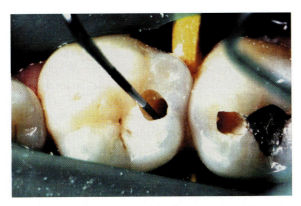

Figure 11-17. A periodontal probe is used to check the depth of the preparation and compare to radiograph of lesion.

Step 6. Place a small piece of metal matrix band proximally to cover the preparation opening. Adapt a new wedge to the proximal surface (see Figure 11-16, D).

Step 7. Clean the preparation with polyacrylic acid (eg, glass-ionomer dentin conditioner), wash, and dry. Some clinicians advocate washing the dentin with a 20% stannous fluoride solution.[54]

Step 8. Using a syringe, fill the preparation to the dentoenamel junction with an autocured glass ionomer. This material is preferred because it is radiopaque and has better physical properties than other glass ionomers. It should completely obturate the proximal access and cover all exposed dentin surfaces (see Figure 11-16, E). Excess glass ionomer is usually extruded proximally, above the wedge.

Step 9. After the base has set (usually 10 min), acid etch both the enamel and the glass ionomer for 30 seconds. Use a bonding agent and place and cure the composite. Remove the wedge and matrix. Immediately remove any proximal glass-ionomer flash, using a Bard Parker blade. Floss any remaining particles from the contact area.

Step 10. Allow the composite to cure for 10 minutes and then finish the occlusal using micron diamonds and other finishing materials. A completed restoration is illustrated in Figure 11-16, F.

Closed-bite filling technique

If the technique is being performed without the use of a rubber dam, completely fill the restoration with a glass ionomer and cover the occlusal surface with dry foil. A large wedge can be used in place of a metal matrix to seal the proximal. The patient can bite on the foil to establish proper occlusion prior to the cement's initial set. Leave the foil in place for 10 minutes, until the restoration can be safely exposed to moisture. Then remove the occlusal portion of the ionomer and place the composite. Finish with micron diamonds and other finishing materials. This method is considerably more messy than the open-bite technique with a rubber dam and is not recommended for routine use.

Amalgam in tunnel preparations

There are advantages and disadvantages to using amalgam as a restorative for tunnel preparations. Amalgam offers a satisfactory mechanical seal, good wear resistance, and is easy to condense into place; but, an amalgam may tattoo the surrounding tooth structure. Use of amalgam also requires removal of unsupported enamel. This may not be desirable in tunnel preparations as this often necessitates removing the marginal ridge such that the tunnel disappears and the preparation becomes a slot. There is also speculation that amalgam blocks the transfer of moisture throughout a tooth and that subsequent dehydration of cusps leads to their eventual fracture.[54]

CLASS II RESTORATIONS

Highly conservative preparations are possible when restoring Class II lesions with composite.[61] When replacing an existing Class II amalgam restoration with a composite, the only alteration required in the preparation is to change the enamel cavosurface margins from 90 degrees to a 45-degree bevel that is 0.5-mm wide. This change improves enamel–resin bonding.

The composite placement steps outlined below apply to teeth undergoing initial preparation for proximal decay.

Armamentarium

The basic setup for composite restorations includes operator items (gown, gloves, mask, face shield, etc), isolation materials (retraction cord, rubber dam materials, and Mylar strips with retention clips), supplies (anesthetic, caries indicator), instruments (explorers, mouth mirror, periodontal probe, small spoon excavators to remove caries, handpiece with assorted burs and micron diamonds, small ball-ended applicator, interproximal carvers, condensers), and placement supplies (cotton forceps and placement brushes).

The basic equipment required includes a curing light, radiometer, tooth dryer, air and water syringes, suction device, and color-corrected light source.

The specific materials needed include the following:

- Suitable dentin liner
- A light-cured minifilled or small-particle composite in compules, or a material that can be loaded into a syringe
- Calcium hydroxide (for pulp capping, if needed)
- No. 1 and No. 2 round-end diamonds (medium-fine grit)
- Regular tapered and pointed 40-μm straight-sided diamond
- Diamond metal strips (eg, G-C Metal Strips [300 and 600 grit], GC America Inc., Chicago, Illinois, or Premier Compo Strips, Premier, King of Prussia, Pennsylvania)
- Bard Parker No. 12 blade and handle
- Metal proximal matrix band
- Transillumination light
- Assorted wooden wedges
- Kelly hemostat
- Conventional amalgam matrix and retainer
- Palodent® matrix band and BiTine Ring (Palodent®, LD Caulk, Milford, Delaware)

Wedges and matrices play important roles in posterior composite restorations. Figure 11–18 shows sample wedges. Figure 11–19 shows matrices and matrix holders appropriate for use in posterior restorations.

Preparation

Make a conservative box preparation with rounded line angles. Figure 11–20 illustrates the box preparations for an amalgam and a composite. Note that in the composite preparation the occlusal is in enamel.

Make a 45- to 90-degree exit angle to expose enamel rod ends for bonding. Studies show that when composite is bonded to the sides of enamel rods, such that polymerization shrinkage forces are perpendicular to the enamel prisms, the stresses can cause the enamel to fracture.[59,62] When these stresses are along the ends of the enamel rods, however, the forces are low compared with the cohesive strength of enamel.[63] Bevels greatly improve but do not eliminate marginal leakage.[64] There is no significant difference in cuspal support,[65] wear rate,[66] or retention[67] between beveled and nonbeveled preparations.

Figure 11–21 illustrates the outline forms of amalgam and composite Class II preparations. Note that the composite preparation is more conservative than the amalgam preparation and that the composite preparation does not break the proximal contact. Depth should be just enough to remove decay. The depths of amalgam and composite preparations are illustrated in Figure 11–22. In the proximal area, the composite preparation enters dentin only to allow access for caries removal. The occlusal portion is finished in enamel if there is no dentinal caries. The gingival floor of a composite should be slightly beveled, whereas the amalgam preparation exits at 90 degrees. Extensions should be minimal. Natural tooth contacts should remain whenever possible. Mark centric contacts with articulating paper and avoid them (see Figure 11–22, B).

Retention is achieved by acid etching. Mechanical retention is unnecessary. Round both external and internal line angles to facilitate placement and adaptation of the composite (see Figure 11–22, B).

Liner
Protect any exposed dentin with a suitable liner (glass-ionomer liner, CaOH or polycarboxylate cement). Remove liner that may be covering enamel that needs to be etched, and complete the preparation. When the gingival floor is below the cementoenamel junction, place the ionomer liner over the entire gingival floor as well as over all internal dentin walls.[68,69]

Variation in preparation design
Each posterior preparation is customized. The use of a proximal slot preparation assumes a radiographic examination has shown caries that cannot be restored with one of the more conservative

Direct Posterior Composites 221

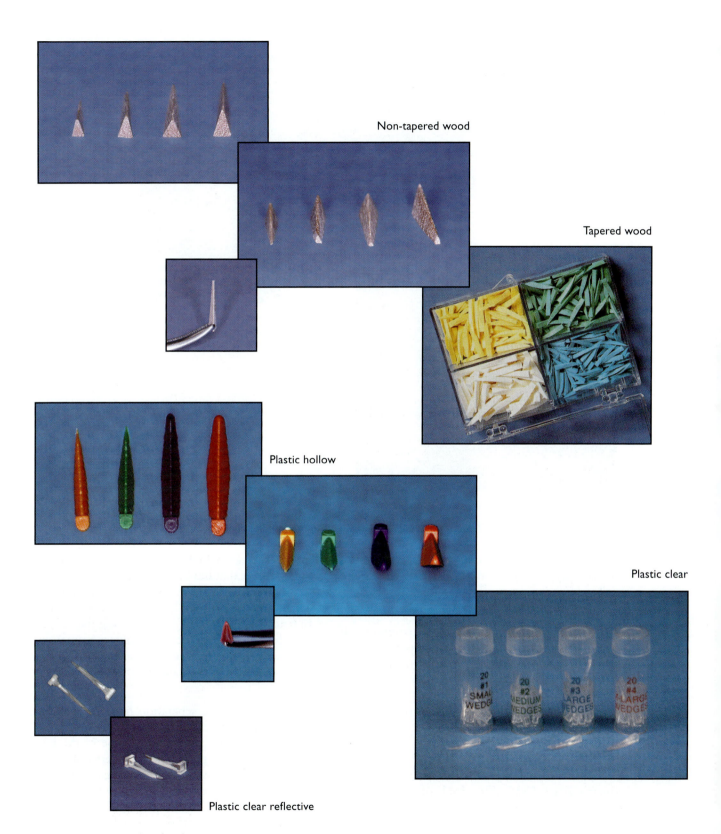

Figure 11–18. Examples of wedges.

222 Tooth-Colored Restoratives

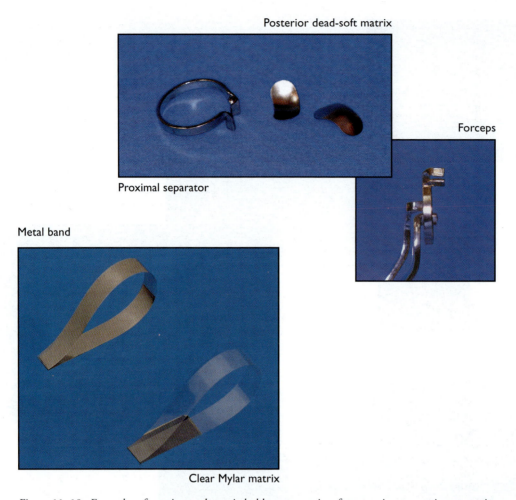

Figure 11–19. Examples of matrices and matrix holders appropriate for posterior composite restorations.

restorations previously discussed (that is, the caries must be approached from the occlusal surface and is too large to preserve the marginal ridge).

Figure 11–23 illustrates the use of a slot preparation to restore proximal caries with composite. If the occlusal surface is sound, the preparation generally does not include it. Figure 11–24 illustrates some common variations in preparation design for posterior composite restorations. A preventive pit and fissure sealant can be placed over the final restoration.

Placement

The proximal contact must be established at the matrix stage. Use a thin, dead-soft metal matrix and a suitable wedge, or a conventional amalgam matrix. The Auto Matrix (LD Caulk) provides excellent proximal adaptation but fits more loosely in other areas, which creates excessive bulk. A metal matrix that has been tempered adapts better to the contact area. To temper a matrix, heat it over a flame and cool it rapidly in alcohol or water. The BiTine Ring (Palodent) has a spring-like action that spreads the teeth for better contact adaptation. Regardless of the matrix used, burnish the proximal area to ensure close adaptation to the adjacent tooth.

Maximum tooth separation must be achieved prior to resin placement to ensure proximal contacts. Using a Kelly hemostat is one of the best ways to place and remove wedges between posterior teeth. Place the wedges before the tooth is prepared so there is time for the teeth to move before the restoration is placed. Separation is particularly important if the restoration cannot be packed with an amalgam condenser.

Direct Posterior Composites

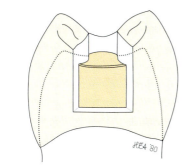 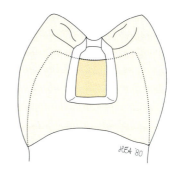

Figure 11–20. The proximal box outline: *A,* for an ideal Class II amalgam preparation, and *B,* for an ideal Class II composite preparation for occlusal and proximal caries.

When filling two proximal surfaces on the same tooth, wedge one side at a time. Filling and curing one box before filling the other one provides maximum tooth separation.

Etch with a gel etchant. To facilitate this application, use a 1-cc tuberculin or diabetic syringe.

Composite placement is best accomplished with a composite syringe or an amalgam carrier. The syringe should have a long neck for good access to posterior teeth and should be able to dispense viscous materials through the tip. Either a metal or a plastic amalgam carrier can be used to place packable composites that come in tubes or tubs. Some clinicians prefer plastic pedodontic carriers that have a syringe-type plugger (eg, Delrin Amalgam Carrier or Gun Type, Premier).

Whenever possible, use a tapered amalgam condenser to compress the material into place. If the composite sticks to the condenser, coat the condenser with a thin amount of bonding agent, or use a heavier bodied composite. Use an explorer or interproximal carver to remove excess material by pulling it toward the margins from the center of the mass.

In light-cured systems, add the composite in increments of 1 to 2 mm. A basic principle is that composite should not bridge opposing margins and should not be mass cured. Condense and cure for 40 to 60 seconds between each addition, depending on the shade. Proper placement in increments controls polymerization shrinkage. Figure 11–25 illustrates two incremental layering methods that effectively reduce contraction gaps. Because of the distance from the curing light to composite on the gingival box, the light intensity drops significantly, resulting in inadequate polymerization. It is important to cure from both

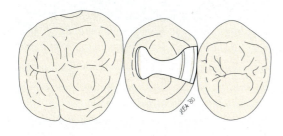 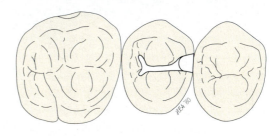

Figure 11–21. Schematic occlusal view of typical Class II preparations: *A,* for amalgam, and *B,* composite restoration of a tooth with occlusal and proximal caries.

224 Tooth-Colored Restoratives

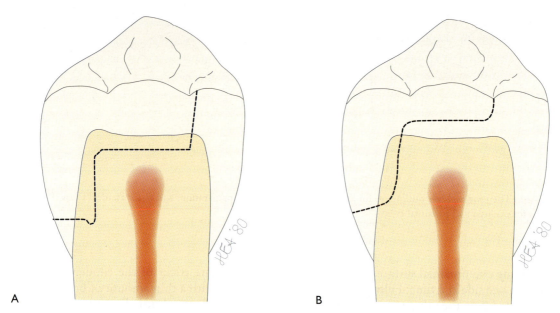

Figure 11–22. Schematic mesial-distal cross-sectional views: *A*, depth of an ideal Class II amalgam preparation, and *B*, depth of an ideal Class II composite preparation for a tooth with proximal and occlusal decay.

proximal surfaces after removal of the matrix to ensure adequate curing of the composite margins. Cuspal tension from polymerization shrinkage is common. Research shows this tension can be minimized if the composite is placed in at least three increments and each increment is sloped up one cavity wall at a time.[70–72]

Finishing
Use fine-grit conventional diamonds for gross reduction and micron diamonds or white stones for final shaping and contouring on the occlusal. Use flexible discs on exposed proximal margins and finishing strips for interproximal and other inaccessible areas.

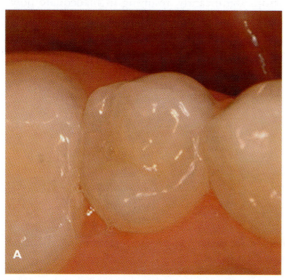
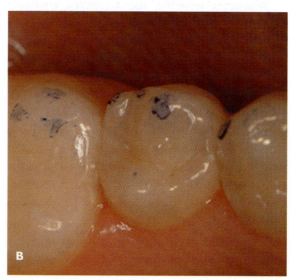

Figure 11–23. Restorative procedure involving an occlusal slot preparation to treat proximal caries. *A*, Preoperative view. *B*, Occlusion is checked using articulating paper.

Direct Posterior Composites 225

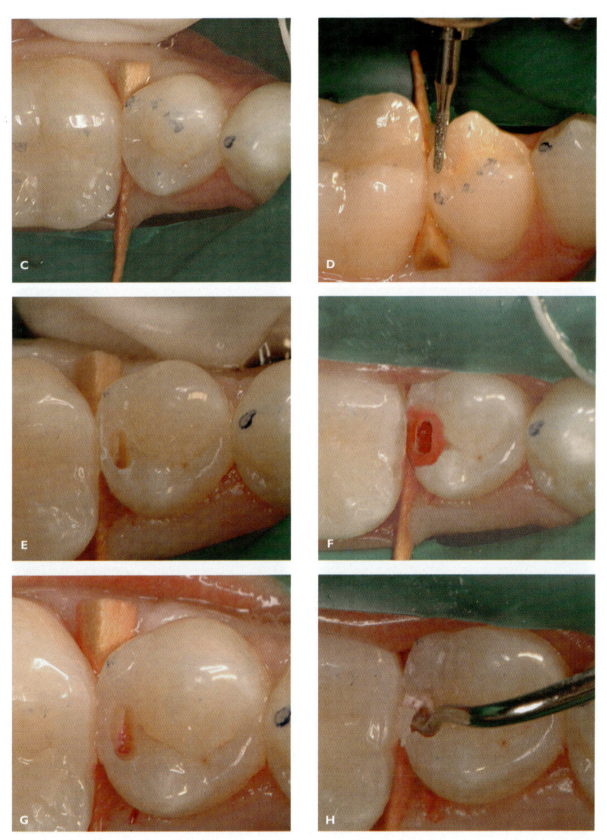

Figure 11–23. *C,* A rubber dam and wooden wedge are placed. *D,* A medium-grit diamond is used to start the preparation. *E,* Initial entry into carious lesion. *F,* Caries detection stain is applied. *G,* The preparation is rinsed and checked for discoloration. *H,* Caries is removed with a spoon.

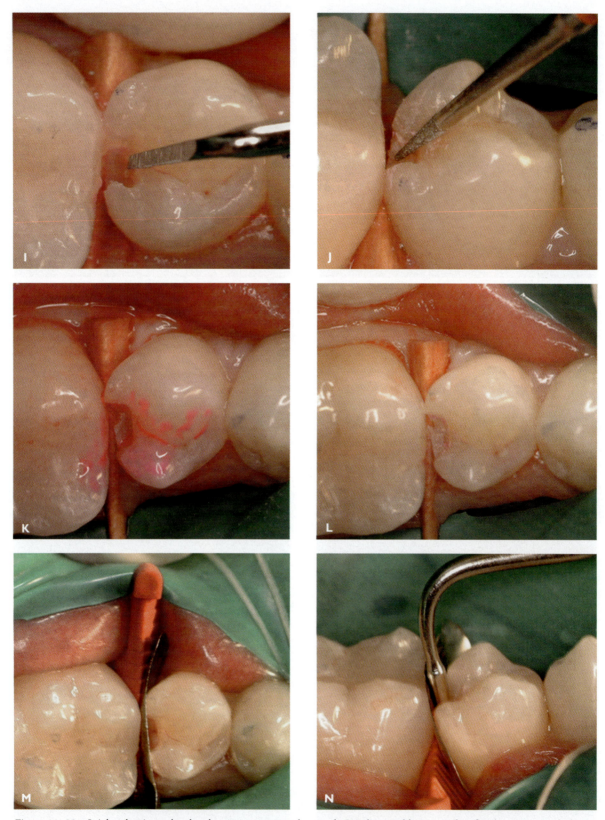

Figure 11–23. *I*, A hatchet is used to break away unsupported enamel. *J*, A diamond bur is used to finish margins and place a slight bevel. *K*, Caries stain is applied again. *L*, The preparation is rinsed and checked for discoloration indicating any caries still remaining. *M*, Dead-soft matrix and a plastic wedge are placed. *N*, The preparation is burnished with a condenser.

Direct Posterior Composites 227

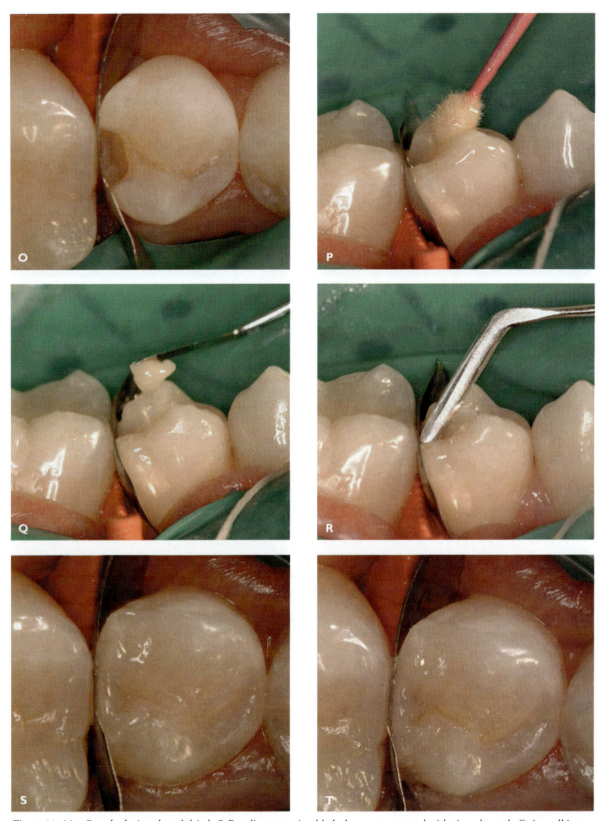

Figure 11–23. *O*, etched, rinsed, and dried. *P*, Bonding agent is added, the excess removed with air and cured. *Q*, A small increment of composite is added. *R*, Composite is adapted to the gingival floor with a condenser and to the proximal walls with an interproximal carver, and then cured. *S*, Composite is added in increments until margins are covered and deep anatomy is established. *T*, The restoration after addition of color modifier to darken the grooves (optional), curing, and placement and curing of final increment of composite.

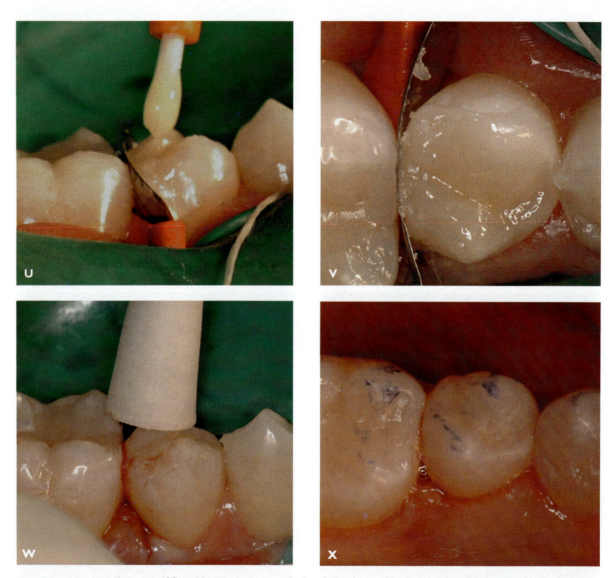

Figure 11–23. *U*, A thin coat of flowable composite is applied and cured to seal margins. A brush is used to create a smooth, even coating, which is then cured. *V*, Restoration just prior to finishing. *W*, The wedge and proximal matrix are removed and margins adjusted with a white stone or micron diamond. Contours are smoothed with a rubber cup. Any proximal flash is removed with a Bard Parker blade. *X*, The rubber dam is removed. Occlusion is checked with articulating paper and adjusted just slightly out of contact to allow for subsequent expansion of composite due to water absorption.

Without proper layering, composite polymerization stresses the enamel interface, which can cause enamel fractures at the margins during finishing.[73] Even with proper layering, these fractures are possible but are less likely. Marginal microfractures can be resealed by etching, drying, and rebonding the margins (ie, adding bonding agent to the finished and polished restorations).[74]

Direct Posterior Composites 229

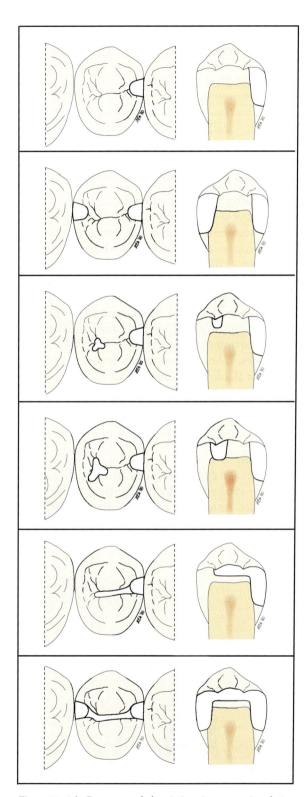

Figure 11–24. Recommended variations in preparation design for composite restorations, depending on extent of caries.

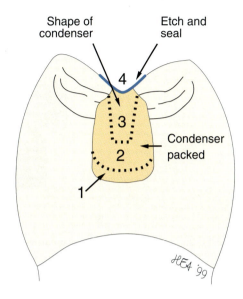

A

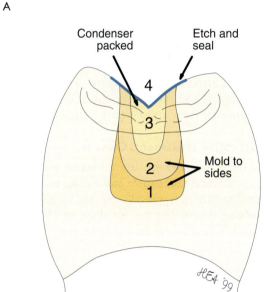

B

Figure 11–25. Incremental layering of composite to restore, A, small and B, large defects.

Composites finished immediately show significantly higher wear rates compared with those finished 24 hours later.[75] Waiting 15 minutes before finishing significantly improves the wear rate.[76]

When checking occlusion, it is generally best to adjust posterior composites slightly out of function. A light centric may be incorporated in larger

230 Tooth-Colored Restoratives

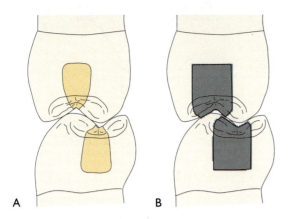

Figure 11–26. *A*, An ideal Class II composite preparation from the proximal. Note the lack of function. *B*, An ideal Class II amalgam preparation from the proximal. Note the central contacts.

restorations. Composite materials expand slightly after placement, which can make restorations too high for correct occlusion. Figure 11–26 illustrates that Class II composites are out of occlusion and that amalgams are stress-bearing restorations.

Restorative treatment, Class II

For these preparations, use a viscous or packable composite and compatible sealant (ie, of the same resin). Anesthesia is generally required for restorations involving dentin but not for those involving only enamel. When two proximal surfaces are involved, wedge and cure one at a time. This ensures the best proximal contact (Figures 11–27 and 11–28).[77]

Dentinogingival margins

Preparations with no enamel at the gingival cavosurface margin should be treated with a glass ionomer, ideally one that is radiopaque. After placement, etch the glass ionomer along with the remaining enamel. Bond the composite to the enamel and glass ionomer in increments.

Maintaining proximal contacts

One of the most difficult problems in posterior resin placement is holding the proximal contact. This becomes more difficult with an increasing size of restoration. A number of techniques can be used. One of the most reliable techniques involves early wedging and careful selection and contouring of the matrix band (see Figure 11–27). Placing orthodontic elastic rings through the contacts before starting the preparation is one way to open the spaces.[78] Another approach is to use an Ivory separator (Columbus Dental).

Restoring cusp stiffness

Some studies show that composites increase cusp stiffness, whereas other studies show no change.[79,80]

Rebonding

Microleakage can be reduced by 60% if unfilled resin is applied to the margins of a finished composite resin.[81] In some studies on Class V restorations, this type of rebonding eliminated leakage.[74]

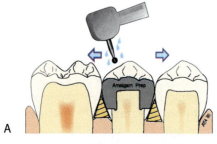
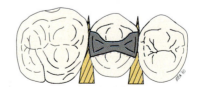
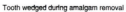

Tooth wedged during amalgam removal

Figure 11–27. The sequence for placing a three-surface posterior composite from a mesial–distal view (*left*) and an occlusal view (*right*). (Modified from technique of Dr. Al Lacy.[77]) *A*, During tooth preparation, both proximal contacts are wedged to gain maximum tooth separation. Amalgam is removed with a diamond.

Direct Posterior Composites 231

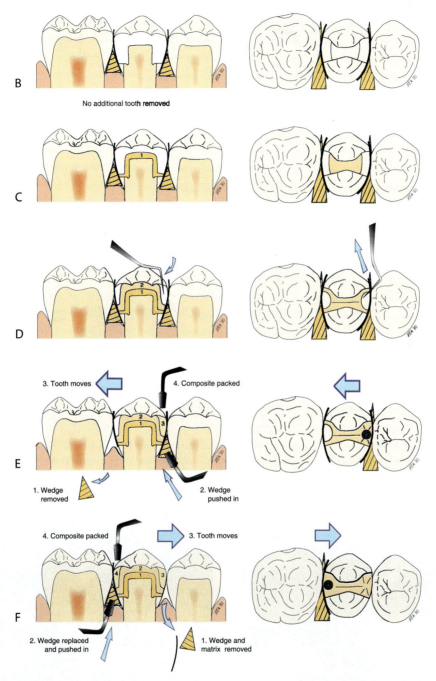

Figure 11–27. *B*, A dead-soft matrix is placed and new wedges are seated firmly with a hemostat. The enamel is etched and washed, and a bonding agent is placed and cured. *C*, A 1-mm layer of composite is applied to the gingival floor and over the axial walls and cured for 60 seconds. *D*, The matrix is burnished in the contact area to improve its adaptation to the adjacent tooth. Another 1-mm layer of composite is added and adapted over the proximal margins with an interproximal carver and cured for 40 seconds. When the composite is cured at the proximal, a condenser is used to hold the matrix firmly against the adjacent tooth. *E*, The wedge at the smallest box is removed and the other wedge is seated more securely to tip the tooth and thereby maximize tooth separation at the largest proximal box. Composite is firmly packed into the proximal box and cured. *F*, The wedge and matrix are removed from the filled and cured side of the tooth and placed next to the remaining and unfilled proximal box. The wedge is placed firmly to achieve maximum tooth separation. Composite is packed firmly and cured in 1-mm thicknesses just short of the final contour.

232 Tooth-Colored Restoratives

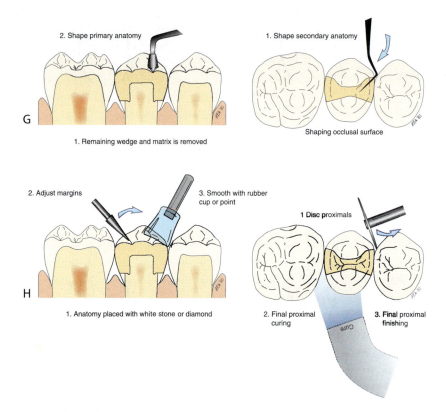

Figure 11–27. *G,* The final layer of composite is placed in the occlusal portion of the restoration. An acorn burnisher is used to place the primary anatomy in the restoration. A half Hollenbeck or interproximal carver is used to place the final anatomy in the occlusal surface, and the restoration is cured. *H,* The wedge and matrix are removed. A Bard Parker blade is used to remove interproximal flash. Initial finishing is done with a white stone or micron diamond and proximal strips. Final finishing is done with rubber cups and points. It is important to cure the proximal surfaces of the restoration from the buccal and lingual for 1 minute to complete polymerization in the areas that had minimal exposure to light.

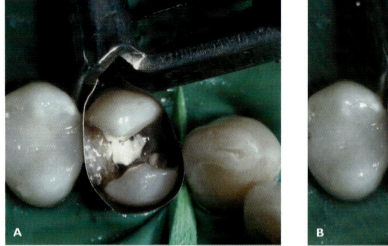 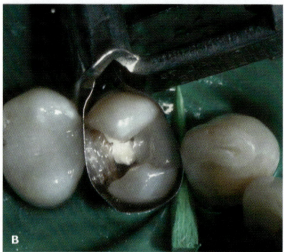

Figure 11–28. Illustration of proper wedging for three-surface posterior composite placement. *A,* The first of two teeth has been restored with a mesial-occlusal-distal composite. The second tooth has been prepared and is ready for initial composite placement. Note that a wedge is firmly placed in the mesial box, which will be filled first. *B,* The first box is filled incrementally.

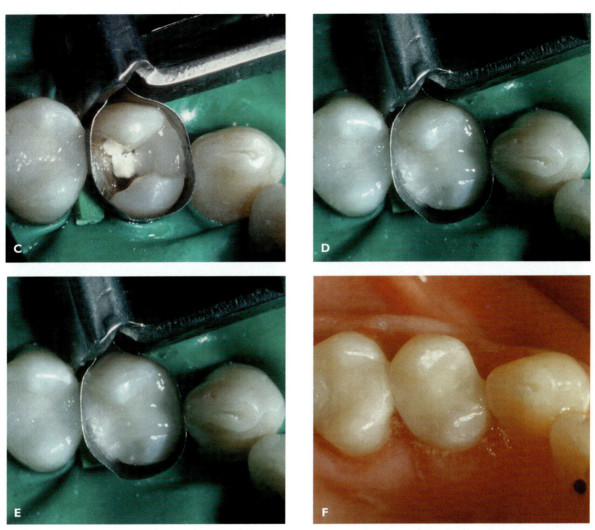

Figure 11–28. *C*, The wedge is removed from the filled box and placed firmly adjacent to the unfilled box. *D*, The distal box is filled incrementally. *E*, The occlusal anatomy is placed. *F*, Postoperative view, after finishing and polishing.

REFERENCES

1. Walls AW, Murray JJ, McCabe JF. The management of occlusal caries in permanent molars. A clinical trial comparing a minimal composite restoration with an amalgam restoration. Br Dent J 1988;164:288–92.

2. Oldenburg TR, Vann WR Jr, Dilley DC. Comparison of composite and amalgam in posterior teeth of children. Dent Mater 1987;3:182–6.

3. Davidson CL, de Gee AJ. Relaxation of polymerization contraction stresses by flow in dental composites. J Dent Res 1984;63:146–8.

4. Hedgahl T, Gjerdet NR. Contraction stresses of composite resin filling materials. Acta Odontol Scand 1977;35:191–5.

5. Masutani S, et al. SEM analysis of marginal adaptation of Class II resin restorations [abstract]. J Dent Res 1983;62(Special Issue):665.

6. Jorgensen KD, Hisamitsu H. Class 2 composite restorations: prevention in vitro of contraction gaps. J Dent Res 1984;63:146–8.

7. Gross JD, Retief DH, Bradley EL. Microleakage of posterior composite restorations. Dent Mater 1985;1:7–10.

8. Johnson GH, Gordon GE, Bales DJ. Postoperative sensitivity associated with posterior composites and amalgam restorations. Oper Dent 1988;13:66–73.

9. Wilson NHF, Wilson MA, Wastell DG, Smith GA. A clinical trial of a visible light-cured posterior composite resin restorative material: five-year results. Quintessence Int 1988;19:675–81.

10. Bayne SC, Tayor DF, Roberson TM, et al. Long-term clinical failures in posterior composites [abstract]. J Dent Res 1989;68(Spec Issue):185.

11. Leinfelder KF, Wilder AD, Teixeira LC. Wear rates of posterior composite resins. J Am Dent Assoc 1986;112:829–33.

12. Derkson GD, Richardson AS, Waldman R. Clinical evaluation of composite resin and amalgam posterior restorations: three-year results. J Can Dent Assoc 1984;50:478–80.

13. Swift EJ. Wear of composite resins in permanent posterior teeth. J Am Dent Assoc 1987;115:584–8.

14. Ripa LW. Occlusal sealants. In: Nikiforuk G, ed. Understanding dental caries. Vol. 2. Prevention: basic and clinical aspects. New York: Karger, Basel, 1985: 145–73.

15. Hicks MJ. The acid-etch technique in caries prevention: pit and fissure sealants and preventive resin restorations. In: Pinkham JR, ed. Pediatric dentistry. 2nd ed. Infancy through adolescence. Philadelphia: WB Saunders, 1994:451–82.

16. Ripa L. Occlusal sealants: rationale and review of clinical trials. Int Dent J 1980;30:127–39.

17. Simonsen RJ. Preventive resin restoration. Innovative use of sealants in restorative dentistry. Clin Prev Dent 1982;4:27–9.

18. Mertz-Fairhurst EJ, Fairhurst CW, Williams JE, et al. A comparative clinical study of two pit and fissure sealants: 7-year results in Augusta, Georgia. J Am Dent Assoc 1984;109:252–5.

19. Simonsen RJ. Retention and effectiveness of a single application of white sealant after 10 years. J Am Dent Assoc 1987;115:31–6.

20. Hardison JR, Collier DR, Sprouse LW, et al. Retention of pit and fissure sealant on the primary molars of 3- and 4-year-old children after 1 year. J Am Dent Assoc 1987;114:613–5.

21. Sveen OB, Jensen OE. Two-year clinical evaluation of Delton and Prisma-Shield. Clin Prev Dent 1986;8: 9–11.

22. Shapira J, Eidelman E. Six-year clinical evaluation of fissure sealants placed after mechanical preparation: a matched pair study. Pediatr Dent 1986;8:204–5.

23. Simonsen RJ. Cost-effectiveness of pit and fissure sealant at 10 years. Quintessence Int 1989;20:75–82.

24. Micik RE. Fate of in vitro caries-like lesions sealed within tooth structure [abstract]. J Dent Res 1972;51 (Spec Issue):225.

25. Handelman SL, Buonocure MG, Heseck DJ. A preliminary report on the effect of fissure sealant on bacteria in dental caries. J Prosthet Dent 1972;27:390–2.

26. Handelman SL, Buonocure MG, Schoute PC. Progress report on the effect of fissure sealant on bacteria in dental caries. J Am Dent Assoc 1973;87:1189–91.

27. Going R, Loeshe W, Grainger D, Syed SA. The viability of microorganisms in carious lesions five years after covering with a fissure sealant. J Am Dent Assoc 1978;97:455–62.

28. Mertz-Fairhurst EJ, Schuster GS, Fairhurst CW. Arresting caries by sealants: results of a clinical study. J Am Dent Assoc 1986;112:194–7.

29. Handelman S, Washburn F, Wopperer P. Two-year report of sealant effect on bacteria in dental caries. J Am Dent Assoc 1976;93:967–70.

30. Mertz-Fairhurst E, Call-Smith KM, Schuster GS, et al. Clinical performance of sealed composite restorations placed over caries compared with sealed and unsealed amalgam restorations. J Am Dent Assoc 1987; 115:689–94.

31. Garcia-Godoy F, Gwinnett AJ. Penetration of acid solution and gel in occlusal fissures. J Am Dent Assoc 1987;114:809–10.

32. Hicks M, Silverstone M. The effect of sealant application and sealant loss on caries-like lesion formation in vitro. Pediatr Dent 1982;4:111–4.

33. Strang R, Cummings A, Stephen KW, et al. Further abrasion resistance and bond strength studies of fissure sealants. J Oral Rehabil 1986;13:257–62.

34. Houpt M, Fuks A, Shapira J, et al. Autopolymerized versus light-polymerized fissure sealants. J Am Dent Assoc 1987;115:55–6.

35. Gerke DC. Modified enameloplasty fissure sealant technique using acid-etch resin method. Quintessence Int 1987;18:337–40.

36. Williams B, Ward R, Winter GB. A two-year trial comparing different resin systems used as fissure sealants. Br Dent J 1986;161:367–70.

37. Charbeneau GT, Dennison JB. Ten-year clinical evaluation of a pit and fissure sealant [abstract]. J Dent Res 1985;64(Spec Issue):209.

38. Sharp HK, Friend GW, Myers DA, Covington JS. Composite reinforced pit and fissure sealants: five-year clinical study [abstract]. J Dent Res 1990;69(Spec Issue):307.

39. Houpt M, Shapira J, Fuks A, et al. A clinical comparison of visible light-initiated and autopolymerized fissure sealant: one-year results. Pediatr Dent 1986;8:22–3.

40. Simonsen RJ, Stallard RE. Sealant-restorations utilizing a diluted filled composite resin: one-year results. Quintessence Int 1977;8:77–84.

41. Simonsen RJ. The preventive resin restoration: a minimally invasive, nonmetallic restoration. Compendium 1987;8:428–32.

42. Houpt M, Shey Z. Occlusal restoration fissure sealant instead of "extension for prevention." Quintessence Int 1985;16:489–92.

43. Hinoura K, Setcos JC, Phillips RW. Cavity design and placement techniques for Class 2 composites. Oper Dent 1988;13:12–9.

44. Sveen O, Buonocore M, Azhdari S. Evaluation of a new restorative technique for localized occlusal caries. J Dent Res 1978;57(Spec Issue): 57.

45. Simonsen RJ. Preventive resin restoration: three-year results. J Am Dent Assoc 1980;100:535–9.

46. Olberding P, Goepferd S. Microleakage of preventive resin, amalgam, and composite restorations. J Dent Res 1989;68(Spec Issue):208.

47. Garcia-Godoy F. Microleakage of preventive glass-ionomer restorations. Compendium 1988;9:88–92.

48. Hicks M. Caries-like lesion formation around occlusal alloy and preventive resin restorations. Pediatr Dent 1984;6:17–22.

49. de Carvalho Oliveira F Jr, Covey DA, Denehy GE. Conservative posterior composite resin preparations. Compend Cont Educ Dent 1986;7:327–32.

50. Kleier DJ, Hicks MJ, Flaitz CM. A comparison of Ultraspeed and Ektaspeed dental x-ray film: in vitro study of the radiographic and histologic appearance of interproximal lesions. Quintessence Int 1987;18: 623–31.

51. Hill FJ, Halaseh FJ. A laboratory investigation of tunnel restorations in premolar teeth. Br Dent J 1988; 165:364–7.

52. Jinks GM. Fluoride-impregnated cements and their effect on the activity of interproximal caries. J Dent Child 1963;30:87.

53. Hunt P. A modified Class II cavity preparation for glass-ionomer restorative materials. Quintessence Int 1984;15:1011–8.

54. Knight GM. The use of adhesive materials in the conservative restoration of selected posterior teeth. Aust Dent J 1984;29:324.

55. Hotz PR, Holzer A. Microleakage and quality of conservative Class II and tunnel restorations. J Dent Res 1989;68(Spec Issue):208.

56. McLean JW. Limitations of posterior composite resins and extending their use with glass ionomer cements. Quintessence Int 1987;18:517–29.

57. Croll TP. Glass ionomer-silver cermet bonded composite resin in Class II tunnel restorations. Quintessence Int 1988;19:533–9.

58. Robbins JW, Cooley RL. Microleakage of Ketac-Silver in the tunnel preparation. Oper Dent 1988;13: 8–11.

59. Bowen RL, Nemoto K, Rapson JE. Adhesive bonding of various materials to hard tooth tissues: forces developing in composite materials during hardening. J Am Dent Assoc 1983;106:475–7.

60. Fusayama T. Two layers of carious dentin: diagnosis and treatment. Oper Dent 1979;4:63–70.

61. Covey DA, Denehy GE. Conservative posterior composite resin preparations. Compend Cont Educ Dent 1986;5:327–32.

62. Jorgensen KD, Asmussen E, Shimokobe H. Enamel damages caused by contracting restorative resins. Scand J Dent Res 1975;83:120–2.

63. Hegdahl T, Gjerdet NR. Contraction stresses of composite filling materials. Acta Odont Scand 1977; 35:191–5.

64. Moore DH, Vann WF Jr. The effect of a cavosurface bevel on microleakage in posterior composite restorations. J Prosthet Dent 1988;59:21–4.

65. Purk J, Eick J, Roberts M, et al. Class II amalgam restoration vs. Class I undermined composite restorations [abstract]. J Dent Res 1989;68(Spec Issue): 211.

66. Isenberg B, Leinfelder K, McCartha C. Efficacy of beveling posterior composite resin preparations [abstract]. J Dent Res 1989;68(Spec Issue):234.

67. Brunson WD, Sturdevant JR, Taylor DF, et al. Analysis of modified retention for posterior composite resins [abstract]. J Dent Res 1988;67(Spec Issue): 221.

68. Kanca J. Posterior resins: microleakage below the cementoenamel junction. Quintessence Int 1987;15: 347–9.

69. Hinkelman KW, Dederich D, Albert A. Microleakage in restorations placed by glass ionomer "sandwich" technique. J Dent Res 1989;68(Spec Issue): 208.

70. Donly KJ, Jensen ME. Posterior composite polymerization shrinkage in primary teeth: an in vitro comparison of three techniques. Pediatr Dent 1986; 8:209–12.

71. Donly KJ, Jensen ME, Reinhardt J, Walker JD. Posterior composite polymerization shrinkage in primary teeth: an in vivo comparison of three techniques. Pediatr Dent 1987;9:22–5.

72. Hassen K, Mante F, List G, Dhuru V. A modified incremental filling technique for Class II composite restorations. J Prosthet Dent 1987;58:153–6.

73. Lutz F, Krejei I, Olderbury TR. Elimination of polymerization stresses at the margins of posterior composite resin restorations. Quintessence Int 1986;17: 777–84.

74. Garcia-Godoy F, Malone WFP. Microleakage of posterior composite resin restorations after rebonding. Compendium 1987;8:606–9.

75. Glasspoole EA, Erickson RL. The effect of finishing time on wear resistance of composites. J Dent Res 1989;68(Spec Issue):207.

76. Wisniewski JF, Leinfelder KF, Bradley EL. Effect of finishing techniques on the wear rate of posterior composite resins. J Dent Res 1990;69(Spec Issue):161.

77. Lacy AM. A critical look at posterior composite restorations. J Am Dent Assoc 1987;114:357–62.

78. Lambrechts P, Braem M, Vanherle G. Evaluation of clinical performance for posterior composite resins and dentin adhesives. Oper Dent 1987;12:53–78.

79. Stampalia LL, Nicholls JI, Brudvik JS, Jones DW. Fracture resistance of teeth with resin-bonded restorations. J Prosthet Dent 1986;55:694–8.

80. Eakle WS. Fracture resistance of teeth restored with Class II bonded composite resin. J Dent Res 1986; 65:149–53.

81. Holan G, Levin M, Bimstein E, et al. Clinical, radiographic, SEM evaluation and assessment of microleakage of Class II composite restorations. Am J Dent 1989; 2:274–8.

Chapter 12

Esthetics

Creative thinking may mean simply the realization that there's no particular virtue in doing things the way they always have been done.

Rudolph Flesch

Artists use a number of illusions to achieve specific visual effects. A classic example is the illusion of a change in the length of a line when it is near other lines (Figure 12–1). Another is the effect of curvature on the appearance of an object's width. For example, a square appears taller and wider than a circle of the same width (Figure 12–2).

In dentistry, the same optical concepts are used to improve the appearance of dentition. By incorporating optical illusion, it is possible to significantly alter the perception of a patient's smile. It is the complex interaction among the features of tooth shape, size, texture, shade, position, and light source that ultimately determine dental esthetics. The basic optical principles applied in dentistry include the following:

- Vertical lines accentuate length
- Horizontal lines accentuate width
- Contrast heightens visibility
- Light reflection increases visibility
- Light deflection decreases visibility
- Shadows create depth
- Light creates prominence

These optical principles are applied by manipulating primarily the contours and color of teeth. Contouring involves the adjustment of incisal edges, line angles, grooves, prominence, and incisal or gingival curvature. Manipulating color involves darkening or lightening teeth or portions of a tooth to affect the appearance of prominence. The perception of contour depends on the reflection or deflection of light. Control of light reflection and color contrast is elemental to creating a desired illusion.

OPTICAL PRINCIPLES

Visual perception depends on cues from which the brain makes assumptions. Mastering production of those cues is the essence of creating illusion. Altering tooth contours can enhance all of the following features.

Embrasure form

Normal incisal embrasure form is shown in Figure 12–3. Altering the embrasure form affects the appearance of tooth width. Smaller embrasures make teeth appear wider whereas large embrasures make them appear narrower (Figure 12–4). Since the embrasure form is in the incisal portion of the teeth, which is the portion most seen during speaking and smiling, changes in incisal embrasure form can have the largest impact on a smile.

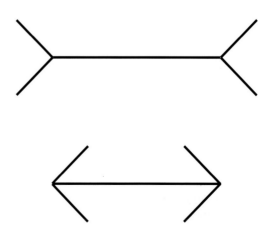

Figure 12–1. Illustration of illusion in line length. The horizontal line is the same length in both illustrations.

238 Tooth-Colored Restoratives

Figure 12–2. Illustration of illusion in straight and curved surfaces. The square and circle are the same width and height.

Light reflection

Ambient light reflection influences the perception of the size and whiteness of teeth. The greater the amount of reflected light, the larger, brighter, and closer the teeth appear. When all the teeth are whitened, the overall dentition appears more prominent than other facial features.

Tooth form

When tooth form is altered, the ambient light changes its direction of reflection. Flatter and smoother surfaces reflect more light directly back to the observer and therefore appear wider and larger. Rounder and rougher surfaces reflect light to the sides, making objects appear narrower and smaller (Figures 12–5, 12–6, 12–7, and 12–8).

Front to back progression

An object positioned closer appears larger than one positioned farther away. Similarly, darker teeth appear farther away and, therefore, smaller and appear to have less detailed features. In contrast, lighter teeth appear closer and larger. Alterations in tooth shade from the front to the back can affect the appearance of the arch form and the size of respective teeth.

Balance

Balance, or equilibrium, is achieved by equalizing opposing forces. Unbalanced objects look transitory, unfinished, and displeasing. In dentistry, left and right balance can be considered in terms of the visual weight of a composition over a centrally located fulcrum (eg, the midline of the maxillary

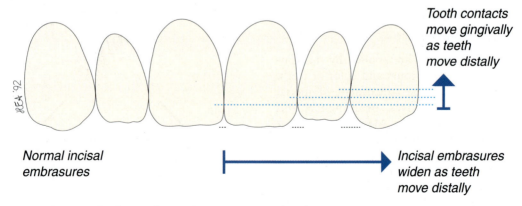

Figure 12–3. Schematic of embrasure form and contacts in normal teeth.

Normal appearing tooth width
Normal incisal embrasures

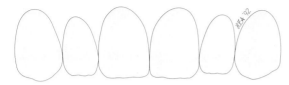

Wider appearing tooth width
Smaller than normal incisal embrasures

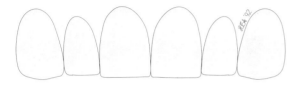

Narrower appearing tooth width
Wider than normal incisal embrasures

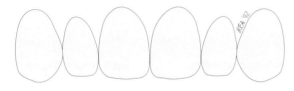

Figure 12–4. Schematic of the impact of altering incisal embrasure form to affect the perception of tooth width. As incisal embrasures are enlarged, teeth appear narrower.

central incisors). Things farther from the center exert more leverage or disharmony than those closer to it. A long cuspid on one side can make the smile look unbalanced, whereas irregularities in the length of laterals or centrals may appear less noticeable to the eye (Figure 12–9). Balance does not require symmetry, but both sides of a composition should have the same overall effect in terms of visual weight.

VENEERS

There are two major categories of veneers, indirect and direct, and many variations within each category. Indirect veneers are made outside the mouth and are bonded into place with a free-flowing composite resin. They are either prefabricated or custom-made. The first indirect veneers were prefabricated acrylic systems. Current custom systems are made of composite or porcelain. Direct veneers are made directly in the mouth, usually of one or more layers of light-cured composite.

Direct composite veneers have gained considerable popularity in recent years. They are especially useful for child or adolescent patients and have become popular as a cosmetic adjunct to adult patient care as well. Direct veneers present a number of advantages, such as minimal tooth preparation and no laboratory involvement. In addition, the technique is flexible, and the dentist has complete control over all aspects of the procedure. The disadvantages of direct veneers are increased chairtime for placement and the physical limitations of direct restorative materials. These physical limitations give the average composite veneer a life span of 4 to 8 years, which is considered short compared with other restorative treatments.

In the past, 10- to 20-year life spans were demanded of all dental restorations. Clinical studies have shown, however, that despite predictions of longevity, most restorations have an esthetic life span averaging only 8 years. Currently, many patients and dentists are willing to accept relatively short-lived restorations. This drop in expectation is justified because newer bonding procedures are noninvasive to oral structures and are often reversible. All bonding materials can easily be replaced, and worn out direct veneers can be refinished or re-veneered.

In many cases, veneers can be placed with little or no tooth preparation. This is particularly true for procedures such as diastema closures and tooth-form modifications. Extension of an incisal edge, however, commonly requires a preparation. Composite veneers that are placed on nonprepared enamel are referred to as extra-enamel restorations, since they are placed outside the confines of the enamel (Figure 12–10). Intra-enamel preparations are those in which all of the margins of the preparation are within the confines of enamel (Figure 12–11). Dentin–enamel preparations involve both dentin and enamel cavosurface margins.

Diagnostic considerations

A number of clinical factors bear review when considering restorative treatment with a composite veneer.

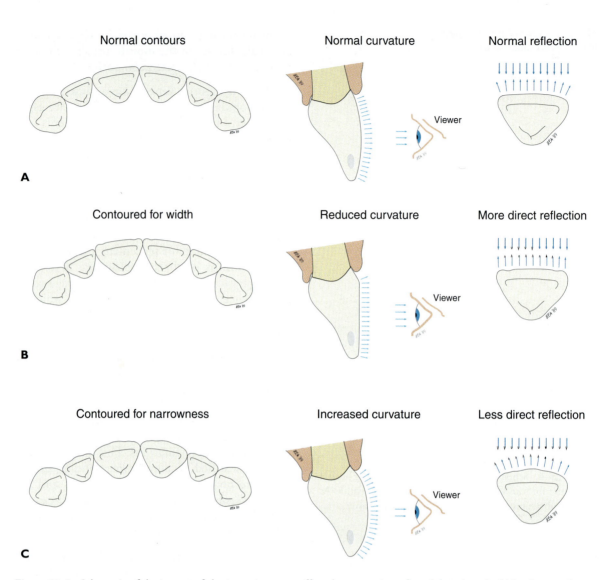

Figure 12–5. Schematic of the impact of altering contours to affect the perception of tooth length and width: *A*, normal contours; *B*, teeth contoured to reduce curvature and light reflection and create the appearance of greater width; and *C*, teeth contoured to enhance curvature and light reflection and create the appearance of less width.

Adequate enamel

Enamel should be present in the incisal portions of the proposed areas of bonding. Dentin bonding should not be relied on to retain the margin area of a composite veneer. When a margin of a veneer extends onto dentin, mechanical retention is necessary in addition to a dentin bonding agent. Veneers are prone to peel from dentin; mechanical retention will maintain the seal long term. Mechanical retention can be as simple as roughening the dentin or as complex as placing a retention groove.

Tooth discoloration

Perhaps the most difficult situation to treat with composite veneers is a badly discolored tooth. In these situations, intra-enamel or occasionally dentin–enamel preparations are needed.

Esthetics 241

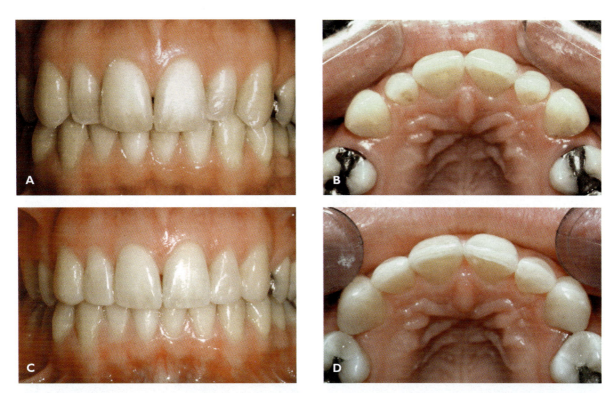

Figure 12–6. Increasing the appearance of width of laterals. *A*, Facial preoperative view of laterals that appear narrow owing to rounded contours; this makes the centrals and cuspids appear oversized. *B*, Incisal preoperative view of laterals showing their rounded contours. *C*, Facial postoperative view. Veneering moved the line angle toward the proximals and created a flatter surface. *D*, Incisal postoperative view showing the flatter surface. Neither the centrals nor the cuspids were changed in width during treatment.

Orthodontic problems
Composite veneers should be considered an adjunct to rather than a substitute for the treatment of misaligned anterior teeth.

Heavy smokers and coffee drinkers
Small-particle composites sometimes stain more than natural teeth, whereas microfilled composites usually stain less. These differences must be considered prior to material selection.

Edge-to-edge occlusion
Composite resins are contraindicated for areas of direct occlusal contact. Lengthening of a central incisor in a Class II occlusion has the best chance of long-term success; a Class III occlusion with centric contacts on the incisal edges has the least chance of long-term success.

Bruxism
Bruxism can cause excessive wear of any composite in function. Composite restorations in occlusal function are contraindicated for patients who brux.

Unusual habits
Patients who routinely hold hard objects between their teeth (eg, pipes, musical instruments, sewing pins, nails, etc) are apt to chip bonding material.

Patient expectations
The patient must understand the limitations of bonding. The use of pictures and models is helpful in demonstrating typical cosmetic results.

Taking and recording shades
With tooth-colored restoratives, it is important to make accurate records of the shades that are used. One goal is to achieve the desired result with as few shade combinations as possible. Complex custom shades may be difficult to duplicate for an adjacent restoration or for repair or replacement of an existing restoration. The use of color modifiers should also be carefully recorded. The best record is a diagram in the patient's chart that shows where the materials were added and includes photographs of

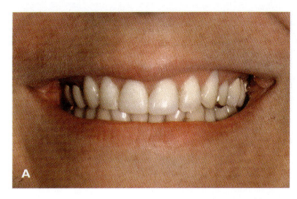
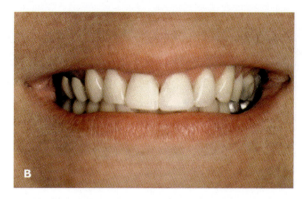

Figure 12–7. Increasing the appearance of width of centrals. *A*, Facial preoperative view of centrals that appear narrow owing to rounded contours. *B*, Postoperative view. Veneering moved the line angle toward the proximals, created a flatter surface, and reduced the width and height of incisal embrasures.

the critical color-correction steps. This information ensures efficiency in making any future repairs or adjacent restorations.

Patient management

It is important to inform patients of the limitations of composite materials. Prior to veneer place-

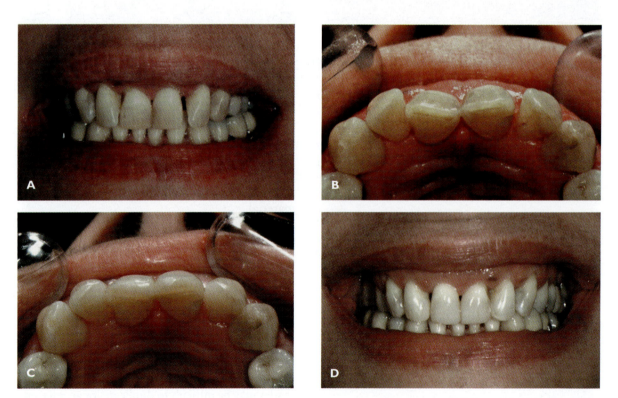

Figure 12–8. Decreasing the appearance of width. *A*, Preoperative view. Teeth appear wide, with extra space between the left central and lateral incisors. *B*, Incisal preoperative view. The flatness of the teeth is enhanced by the Class II, Division II occlusion. The patient did not want the teeth to look wider following diastema closure. *C*, Incisal postoperative view. The accentuated rounding of the teeth gives them a narrower appearance, despite their actual increase in width. *D*, Facial postoperative view. The accentuated rounding does not look unnatural and yet has a large impact on creating the illusion of narrowness.

Esthetics   243

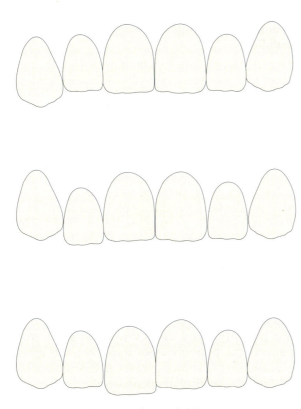

Figure 12–9. Schematic of vertical disharmony.

ment, problems concerning staining and fracture should be discussed, as well as maintenance requirements.

The patient must be informed that

- veneers are not permanent restorations,
- checkups are required,
- repairs may be required at any time,
- bonding material is softer than tooth structure,
- hygiene is important,
- composite veneers are less costly than crowns but not necessarily more cost effective, and
- the cost of future repairs and replacements is the responsibility of the patient.

Bonding checkups

Bonding checkups are an important aspect of patient management. Two-week, 3-month, and 6-month checkups aid in catching problems early. During each checkup, the work should be evaluated in terms of occlusion, esthetics, color stability, marginal integrity, and gingival health. The sooner a potential problem in material or placement is corrected the better.

Fees

Composite veneers are typically billed on an hourly basis. Since they usually require half the time needed for an anterior crown, the fee charged is generally half that charged for a porcelain-bonded-to-metal crown. Difficult and time-consuming cases involving extensive use of color modifiers and opaquers would warrant a higher fee. A higher fee should also be charged if maintenance beyond 12 months is included with the restoration. Esthetic contouring, if needed, is generally considered a separate service.

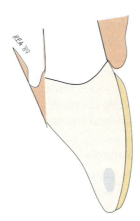
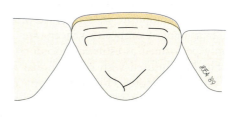

Figure 12–10. An extra-enamel preparation is ideal for teeth that are undercontoured or have lost substantial amounts of their enamel surface.

244 Tooth-Colored Restoratives

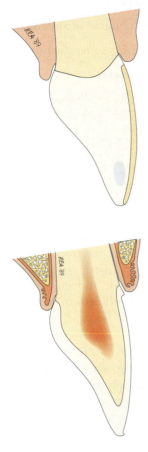

Figure 12–11. Intra-enamel preparations are finished supragingivally and, ideally, remain completely in enamel. A peripheral seal of enamel should be retained.

Third-party payment

Most insurance carriers and health maintenance organizations do not cover the placement and maintenance of composite veneers, since they are elective treatment. Composite veneers are most commonly performed as esthetic procedures and should not be confused with conventional treatment of caries or fractures. However, in some cases, a composite veneer is an appropriate alternative to an anterior crown. If this is explained to the responsible party, they will often cover the procedure, as it is in their best interest financially to do so. Before and after photographs are helpful in conveying the nature of the treatment to the parties involved.

Using direct composite veneers in practice-building

Dental practices are often built by providing treatment that enhances a person's self-image. Bonding procedures create healthy-looking teeth, which may impart to a patient a feeling of being healthier, younger, and more attractive. Nonetheless, patients quickly forget how their teeth appeared prior to dental treatment once the dental work has been completed. Photographs are the best way to substantiate the benefits of treatment. It is advisable to take before and after photographs of each patient undergoing treatment. Make three copies of the before photo and give one to the patient; their smile will act as their post-treatment record. The before photo establishes in the patient's mind the benefits of their dental treatment. The two other sets of before and after photos are for patient records and third-party purposes. Photographs in the patient record can be used to show new patients the possibilities of treatment. An office picture album showing cases before and after treatment is particularly persuasive.

Treatment planning

There are two common methods of planning a case for composite veneers: a waxup on a diagnostic model and a trial buildup of composite directly in the patient's mouth. The former is useful in large restorations where direct application of composite would consume excessive chairtime and materials, and in cases that involve contouring, which is irreversible. Trial buildups are useful with large restorations to check shade combinations and allow the patient to feel the changes in thickness that may be planned for some teeth. In small cases, direct buildups allow the patient to quickly see the type of changes planned. Some dentists use color imaging. It is fast, and projects can be printed immediately. A severe limitation, however, is that what is achievable electronically may not be achievable through dental treatment.

Diagnostic models

Some esthetic procedures are irreversible. Diagnostic (study) models are ideal to establish any tooth preparation or esthetic contouring that may be necessary to achieve an optimum esthetic result.

To prevent unnecessary tooth reduction, it is best to use two sets of diagnostic models as an aid in treatment planning. One should remain untouched, as a reference point. This control model makes it easy to gauge the amount of tooth structure that has been removed from the working model.

Once the working model has been trimmed to closely match esthetic contouring procedures, white inlay wax can be added to represent areas to be bonded. The use of white wax and white stone for the model produces a treatment mockup suitable for sharing with the patient.

A third model may be helpful for the novice operator. Two colors of wax might be used on this model to indicate placement of microfilled and heavily filled materials. Tooth lengthening or diastema closure restorations may require a heavily filled material covered with a thin microfilled veneer. Areas potentially needing color modifiers can be marked on the diagnostic cast.

When restorative treatment will change a patient's natural smile, the patient should see a preoperative and planned postoperative model prior to the start of treatment, and should hear again the limitations of bonding procedures. Too often, patients have expectations that cannot be achieved with these procedures. The use of study models helps limit disappointment and re-treatment. Patients should also be advised of potential repairs and adjustments that may be needed during the life of the restoration.

Tooth-form templates

A template is a dentist's aid that transfers the planned lingual contour, tooth width, and incisal edge shape and position from a study model to the patient's tooth. Once a diagnostic model has been completed, the new incisal edge form and thickness can be recorded by taking a silicon putty impression that covers the lingual and incisal surfaces and leaves the facial area exposed. When the impression material has set, the material is trimmed with a blade to the facial–incisal line angle. The template is then removed from the model, the lingual and gingival excess trimmed away, and the template placed in the patient's mouth to act as a positioning guide for the composite. The composite can be packed directly against the template to ensure proper location and incisal edge form. Esthetic contouring should not be done on the model surfaces, since it would interfere with the template's adaptation to the tooth. Once the composite has been adapted to the template and cured, the template can be removed and the restoration completed, including any necessary contouring.

Trial buildups

Trial buildups, also known as esthetic mockups, are valuable patient education tools. Unlike a study model, a trial buildup allows a patient to see proposed changes in his or her mouth rather than on a plaster model. Usually only a simple composite addition is necessary to allow a patient to preview possible improvements. Although dentists are comfortable with study models, patients respond with considerably more enthusiasm when they can experience proposed changes directly.

Trial buildups are essential in determining the correct use of color modifiers. To check a color, place the modifier directly on the tooth and cure it. Then place the appropriate shade and thickness of composite over the modifier and cure (Figure 12–12). If these materials are placed on slightly moist nonetched enamel they are easy to remove by tugging firmly with an explorer or spoon excavator. Repeat this procedure until the desired result is achieved. Varying the intensity of the color modifier with the composite shade can result in almost limitless shading possibilities. Record the final selected combination in the patient's record.

From a technical standpoint, a trial buildup is useful because all currently available light-cured composites exhibit a different color and opacity after polymerization (usually lighter and less opaque). Trying the selected combination of shades and color modifiers on the tooth prior to treatment maximizes the color match and esthetic result.

Procedure for trial buildup

Step 1. Clean stained teeth with pumice and water. Do not excessively dry the tooth.

Step 2. Do not acid etch the tooth. Trial buildups are done on unetched enamel.

Step 3. Use the manufacturer's shade guide or a customized office shade guide made from the restorative to select the appropriate color.

246   Tooth-Colored Restoratives

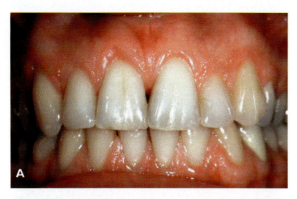

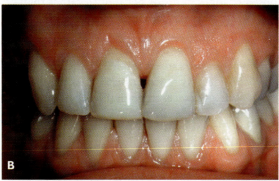

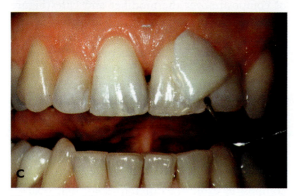

Figure 12–12. The trial buildup process allows the patient to preview a proposed esthetic change: *A,* preoperative, *B,* trial buildups in place, *C,* trial buildups being removed.

Step 4. Place the desired amount of color modifier on the tooth and cure.

Step 5. Contour the composite to the ideal shape with a hand instrument.

Step 6. Cure for a minimum of 20 to 40 seconds to establish the true color of the composite.

Step 7. Show the patient the result. Ask if he or she is satisfied with the proposed new look. If not, find out what changes the patient would like to make.

Step 8. Record the results. Specifically, note how improvements in shade and contour could be made during the actual composite placement.

Step 9. With a spoon excavator or sharp instrument, remove the resin. It will usually pop off with a firm tug.

Step 10. Repeat as necessary.

Trial buildups can be left on a patient to wear home. They often stay in place for a day or so depending on the dryness of the tooth when applied. If they are removed intact, the patient can try them on at home with Vaseline to show family members the type of result possible.

Considerations in veneer placement

Veneer placement is a highly technique-sensitive procedure. Rigid adherence to the principles of placement is essential to achieve optimal results. Unlike amalgam, composite resin is not a forgiving restorative material. The following principles are offered as helpful starting points for the novice operator.

What to do when placing composite veneers

- Do esthetic contouring prior to veneering.
- Do check the shade prior to treatment when the tooth is hydrated.
- Do disc enamel prior to acid etching.
- Do place and cure a bonding agent over etched enamel.
- Do use heavily filled composites in stress-bearing areas (eg, incisal edges).
- Do use a composite with very fine particle size on the surface (preferably a microfill).
- Do make the final outer layer continuous whenever possible to avoid irregularities or voids in the surface.
- Do finish above tissue whenever possible.
- Do look for adverse tissue responses at recall.

What not to do when placing composite veneers

- Do not start treatment unless the patient has seen a waxup or trial buildup of the desired results.

- Do not start treatment unless the patient has a full explanation of the limitations of treatment. Provide written documentation.
- Do not take or check the tooth shade with a rubber dam in place.
- Do not remove natural tooth contacts in preparation, if possible.
- Do not contaminate an etched enamel surface with water, saliva, or handpiece oil.
- Do not overcontour the restoration.
- Do not leave thin areas of composite at the margins.
- Do not attempt to make large color changes with surface glazes.

Esthetic contouring

Esthetic contouring is one of the most practical ways of improving a person's smile. The smoothing and rounding of chipped incisors is not only esthetically pleasing but also reduces further chipping and soft-tissue irritation. A major disadvantage of esthetic contouring is its irreversibility; therefore, a study model indicating planned changes must be shown to the patient prior to treatment. Another disadvantage is that teeth generally appear darker since removal of enamel allows the darker toned dentin to show through. When planning esthetic contouring for a case, avoid taking more than 0.5 mm from the surface of a central incisor and 0.75 mm from the surface of a cuspid. Larger reductions can result in adverse color changes in the tooth surface as well as dentin exposure or tooth hypersensitivity.

Discolored teeth

For many patients with discolored teeth, restoration to a lighter shade is relatively simple: one shade of composite is applied and the natural color distribution of the tooth shows through, yielding a lighter, natural-looking effect. However, some teeth are so discolored their natural shade distribution has been lost. In these more complicated cases, more than one shade of composite or color modifier is required.

Altering the shade of a tooth with more than one shade can be difficult. The limitations of veneer thickness and the lack of the masking ability of composite typically require the use of color modifiers. Use of color modifiers in turn dictates greater thickness of the veneer to avoid losing tooth vitality. The appearance of natural shade distribution across a tooth is achievable by combining different shades of color modifiers and composite. The major disadvantage of this technique is a discontinuous outer layer of composite, which creates the possibility of voids at junctions. The more viscous the composite the greater the likelihood of voids.

Multiple shades of composite can be used in an overlapping fashion on the full labial composite veneer (Figure 12–13). The body shade should overlap both the gingival and incisal shades. Failure to properly overlap results in a sharp, unnatural demarcation between the layers. The total thickness of the superficial layer should be at least 0.2 mm. Overlapping becomes difficult when making thinner additions. If thinner layers are necessary, use a flowable composite.

Shade distribution for color modifiers

Color modifiers can be used between layers of composite. This is particularly convenient between the supportive and surface layers of larger composite restorations. It is also advantageous, because the use of a color modifier allows space for a continuous outer layer of resin. This reduces the possibility of facial voids.

Color modifiers are best placed over a cured bonding agent and then covered with composite. Brown and orange shades are appropriate for characterization near the gingiva; blue and gray shades in the incisal area create the appearance of incisal translucency. Color modifiers should always be cured prior to covering with composite. Regardless which combination of materials is used, the shades and their locations should be recorded in the patient's dental record to aid in making future repairs and adjacent restorations. Figure 12–14 shows the areas where color modifiers are commonly applied.

Restorative treatment of discolored teeth

Tooth preparation is not the preferred method of treating generalized tooth discoloration. It is effective, however, in the treatment of isolated areas of enamel discoloration. Removing these areas and restoring them with bonding material is the most practical method of treatment. Cases of generalized discoloration are often best treated with bleaching.

248 Tooth-Colored Restoratives

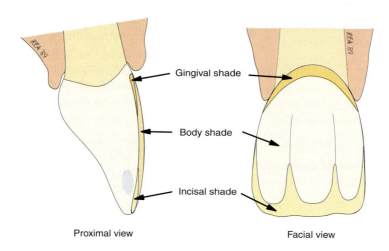

Figure 12–13. Schematic representation of composite shade distribution for a typical full facial composite veneer. A brown shade is used for gingival color, a universal shade for body color, and a lighter shade for the incisal edge color.

In some cases, these conservative treatment methods fail and enamel preparations are needed. The following preparation techniques provide guidance for such a situation. These preparations are intra-enamel: all the cavosurface margins are confined entirely within enamel. These are the most commonly used preparations for the placement of direct composite veneers. When the facial surface is to be veneered for cosmetic reasons secondary to discoloration, it is best to use color modifiers under the composite veneer surface.

Many discolored teeth are uniformly discolored (eg, stains attributable to age) and removal of enamel creates space for composite with minimal tooth darkening. With other discolored teeth, the stain is primarily in the dentin (eg, stains attributable to use of tetracycline) and removal of enamel results in a darker tooth. Some discolored teeth are discolored only superficially (eg, stains attributable to fluorosis) and removal of enamel immediately removes the stain. With such superficial staining, tooth surface removal may comprise the only treatment needed.

Armamentarium

The basic setup for placing composite veneers includes operator items (gown, gloves, mask, face shield, etc), isolation materials (retraction cord, rubber dam materials, Mylar strips with retention clips), basic supplies (anesthetic, caries indicator), instruments (explorers, mouth mirror, periodontal probe, handpiece with assorted diamonds, interproximal carvers, condensers), and placement supplies (cotton forceps and placement brushes).

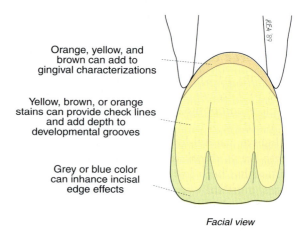

Figure 12–14. Schematic map of color modifier usage under a full facial composite veneer.

Esthetics **249**

The basic equipment required includes a curing light, radiometer, tooth dryer, air and water syringes, suction device, and color-corrected light source.

The specific materials needed include the following:

- Light-cured composite
- Resin-compatible bonding system
- Color modifiers
- Round-ended cylinder diamond, medium grit
- Quarter-round bur
- Flame-shaped finishing burs and micron diamonds
- Finishing discs and strips
- Composite placement instrument
- Bard Parker No. 12 and No. 15 blades
- soft plastic tape (eg, plumber's tape)

Intra-enamel preparations

Outline

Using a round-ended diamond, prepare a labial chamfer in enamel. This chamfer extends gingivally just short of the gingival tissue and short of the dentin–enamel junction. The mesial and distal proximal borders of the preparation stop just slightly labial to the contact areas (Figure 12–15).

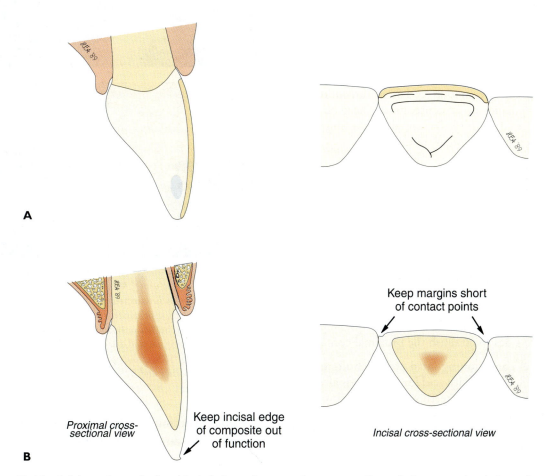

Figure 12–15. *A*, Schematic proximal and incisal views of a composite veneer outline and, *B*, cross-sectional views of a composite veneer preparation not involving the incisal edge.

250 Tooth-Colored Restoratives

This type of preparation enhances resistance form and results in a clearly defined periphery to which the composite resin can be finished.

Depth
The depth of the preparation should be approximately one-quarter to three-quarters the thickness of the enamel, depending on the extent of the discoloration. A quarter-round bur may be used to provide a 0.5-mm depth measurement. This depth allows for the labial thickness of composite needed to cover most discoloration without significant overcontouring. In severely discolored teeth, it allows space for color modifiers to mask stains and alter the shade of the underlying tooth. Leave nondiscolored portions of the tooth untouched.

Retention
All retention comes from acid etching the enamel on the labial surface. No additional mechanical retention is used.

Pulp protection
No pulp protection is used, because the labial enamel layer should be intact. If dentin is exposed during the preparation and it is surrounded by etched enamel, no extra precautions need be taken; however, if dentin is exposed at the margin, a dentin bonding system should be used.

Placement of light-cured composite
Light-cured composites allow adequate time to work with the material prior to curing.

Sculpting
Use a heavy-body material. Place the material directly on the tooth and shape it using the appropriate hand instruments. Use an interproximal carver to shape the material proximally and a half-Hollenbeck carver to shape the labial surface. Compress the material from both the labial and lingual sides to establish the proximal contacts.

Enamel conditioning (acid etch technique)
Etch the enamel with acid for 20 seconds after protecting the adjacent teeth with Mylar strips (120 s is necessary for substantial enamel fluorosis and primary teeth). Rinse with water for a minimum of 10 seconds, and dry thoroughly with air.

Bonding agent and color modifiers
Wet the etched enamel with bonding agent as thinly and as evenly as possible. Polymerize using

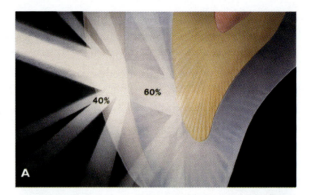
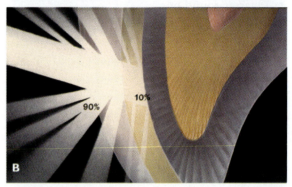
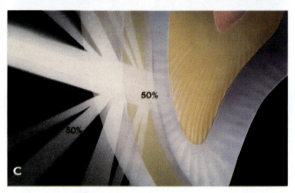

Figure 12–16. Schematic illustrations of *A*, normal light reflection in a young tooth: 40% of the light is reflected off the surface and 60% is reflected off the dentin–enamel junction, yielding a vital appearance; *B*, masking of the facial surface with a color modifier or opaque composite, resulting in 90% external reflection and a lack of tooth vitality; *C*, distributed masking: 50% of the opaquing is achieved internally with a color modifier and 50% through composite.

a visible light source. Place a color modifier, if needed. Use it over the entire surface or in specific areas to mask out discoloration. If one thin coat does not mask the discoloration, polymerize it and apply a second coat. Do not apply a thick layer of color modifier. With defects such as yellow check lines, it is best to block out only 50% of the defect with a color modifier, allowing the restorative to do the rest (Figure 12–16). Overmasking with color modifier can result in an opaque restoration with less than ideal vitality (Figure 12–17). The hint of check lines, visible through the composite, retains the natural character of the tooth; this is more desirable than a uniform white surface (Figure 12–18). Cure any opaquer or color modifier used.

Layered placement
Squeeze from the tube a piece of putty-like composite slightly larger than needed for the restoration. Form it into a disc slightly smaller than the restoration. Place this pre-formed disc of uncured composite over the cured bonding agent. Use a plastic instrument, explorer, or half-Hollenbeck to mold the material into the desired contour, adapting it to the margins. Prior to curing, remove the flash from the margins and proximal areas. Cure the composite at the margin areas; avoid the center of the restoration as much as possible. (This may require masking a portion of the light rod.) Once the margins are polymerized, check the seal with an explorer. If necessary, place a flowable material at any margin that has lifted from the tooth. Cure the entire restoration for 40 to 60 seconds.

Bulk placement
Put a mass of composite on a pad; transfer it to the tooth. Use two instruments to tease it over the cured bonding agent in all directions. Use a plastic instrument, explorer, or half-Hollenbeck to mold the material into the desired contour. Slowly pull the Mylar toward the lingual to help adapt the material into the proximal areas. Composites typically adhere to the matrix; using an interproximal carver, gently transfer the composite from the matrix to the lingual surface, and then contour. Once the composite is contoured on both facial and lingual, score the junction between the composite and the matrix until a minimum amount of composite remains attached. Rapidly pull the matrix away from the tooth. The matrix should separate freely, leaving the

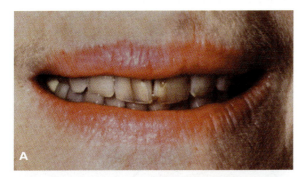
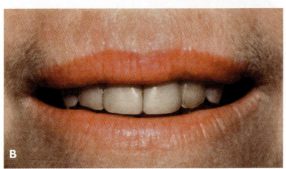
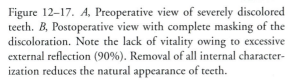

Figure 12–17. *A*, Preoperative view of severely discolored teeth. *B*, Postoperative view with complete masking of the discoloration. Note the lack of vitality owing to excessive external reflection (90%). Removal of all internal characterization reduces the natural appearance of teeth.

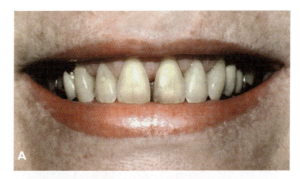
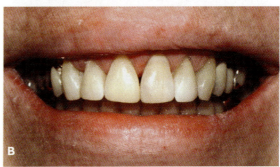

Figure 12–18. *A*, Preoperative view of discolored teeth (classic case). *B*, Postoperative view. Correct use of color modifier: 50% of discoloration is masked by color modifier and 25% by opaque composite, which allows 25% of natural internal characterization to show through.

composite in place. Now mold the composite to the desired contour. Reestablish the proximal contact by compressing the composite from the facial and lingual. Prior to curing, remove any flash from the margins. Cure as described for layered placement.

Finishing and polishing

Wait at least 10 minutes following polymerization before finishing. Remove the gingival retraction cord by pulling it toward the tissue. If the restoration is overcontoured, reduce the contour with a flame-shaped diamond or coarse disc. Use a safe-end diamond to eliminate any gross excess of composite that has been cured past the margins of the preparation. View the restoration from the incisal edge and evaluate the facial thickness and contour in the gingival body and incisal areas by rotating the mirror. For final contouring and margin adaptation, use finishing diamonds (or white stones) with water and a handpiece. Blend the final contours using a rubber finishing cup. Polish the restorative using flexible discs. For a final polish, use a soft rubber cup and polishing paste. Check occlusion to ensure the restorative does not function in protrusive or lateral movement.

Restorative treatment of severely discolored teeth

Occurrences are rare, but some discolored teeth do not respond well enough to bleaching to permit masking them with a composite veneer the thickness of enamel. The underlying dentin is too extensively involved and more generous facial tooth reduction may be necessary. Tooth preparation into dentin is a method of last resort prior to proceeding with more invasive crown and bridge procedures. Less than 1% of the teeth treated with veneers require this type of tooth reduction. As always, prior to performing any preparation, inform the patient of the invasiveness and irreversibility of the treatment. The patient must be prepared to accept crowns as an alternative if these procedures do not provide acceptable results.

The following preparations are dentin–enamel preparations. They have both dentin and enamel cavosurface margins (Figure 12–19). These preparations require careful tissue management to avoid the periodontal problems that can result from the placement of subgingival margins.

Armamentarium

The basic setup for a dentin–enamel preparation includes operator items (gown, gloves, mask, face shield, etc), isolation materials (retraction cord, rubber dam materials, and Mylar strips with retention clips), basic supplies (anesthetic and caries indicator), instruments (explorer, mouth mirror, periodontal probe, small spoon excavators to remove caries, handpiece with assorted burs and

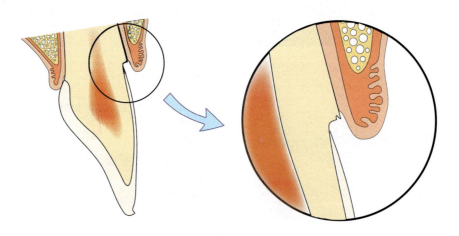

Figure 12–19. Schematic representation of the relation between the composite preparation and the tissue in a dentin–enamel preparation that required masking of discoloration in the gingival one-third.

diamonds, small ball-ended applicator, interproximal carvers, condensers), and placement supplies (cotton forceps and placement brushes).

The basic equipment required is a curing light, radiometer, tooth dryer, air and water syringes, suction device, and color-corrected light source.

The specific materials needed include the following:

- Light-cured composite
- Resin-compatible bonding kit
- Color modifiers or color opaquers
- A dentin–enamel bonding agent
- Dentin liner (eg, glass-ionomer liner or CaOH)
- Braided retraction cord, No. 9
- Fine flame diamond
- Burs: No. 169L, 1/4-round, 33-1/3 inverted cone
- Round-ended cylinder diamond, medium grit
- Finishing burs and micron diamonds
- Flexible finishing discs
- Composite strips
- Composite placement instrument
- Bard Parker No. 12 and No. 15 blades
- Cheek retractors

Dentin–enamel preparations

Place cheek retractors and a braided or knitted retraction cord to retract the gingiva. An alternative approach is to use a rubber dam and a No. 212 rubber dam clamp. However, this approach restricts work to one central incisor at a time, which could compromise achieving a good match among multiple teeth. It is difficult to opaque two teeth in an identical fashion when they are not done at the same time.

Outline

Using a round-ended diamond or No. 169L bur in the gingival one-third, prepare a 1-mm labial shoulder. This shoulder extends gingivally just short of the gingival retraction cord. The mesial and distal proximal borders of the preparation stop just slightly labial to the contact areas (see Figure 12–19). The cavosurface exit is 60 to 90 degrees. This type of preparation results in a clearly defined periphery to which the composite resin may be finished.

Depth

In the incisal two-thirds, the depth of the preparation should be approximately one-quarter to three-quarters the thickness of enamel, depending on the extent of the discoloration. This depth provides space for color modifiers and composites to alter the shade of the original tooth. It does this at both the incisal and gingival areas without overcontouring of the final restoration. A retention groove enhances the attachment and seal at the dentin margin.

Retention

In the incisal two-thirds, retention is achieved by acid etching the enamel on the labial surface. In the gingival one-third, a 1/4-round bur (or a 33-1/3 inverted cone bur) is used to place a 0.5-mm retention groove just inside the cavosurface margin.

Placement of color modifiers

An opaquer (a tinted white modifier that masks 100%) is needed for severely discolored teeth; it is sandwiched between two layers of bonding agent prior to addition of the restorative. An opaquer may be used in place of or in addition to a color modifier. For lighter discoloration, use a conventional white color modifier over the entire surface or in specific areas. If one thin coat does not mask the discoloration, polymerize it and apply a second coat. Do not apply a thick layer of color modifier. With defects such as yellow check lines, it is best to block out only 50% of the defect with a color modifier, allowing the restorative to do the rest. Thus, dark check lines are converted into subtle characterizations. As discussed in the previous section, overmasking with color modifiers can result in an opaque restoration with less than optimum vitality.

A color modifier should be used as a trial buildup prior to treatment to determine the proper amount of opaquing. Figure 12–20 shows a typical procedure for evaluating the use of a color modifier.

Procedure

Enamel bonding (acid etch technique)

Etch with acid for 20 seconds after protecting the adjacent teeth with Mylar strips (120 s is necessary

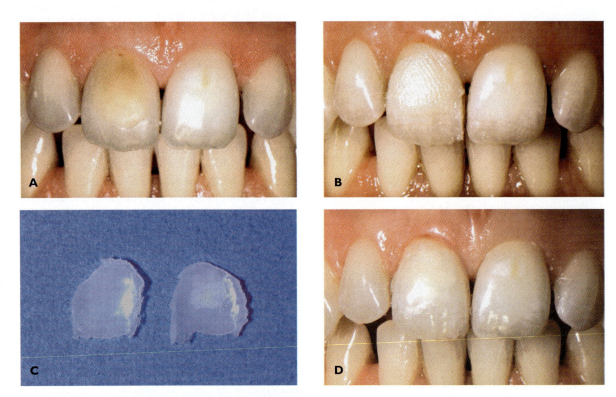

Figure 12–20. *A*, A stain prior to masking; *B*, a test coat of color modifier and composite placed on the tooth and cured; *C*, two test samples that have been applied and removed; and *D*, the correct combination needed to restore the tooth.

for substantial enamel fluorosis and for primary teeth). Rinse with water for a minimum of 10 seconds, and dry thoroughly with air.

Bonding agent
Wet the etched enamel with a bonding agent, applying it as thinly and evenly as possible. Polymerize using a visible light source. Place a color modifier, if needed. Cure any opaquer or color modifier used.

Layered placement
Squeeze from the tube a piece of putty-like composite slightly larger than needed for the restoration. Form it into a disc slightly smaller than the restoration. Place this pre-formed disc of uncured composite over the cured bonding agent. Use a plastic instrument, explorer, or half-Hollenbeck to mold the material into the desired contour, adapting it to the margins. Prior to curing, remove the flash from the margins and proximal areas. Cure the composite at the margin areas; avoid the center of the restoration as much as possible. (This may require masking a portion of the light rod.) Once the margins are polymerized, check the seal with an explorer. If necessary, place a flowable material at any margin that has lifted from the tooth. Cure the entire restoration for 40 to 60 seconds.

Bulk placement
Put a mass of composite on a pad; transfer it to the tooth. Use two instruments to tease it over the cured bonding agent in all directions. Use a plastic instrument, explorer, or half-Hollenbeck to mold the material into the desired contour. Slowly pull the Mylar toward the lingual to help adapt the material into the proximal areas. Composites typically adhere to the matrix; using an interproximal carver, gently transfer the composite from the matrix to the lingual surface, and then contour. Once the composite is contoured on both facial and lingual, score the junction between the composite and the matrix until a minimum amount of composite remains attached. Rapidly pull the matrix away from the tooth. The matrix should separate freely, leaving the composite in place. Now mold the composite

Esthetics

to the desired contour. Reestablish the proximal contact by compressing the composite from the facial and lingual. Prior to curing, remove any flash from the margins. Cure as described for layered placement.

Finishing and polishing

Wait at least 10 minutes following polymerization before finishing. Remove the gingival retraction cord by pulling it toward the tissue. If the restoration is overcontoured, reduce the contour with a flame-shaped diamond or coarse disc. Use a safe-end diamond to eliminate any gross excess of composite that has been cured past the margins of the preparation. View the restoration from the incisal edge and evaluate the facial thickness and contour in the gingival body and incisal areas by rotating the mirror. For final contouring and margin adaptation, use finishing diamonds (or white stones) with water and a handpiece. Blend the final contours using a rubber finishing cup. Polish the restorative using flexible discs. For a final polish, use a soft rubber cup and polishing paste. Check occlusion to ensure the restorative does not function in protrusive or lateral movement.

Diastema closure

Closing spaces between teeth is a common cosmetic dental treatment. This section discusses the most common methods for closing a diastema with a direct restorative. Figure 12–21 illustrates some of the typical spaces that dentists are asked to treat.

Light-cured composite resin is the typical restorative for diastema closure. Approximately 25% of the adult American population has a midline diastema. Cultural differences exist, but the trend in the United States suggests that more people would have their diastemas closed if they could do so without damaging their existing teeth. Use of direct veneers for diastema closures offers the advantages of a conservative, reversible restoration with essentially no tooth structure removal. The disadvantages of using direct veneers include less durability and less color-stability than ceramic restorations. In addition, periodontal problems can result from the addition of the proximal contour needed to close the space.

Proximal restorations

Proximal restorations can work well for 1- to 2-mm spaces. These restorations are done with a single restorative that is finished facially in a developmental groove (Figure 12–22, *A*). In some arches, a larger space (2–3 mm) can be closed in the same way. In these cases, the teeth can appear unusually wide, making a rounded contour important (see Figure 12–22, *B*). Many of these restorations can be done with little or no tooth preparation. Since the facial enamel–restorative interfaces are in highly visible areas, finishing these in the developmental groove provides a more cosmetic finish line.

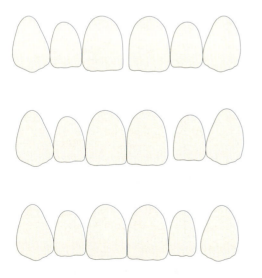

Figure 12–21. Schematic representation of some common types of space closures.

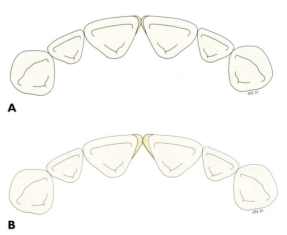

Figure 12–22. An incisal view of proximal restorations used to close spaces: *A*, a small diastema; *B*, a medium diastema.

Unprepared tooth. Veneering the facial surface can minimize the appearance of width in a diastema closure. Altering the contour yields a narrower appearance (Figure 12–23). This effect can be further improved by rounding the distal contacts of the teeth. The total effect of these procedures is to move the bodies of the teeth to the center and improve the appearance of the midline contours (Figure 12–24).

With direct systems, a larger restoration is stronger and more esthetic if 1 mm of a polishable material is used over a more durable material to provide support. A heavily filled material (which is often not very polishable) provides the necessary durability to reduce fractures, whereas a microfill or submicron hybrid composite allows for a higher polish that would reduce external staining.

Prepared tooth. In larger diastemas (3 to 4+ mm), a preparation is often required to provide the resistance form to avoid displacement. A conservative restoration is demonstrated in Figure 12–25. Enamel contouring opposite the diastema closure can result in the illusion that the restored teeth have not been excessively increased in mesial-distal width.

Full coverage. One of the easiest ways to close a diastema is to make the teeth larger through full-coverage restoration (Figure 12–26). The increase in central incisor dominance can provide good esthetics in many patients, and this technique provides the dentist excellent control over contours. Full-coverage preparations can be done where all of the preparation is in enamel. A typical result with full-coverage composite restoration is shown in Figure 12–27.

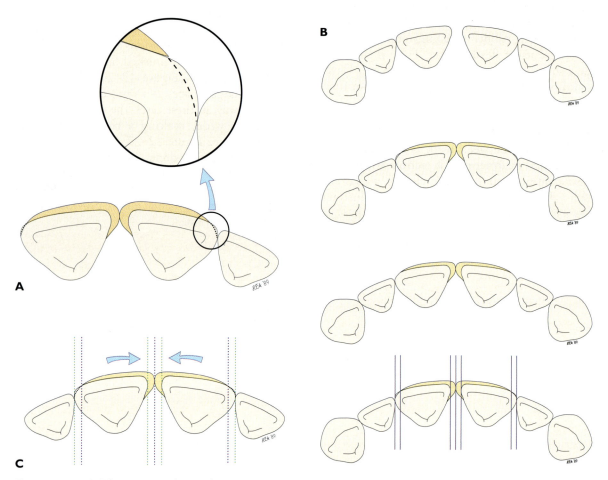

Figure 12–23. *A,* Schematic incisal view of two veneer preparations used to close a large diastema. The distal proximal rounding gives the appearance of increased width; *B,* restorative sequence in diastema closure; and *C,* movement of line angles toward the midline.

Esthetics 257

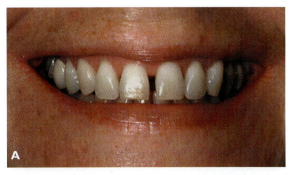

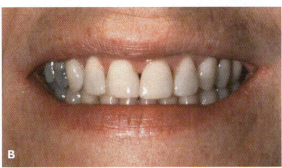

Figure 12–24. The overall effect veneers can produce when used to move the body of a tooth to the midline.

Diastema closure restorative technique

In simple cases, a trial buildup may be adequate to provide diagnostic information and to obtain a patient's consent for treatment. More pronounced cases, or those involving multiple teeth, require a more comprehensive treatment plan. A good approach is to use a study model from an earlier appointment in which a diagnostic waxup was completed. A template is used to provide guidance during placement.

If esthetic contouring is needed, it should be completed during a preliminary appointment, because contouring changes the shade of a tooth.

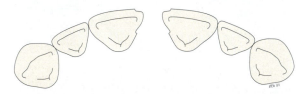

Figure 12–25. Schematic representation of a conservative preparation used to increase marginal thickness and provide resistance form.

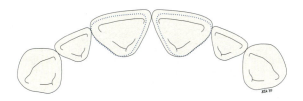

Figure 12–26. Schematic of the outline of a full-coverage treatment; the outline of the natural teeth is shown in dotted lines.

It is possible that a patient will decide to stop treatment following contouring because the esthetic improvement it achieves is adequate for them.

Two-phase direct technique

The following procedure outlines a two-phase technique for placing a microfilled composite over a heavily filled composite base (Figure 12–28). Note that it follows the guidelines of other direct restorative procedures.

Step 1. Determine correct shade. Place and cure together the combination of composites to be used; compare with the teeth.

Step 2. Decide which tooth is to be restored first. Protect the adjacent teeth with Mylar or a smooth plastic tape. Disc, etch, wash, and dry the tooth. Place a bonding agent and distribute it evenly with a brush. Cure the bonding agent. Add color modifier, if needed, and cure.

Step 3. Extend a heavily filled composite from the proximal portion of the tooth and shape it to ideal contour lingually, 1 mm short of the labial contour. This should be done freehand. Cure the restorative for 40 seconds.

Step 4. Place a polishable composite over both the facial enamel of the tooth and the previously cured heavily filled composite. Stop just short of the distal proximal contacts.

Step 5. Use an interproximal carver and an explorer to shape and contour the restorative. Use of different shades of the composite may assist in simulating the natural coloration of gingival and incisal areas.

Step 6. Contour as needed. Once contoured, cure the composite for 40 seconds (60 s for dark shades).

258 Tooth-Colored Restoratives

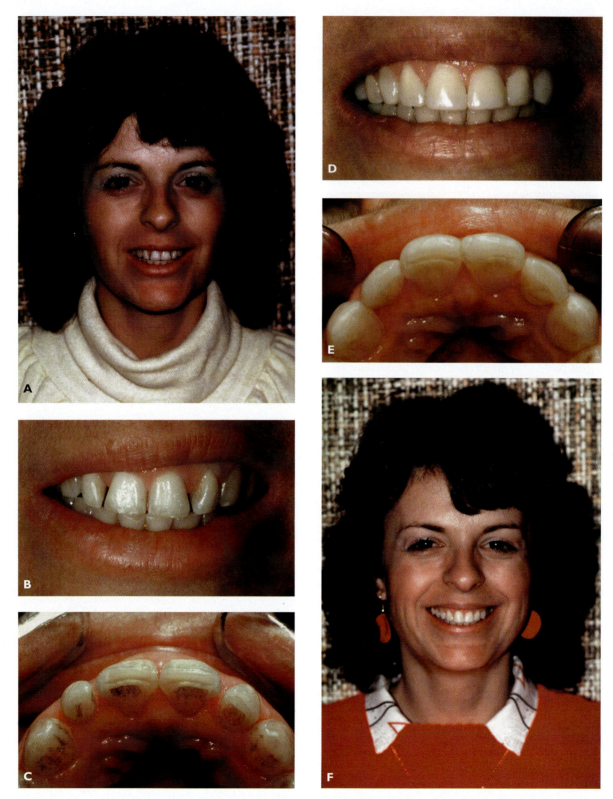

Figure 12–27. *A*, Preoperative facial view of misshapen teeth that were treated to close diastemas on both sides. *B*, Preoperative close-up of smile. *C*, Preoperative incisal view. *D*, Postoperative smile view. *E*, Postoperative incisal view. *F*, Postoperative facial view.

Esthetics 259

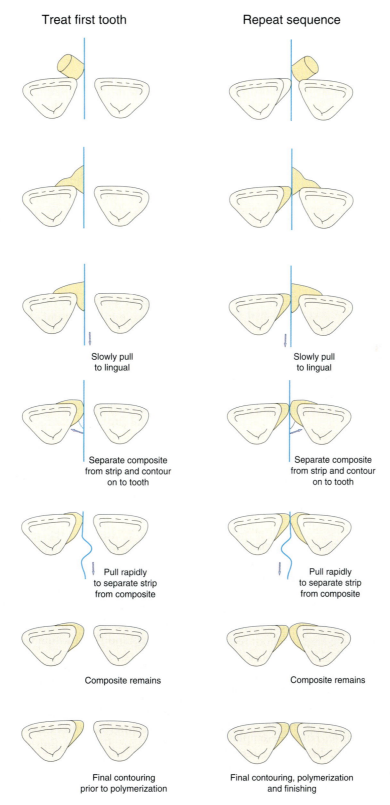

Figure 12–28. Schematic representation of the procedure for placement of composite to close a diastema.

Step 7. Finish the restoration with the appropriate burs and discs.

Step 8. Establish the proper midline. It is important that the mesial surface of the restoration does not tip to either side of the midline. The width of the tooth and the distance between the finished mesial–proximal surface and the distal of the untreated tooth should be exact. Also carefully examine the proximal gingival embrasures to ensure properly rounded contours that do not impinge on the gingival tissues.

Step 9. Once the first restoration is correctly placed, restore the contralateral tooth in a similar fashion. Pay attention to matching the gingival embrasure form to the previously restored tooth.

Step 10. Round the proximal contours opposite the diastema closure to create the illusion that the restored teeth have not been widened excessively. Do not remove more than 0.5 mm of enamel. Excess tooth reduction can darken a tooth or expose dentin. (Ideally, this step is done prior to the addition of composite, since it can affect tooth shade; however, the need for this procedure may not be apparent until after the veneers are placed.)

Two-phase direct technique with template
There are many ways to make a template; this is one suggested method: mix silicon putty as directed by the manufacturer (bite-registration material is an acceptable alternative). Place the putty on a lubricated model of the arch from the lingual to at least 6 mm beyond the gingival margin to the palate. Adapt the putty to the lingual surface and over the incisal edges by about 1 mm. Allow to set, then score the incisal embrasures with a Bard Parker knife (without damaging the model) to a depth of at least 1 mm. Remove the template from the model and trim the facial surface to the incisal–facial line angle without removing the score lines. On each side of the tooth to be restored, using a Bard Parker blade, make clean cuts from the score marks through the interproximal area and past the lingual margin, without separating the putty. A Mylar strip should easily fit into the gap left by the knife. Trim the template to remove any awkward bulk. Ideally, the template should mechanically lock back onto the diagnostic model. Try the template in the mouth. It should lock on in the mouth the way it does on the model; make any adjustments needed to achieve this fit.

Step 1. Determine correct shade: Place and cure together the combination of composites to be used; compare to the teeth.

Step 2. Decide which tooth is to be restored first. Protect the adjacent teeth with Mylar or a smooth plastic tape. Disc, etch, wash, and dry the tooth. Place a bonding agent and distribute it evenly with a dry brush. Cure the bonding agent. Add color modifier, if needed, and cure.

Step 3. Disc the surfaces that will be restored. Place the template in the mouth. Insert Mylar through the template into the interproximal spaces. An interproximal carver may be useful to separate the silicon putty and facilitate Mylar placement. Trim the Mylar to 3 mm past the facial surfaces.

Step 4. Place a heavily filled composite into the template 1 mm short of the labial contour. This should be done freehand. Cure the restorative for 40 seconds.

Step 5. Place a polishable composite over both the facial enamel of the tooth and the previously cured heavily filled composite. Stop just short of the distal proximal contacts.

Step 6. Use an interproximal carver and an explorer to shape and contour the restorative. Use of different shades of the composite may assist in simulating the natural coloration of gingival and incisal areas of the tooth.

Step 7. Remove the template and the Mylar strips. Finish the restorative with the appropriate burs and discs.

Step 8. Evaluate the midline placement established by the template. It should match that of the study model. Establish the proper mesial–proximal contours and the midline with a thin disc.

Step 9. Once the first restoration is correctly placed, restore the contralateral tooth in a similar fashion. Use a football-shaped diamond to remove lingual flash. Use a No. 12 Bard Parker blade to remove interproximal excess lingually and proximally. Use diamond finishing strips to establish proper embrasure form.

Step 10. Add enamel contouring, if needed. (Since contouring cannot be done in the diagnostic waxup or template, it is done at this point.)

Esthetics 261

Correction of malposed teeth

A variety of tooth formation or positioning problems occur that affect esthetics and can be appropriately treated with direct restorations: teeth can be facially out of plane, rotated, vertically out of symmetry, angled, and overlapping.

Moving teeth facially

Teeth can be "moved" facially by adding a thickness of composite to the facial surface. This addition gives the teeth more appropriate positioning (Figure 12–29). These are referred to as extra-enamel restorations since they are placed outside the confines of the enamel. Care is taken to avoid involving the gingival areas of the teeth and thus any adverse periodontal effects.

Dealing with the proximal area of these restorations can be difficult since the proximal contact is usually widened from lingual to facial. In addition, access to the proximal margins is compromised, making hygiene problematic. Whenever possible, attempts should be made to keep these margins in cleanable areas just short of the natural tooth contact. Over time, chipping can result in staining or caries, which further compromises hygiene and encourages decay.

The correction of these malposed teeth may produce less than favorable tooth contours. Excellent oral hygiene is mandatory as well as follow-up care to ensure that bonded areas are tolerated by the periodontal tissue. Figure 12–30 shows a common correction for Class II, Division II occlusions.

Correcting rotations

Veneering to change contours can visually correct rotated anterior teeth. This technique is best used as an adjunct to rather than a replacement for orthodontics. By bonding only a portion of a tooth, it is possible to rotate the facial surface of an incisor. This rotation is enhanced by contouring on the opposite side of the tooth (Figure 12–31). Be

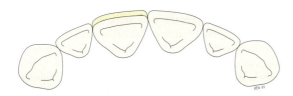

Figure 12–29. Schematic incisal view of the correction of a lingually inclined central incisor.

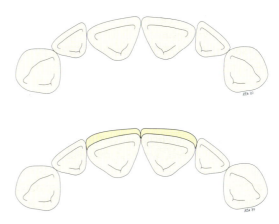

Figure 12–30. Schematic incisal view of a typical Class II, Division II occlusion (*top*), which is typically corrected by adding to the facial of the centrals (*bottom*). The major disadvantage of this approach is increased incisal width; however, many patients tolerate this well.

aware, however, that correcting a rotation widens a tooth from facial to lingual, often in just one area. Many patients find this produces an unnatural feeling. With esthetic contouring, the tooth is narrowed facial–lingually from its original thickness in

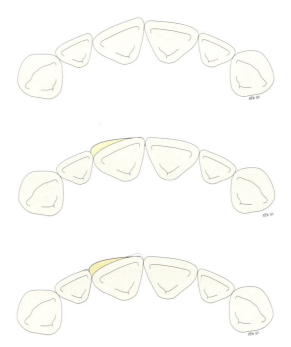

Figure 12–31. Schematic incisal view that demonstrates the correction of a rotated central incisor with a restorative and enamel contouring; *top*, before; *middle*, after; *bottom*, natural tooth outlined by dotted lines.

other areas. Bonding on the lingual side of the tooth to balance the width of the incisal table often compensates for this change (Figure 12–32). When the treatment plan is to add to the lingual surface of a central incisor, care should be taken to avoid occlusal interferences. Figure 12–33 shows a typical clinical case.

As previously mentioned, esthetic contouring can darken a tooth, because removal of enamel brings the darker shaded dentin closer to the surface. This effect is more noticeable in more mature patients because of their naturally darker teeth. Therefore, it is important to delay determination of composite shade until after esthetic contouring is finished; ideally, during a later appointment.

An alternative to removing enamel is to bring the teeth forward facially. In some dentitions this may be a suitable option. A diagnostic waxup is an important aid in exploring these options.

When cuspids are rotated, a diastema can result; correction of the rotation and the diastema involves placing a restorative on the lingual and discing the

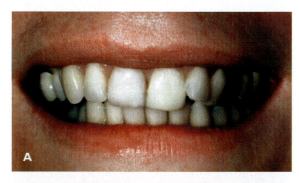
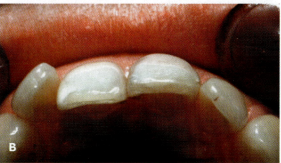
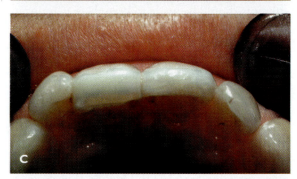
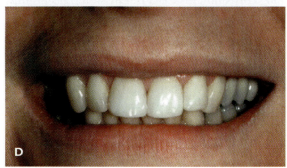

Figure 12–33. *A*, Preoperative facial view of misaligned teeth. *B*, Preoperative incisal view. *C*, Incisal view showing the correction of a rotated central incisor. *D*, Postoperative facial view. After enamel recontouring, restorative materials were placed on the facial and incisal to correct the alignment of the arch form. Note the wider incisal table needed to accomplish this.

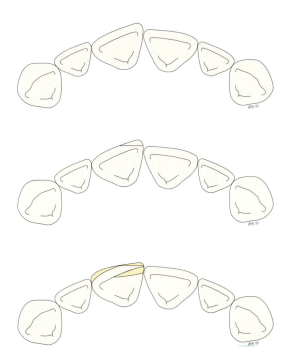

Figure 12–32. Schematic incisal view of the addition of composite to the lingual and facial to correct a rotation.

facial to the proper contour (Figure 12–34). Because the enamel on cuspids is thick, relatively large esthetic changes can be made. A typical result is shown in Figure 12–35. A larger case, involving both cuspid reshaping and closure of a diastema, is shown in Figure 12–36. The combination of these techniques can significantly improve a patient's appearance.

Correcting vertical problems

Correction of vertical gingival asymmetries often requires periodontal and or orthodontic intervention. Periodontal surgery to remove bone and reposition gingival tissues can provide excellent results, especially when performed in conjunction with provisional restorations and given adequate healing time. In patients with high lip lines, the gingival outline can have as much or more of an effect on esthetics than the treatment of teeth.

Incisal asymmetries are easier to treat (Figure 12–37). A recessed incisal edge is shown in Figure 12–38. These asymmetries, which can have a profound effect on a smile, usually can be treated effectively with restorative treatment alone. They are sometimes the result of trauma. More commonly, they are caused by a wear pattern. Special attention should be paid to the occlusion, since protrusive and lateral movements could fracture restorations that lengthen the teeth. Sometimes these movements are parafunctional and difficult to detect on routine examination. If a wear pattern

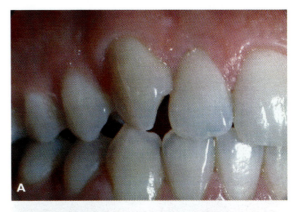
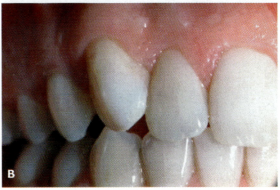

Figure 12–35. *A,* Before and, *B,* after photographs of a restored rotated cuspid.

exists, that movement will most likely occur again, even if the patient cannot reproduce it during an office examination.

Correcting angled teeth

Angled teeth can be among the most difficult to treat without full-coverage restorations. They are best treated with orthodontics. If treated restoratively, a contoured veneer can "straighten" teeth by altering the embrasure form to make the line angles more prominent on one side and more rounded on the other. This gives the tooth the appearance of tipping toward the rounded side. This type of contouring requires a good understanding of the optical effects of contour (Figure 12–39).

Angled teeth are more visible with a high lip line. If half or more of the facial surface is exposed during smiling, the correction of angled teeth with direct restorations can be difficult. The simplest approach is to correct the incisal silhouette to improve the vertical symmetry. Aligning

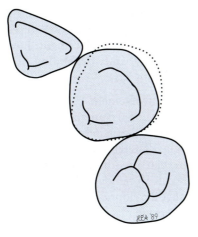

Figure 12–34. Schematic representation of the addition of composite to the lingual to correct a rotated cuspid.

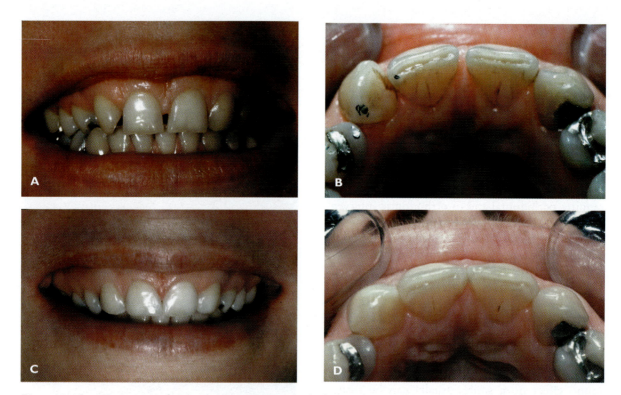

Figure 12–36. *A*, Preoperative facial view of teeth with multiple diastemas, rotated cuspids, and missing laterals. *B*, Preoperative incisal view. *C*, Postoperative facial view of restoration. *D*, Postoperative incisal view showing enamel contouring of cuspids and diastema closures with proximal restorations.

the facial incisal edges can provide excellent esthetic results without an invasive full-coverage restoration (Figure 12–40).

Correcting overlaps

Of all esthetic problems, correction of a crowded arch is the most difficult, particularly if it includes the formidable challenge of overlapping teeth at the midline (Figure 12–41). Severe cases call for tooth extraction followed by orthodontics, but such treatment is not always practical. Generally, the alternative treatment for severe overlapping is full-coverage restoration. This can result in narrow teeth that may not meet the esthetic demands of the patient. Minor overlapping can sometimes be corrected with direct composite additions or veneers. Careful diagnosis and treatment planning with the aid of waxups on models with and without tooth removal results in the most predictable treatment.

Veneer maintenance and failure

Unlike most small composite resin restorations (eg, Classes I, III, and V in enamel), larger composite veneer restorations require maintenance. Because of their large size and thinness, the margins of these restorations break down, chip, and stain more than others. When they are placed under stress, failure is also more common than with smaller restorations. Owing to the flexure of composite during function, crack propagation in a matrix increases over time, leading to catastrophic failure. These types of failures generally occur 2 to 5 years after placement; however, they can occur at any time, depending on the forces placed on the material.

Periodontal involvement

Unlike conventional composite restorations, composite veneers are generally finished near the gingival margins. Therefore, the length of the margin is greater than in other restorations, making it more difficult to remove all of the flash or excess material that develops near the margin. Since most direct veneers are placed without the use of a rubber dam, bonding materials can easily attach at or underneath the gingival crest.

Excess bonding agent that is blown off a tooth with an air syringe during placement can result in

Esthetics

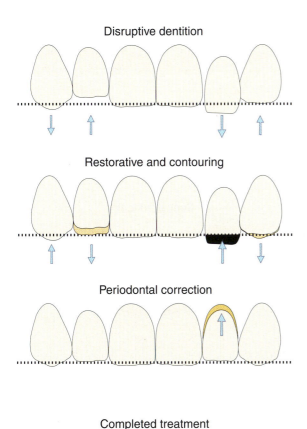

Figure 12–37. Schematic representation of a typical asymmetric vertical tooth pattern.

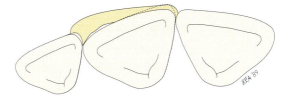

Figure 12–38. Schematic representation of a typical asymmetric incisal edge and its connection with composite.

a thin layer of resin at the gingiva, which can cause an adverse tissue response. Bonding agent is difficult to see in the presence of saliva. Evidence of gingival inflammation during a follow-up visit can lead a dentist to detect these small pieces of flash (Figure 12–42).

Marginal breakdown

White lines. Composites often tear at the margins during the finishing process. This is partly attributable to the effect of polymerization shrinkage over a large surface area, but a significant factor is the trauma to the restoration–tooth interface during the finishing process. Finishing procedures, which produce heat and friction, are damaging to a newly place composite.

A white line margin is an open margin that is visible immediately after finishing (Figure 12–43). A few days after placement, the composite swells and moisture fills in the gap and makes the white line disappear. However, the margin is still open and will stain over time. Such marginal stains usually go deep into the tooth–restorative interface and resist removal by discing.

Occlusion-related chipping. The most common reason for early breakage of direct veneers is occlusion, especially parafunctional habits (Figure 12–44). When placing a composite resin in an area that extends the incisal edge of a tooth, it is necessary to ensure that occlusal movement was not the factor determining existing tooth length. When tooth movement has shortened a tooth, it may be necessary to make changes in incisal guidance, such as to increase the height of the cuspid, to allow space for a longer tooth. Remember that an anterior veneer is rarely able to guide the occlusion when the composite is placed in tension; however, a composite can undergo considerable loading in compression. The best approach is to increase the cuspid rise by adding material to the lingual of the maxillary cuspids, which places the material in compression during jaw movement. Increasing the incisals of the cuspids would put the material in tension. When cuspid length is increased, the occlusal table must be widened to make a larger amount of material available to resist sheer forces.

Chipping at non-contact areas. All composites show the wear of age caused by thermal cycling, tooth movement, and fatigue. The margins, where the composite undergoes the most stress from expansion and contraction cycles, break first, owing to postoperative chipping. These chipped areas can stain, collect plaque, and, in some cases, result in recurrent decay (Figure 12–45).

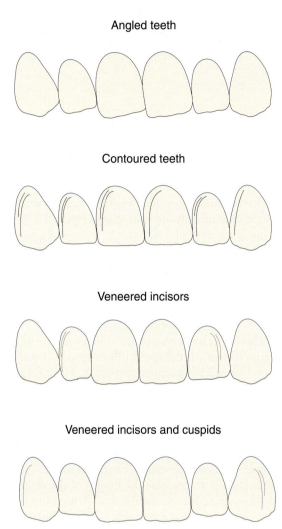

Figure 12–39. Schematic representation of vertically angled arch and the effect of contouring and veneering.

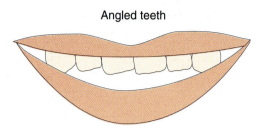
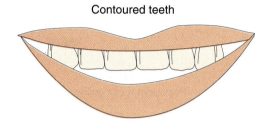
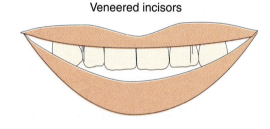
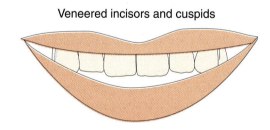

Figure 12–40. The effect of lip line on the appearance of a vertically angled arch.

Pits. Singular pits are generally associated with voids in the restorative, which occur during placement. Widespread pitting is less common and is associated with the use of dry or expired composite (Figure 12–46).

Chipping at contact areas. Chipping can result from occlusal trauma (eg, accidents or bruxing) or fatigue caused by cyclic loading (ie, constant low forces over a long time, such as chewing). Contact area chipping is most common on the incisal edge and is often related to parafunctional habits (Figure 12–47). The preparation design can affect occlusal chipping. A chamfer or rounded shoulder margin is more durable than a slightly beveled margin (less than 45 degrees). In smaller restorations where tension from occlusal loading is low, butt joint margins are acceptable.

Esthetics 267

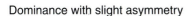
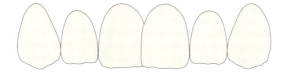
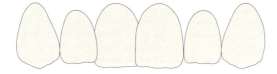
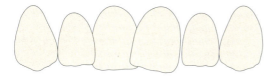
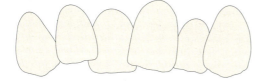

Figure 12–41. Schematic representation of the increasing severity of tooth overlap in progressively more crowded arches.

Layer separation. Separation between layers of composite occurs when one layer does not adequately bond to an underlying layer during initial placement or later repair. The latter is the most common cause, especially when a smoother composite is layered on top of a rough one during a repair. Since the outer layer is repaired by a delayed resin–resin bonding process, the bond is generally 20 to 50% at placement and deteriorates over time (Figure 12–48).

Maintenance and repairs

Minor marginal breaks can often be treated with discing. This removes the damaged area and

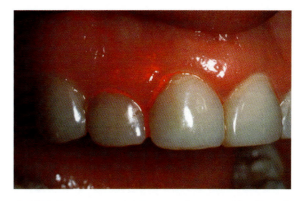

Figure 12–42. Gingival inflammation and bleeding from residual resin remaining subgingivally.

exposes the sound restoration underneath. A small amount of discing reduces the contour only slightly (Figure 12–49). Such discing must be repeated periodically. Eventually, only a small amount of restorative remains on the tooth. At this point the entire veneer must be removed and replaced.

Composite should not be repaired by attempting to bond new composite to old composite. If a restoration needs repairing, the old composite should be removed and new material added to clean tooth structure. If complete removal is not practically feasible, as might be the case with a large restoration, an option is to bond a portion of the restoration to new tooth structure and attach the remainder of the material to mechanical undercuts and rough surfaces on the older restoration.

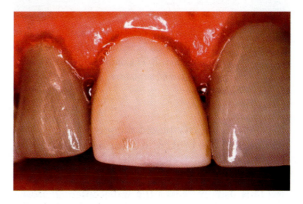

Figure 12–43. A pronounced white line margin on the facial of an incisor. The composite is thin in this area and is easily damaged by polymerization stress and the normal traumas associated with final finishing.

268 Tooth-Colored Restoratives

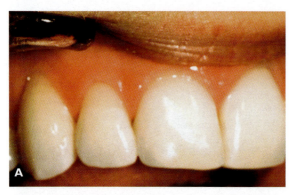
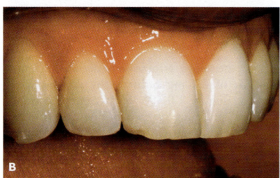
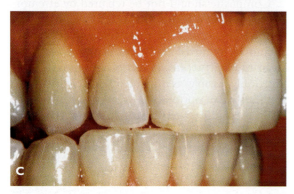

Figure 12–44. *A,* A direct composite veneer restoration that included lengthening the distal incisal edge of the upper right central to improve esthetics. *B,* The restoration broke shortly after placement. *C,* A lateral protrusive movement was the cause of the fracture.

When a properly placed composite in a stress-bearing area has broken, it must be replaced with a stronger material; that is, the replacement composite must be stronger than the existing composite. This usually means the replacement material must have a higher filler loading. If the strongest composite available was used in the original restoration, a porcelain-bonded restoration should be considered as a replacement.

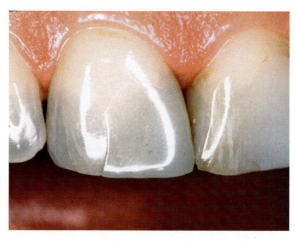

Figure 12–45. A large chip on the facial of a microfilled composite veneer.

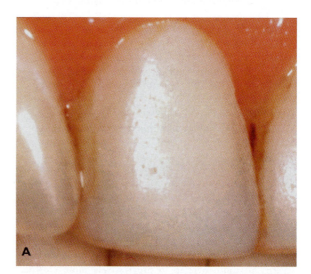
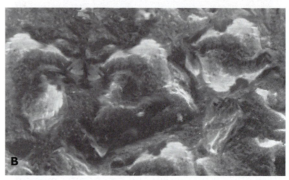

Figure 12–46. *A,* Close-up view of generalized surface pitting. The tooth was treated with a dried out, expired, microfilled composite material. *B,* Electron micrograph of the surface of large prepolymerized particles of resin (50 to 100 mm) used as a filler in a microfilled composite resin.

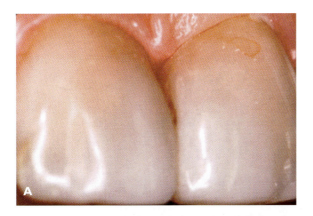
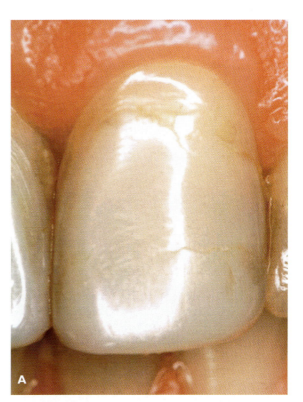

Figure 12–47. *A*, The proximal breakdown of the margins of a microfilled composite resin veneer on a central incisor, and *B*, a magnification of the breakdown area.

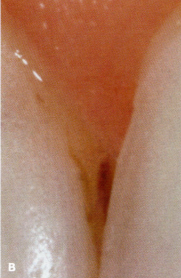

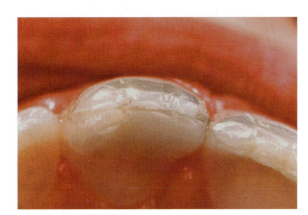

Figure 12–48. Layer separation of a microfill bonded to a macrofill material 4 years after the original placement. The repair failed about 18 months after the restoration was re-veneered.

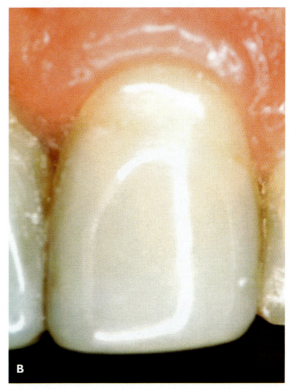

Figure 12–49. *A*, A composite veneer at 5-year recall, and *B*, the same restoration after discing to smooth.

Appendix A

Nomenclature for Curing Composite Resins

This section summarizes the key principles behind each new dental term for the polymerization of resins.

The term spectral requirements (SR) for photopolymerization describes the wavelength range of energy that is absorbed by the photoinitiators within the polymerizable material. Each composite material should list the SR at a specific range of wavelengths. A term for this already exists in physics: the "full width at half maximum" (FWHM). The dental term spectral requirements (SR) for photopolymerization is the same and is defined as that point 50% down each curve of a graph depicting resin absorption as a function of the wavelength applied. In this graph, the x-axis is absorption and the y-axis is wavelength. Although FWHM could be used, SR is more readily understood in relation to dentistry; thus, SR is the preferred dental term and FWHM should be used to establish this number.

The term spectral emission (SE) for photopolymerization describes the spectral output of the curing unit over a range of frequencies (typically 400 to 500 nm). The bandwidth should allow for spectral overlap of the spectral absorption ranges (SR) of the photoinitiators. Otherwise, initiation and resulting polymerization is inefficient. The term for this in physics is "energy density" (ED), which is the energy emitted from a light source, generally over all bandwidths. This emission is concentrated by collimation to a specific spot size. Some light rods collimate the light to a smaller diameter, called the spot size, to increase the power density. Generally, the curing tip diameter or spot size should be the size of the typical tooth, which is 9 mm by 11 mm for a central incisor. Too small a spot size necessitates overlapping curing cycles. In addition, curved light guides generally lose some intensity and uniformity compared with straight light guides.

The term energy density (ED) has been used in dentistry to define the energy emitted at specific wavelengths (commonly 400 to 500 nm or more) and should be kept. The new term, SE for photopolymerization, is proposed as a dental term for the bandwidths needed for the photoinitiators found in dental resins (and, intentionally, the bandwidths emitted by dental curing units), because it is more precise and fits in with the other nomenclature. It is important that the bandwidth of the spectral emission for photopolymerization of a curing unit is broad enough to ensure effective spectral overlap with all the photoinitiators used in current composite resins.

The SE for photopolymerization should include the output from the tip of all wavelengths a curing unit emits. These may have an effect on the pulp as well as on the cure of the composite. This would be expressed as SE/450 to 475 nm = 12 joules/cm^2 of a total of 18 joules/cm^2. Abbreviated, it would read 18 J/SE: 450 to 475 nm = 12 J.

The term power density (PD) refers to the power setting on the curing unit. Most units have just one setting, "on" or "off," whereas newer units have many power settings. Power density is expressed in milliwatts per square centimeter (mW/cm^2). A square centimeter is used because it is the size closest to that of the typical veneer or posterior restoration. Power output is determined by using a laboratory-grade spectral radiometer within the desired bandwidth (usually 400 to 500 nm). The energy outside the desired bandwidth, such as infrared, which heats the tooth, should also be reported.

Power range (PR) indicates the range of power densities of a particular curing unit. PR = 400 mW/cm^2 for many older units; new units could be PR = 25 to 800 mW/cm^2.

Energy density for optimal polymerization at a specified depth (EOP@D) refers to the total energy needed to optimally polymerize a composite at a specific depth. The required wavelength must be specified and both light and dark reactions at 24 hours should be included. The term EOP@D, where D is the measurement in millimeters for the depth of cure, should be expressed in joules per square centimeter (J/cm^2). Future composites will probably require less energy for initiation, and the common abbreviation will be EOP@Xmm. For example, currently, EOP@2mm would be the most commonly used term: a composite cured for 40 seconds at 400 mW/cm^2 would be EOP@2mm = 16 J/cm^2 at a required wavelength of 400 to 500 nm.

No "D" after EOP indicates that the depth information has not been included and describes only the energy needed for optimal polymerization at the surface. Energy for optimal polymerization (EOP) can be used alone for bonding agents where there is no significant depth.

An EOP@2mm: 8 J/cm^2 composite, abbreviated EOP@2 8, would be cured in 20 seconds at 400 mW/cm^2, or in 10 seconds at 800 mW/cm^2, and would reach optimum polymerization at a thickness of 2 mm. Both composites and lights of this power are now on the market. Unfortunately, resin polymerization is not this precise, but this is a reasonable calculation for clinical use.

As depth of cure improves in the future, the protocol would still apply. For example, it may be possible to bulk cure, making a term such as EOP@5mm useful (indicating a 5 mm depth of cure requirement).

Energy application sequence (EAS) is the practice by which the energy is applied to the resin. It is the curing technique used by the dentist to initiate the resin. The precise bandwidth (within 10 nm), the power density, as well as any time between additional curing steps should be stated. The EAS describes the way in which the amount of power density and time are applied.

When the configuration factor (C-factor) is small, the EAS may not have much clinical significance. The C-factor is related to the number of tooth surfaces to which a composite is bonded (Figure A–1).

The greater the number of opposing walls, the higher the C-factor and the more significant the effect of polymerization shrinkage. When the C-factor is high, the EAS can make a large difference in marginal seal and suggested placement technique.

The EAS can also be described in classes; the most common would be type I, followed by type II, and so on. Potential future advancements and improved systems can be built on these concepts.

Types of EAS are

1. uniform continuous: traditional linear curing at one power density.

2. ramp: a slow, steady increase in intensity, from a low (50 to 100 mW/cm^2) to high (800+ mW/cm^2) power density.

3. step: a low power density for a short time followed by a high power density for a longer time.

4. high-energy pulse: a short curing time that is only a portion of the EAS.

5. pulse delay: a low power density for a short time, followed by a waiting period and then high power density.

The EAS can be abbreviated as: time@PD – time@PD for single cures (step) or time @ PD–(wait in brackets)–time@PD for double curing (pulse), and so on. Creating a soft cure means working with the material at a low conversion rate and then completing the polymerization later. It is important to understand that all composites appear normal after a short curing cycle, but visual evaluation is a poor judge of actual effect.

For example, some units (eg, ESPE) use a step curing sequence of 10@100 to 30@800, which means 10 seconds at 100 mW and 30 seconds at 800 mW in immediate sequence, or, in a more understandable abbreviation, 10 s/100 mW– 30 s/800 mW.

Another unit (eg, Bisco) uses pulse curing: 3@200–(3–5 min)–10@600; which means 3 seconds at 200 mW, and then wait 3 to 5 minutes, then 10 seconds at 600 mW. This can also be abbreviated as 3 s/200 mW/wait 3 min/10 s/600 mW.

Many units (eg, Demetron) use ramp curing of 100 to 1000 mW/cm^2 over 10 seconds, which is

Appendix A: Nomenclature for Curing Composite Resins 273

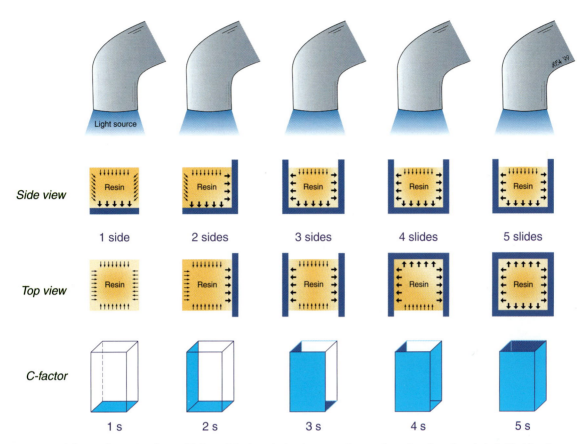

Figure A–1. The configuration factor (C-factor) is the relation between the number of surfaces bonded divided by the number of surfaces unbonded. As the configuration factor goes up, the effects of polymerization stress and strain become more significant in maintaining marginal seal. (Adapted from Feilzer AJ, de Gee AJ, Davidson CL. Relaxation of polymerization contraction shear stress by hygroscopic expansion. J Dent Res 1990;69:36–9.)

described as 10@100–1000. A 10-second pulse cure (1000+) (they call burst cure) is a continuous 10@1000.

Pulse energy (PE) is a specific combination of time and power density (such as 3 s @200 mW/cm², etc.) used for each curing step to cure a resin. Pulse energy would be part of the entire EAS used to initiate a resin system. It would not apply to continuous curing. The first pulse is the initial cure (soft cure is technically incorrect) and the second pulse is the final cure. The ESPE, Bisco, and Kerr lights all use pulse energy in different modes.

APPENDIX B

Universal Restorative Tray

A dentist's armamentarium setup greatly influences his or her ability to produce quality restorations efficiently. A universal tray setup is advantageous since it provides the instrumentation for most restorative procedures (Figure B–1). The universal tray minimizes per appointment setup time and facilitates the accomplishment of multiple procedures in a single visit, either according to plan or as unexpected needs present themselves. Although a universal tray does not contain every instrument that might be needed for any restorative procedure, it can supply the majority of instruments at great convenience to the dentist.

In addition to swift access to instruments, a significant ancillary advantage of the universal tray is ease of sterilization. To sterilize the instruments in the two-part tray shown, the instruments are left in place, the tray is folded closed and cleaned ultrasonically, rinsed in water, mechanically air dried, wrapped in autoclave wrap, and autoclaved (Figure B–2). The simplicity of the procedure helps ensure proper follow through by staff and also dramatically reduces the amount of staff time required for sterilization.

The universal tray setup shown is designed for a dentist performing composite, glass ionomer, veneer, onlay, post-and-core buildup, crown, bridge, and other common restorative procedures. Table B–1 lists the instruments included and provides identifying information to assist in ordering these supplies from their manufacturers.

A universal diamond block is also helpful (Figure B-3). Ideally, all diamond cutting instruments are stored together and sterilized as a group. Burs should be used only once and disposed of; therefore, they are not included in a reusable universal cutting block. Burs can be purchased in individual packages and dispensed as needed.

Rubber dams are highly recommended for every restorative procedure, except where they prohibit operator access (eg, root caries). To facilitate their use, rubber dam clamps, forceps, and frames are included in the universal setup (Figure B–4). A reflective svedopter (optical saliva ejector) is the recommended alternative, because it displaces the tongue, removes excess saliva (when attached to an evacuator), and has a mirror surface that increases illumination (Figure B–5).

Depending on a dentist's breadth of practice, auxiliary trays can be assembled for specific restorative procedures that require additional instrumentation, such as endodontic, periodontic, orthodontic, and implant procedures. The universal tray setup is not appropriate for oral surgery procedures.

A universal set of consumables can also enhance procedural efficiency. Pre-packing consumables into sterilization bags is a task an assistant can perform before or after office hours, or when there are breaks in the schedule. A universal set of consumables might include anesthetic and needle, topical anesthetic, cotton gauze, cotton rolls, pre-punched rubber dam, rubber dam napkin, syringe needle, dry angles, cotton swabs, cotton pellets, floss, mixing pad, dispensing well, Mylar strips, wedges, brushes, disposable applicators, suction tips, disposable air and water syringe tips (if used), finishing discs and strips, Bard Parker blade, rubber cups and points, and articulating paper (Figure B–6).

Figure B–7 shows a typical operatory setup, including a universal restorative tray and unpacked consumables.

276 Tooth-Colored Restoratives

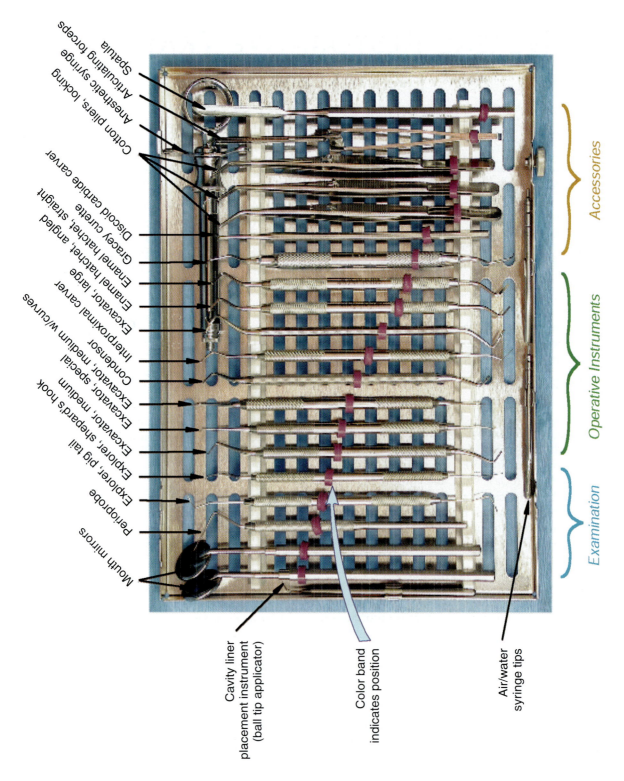

A

Appendix B: Universal Restorative Tray

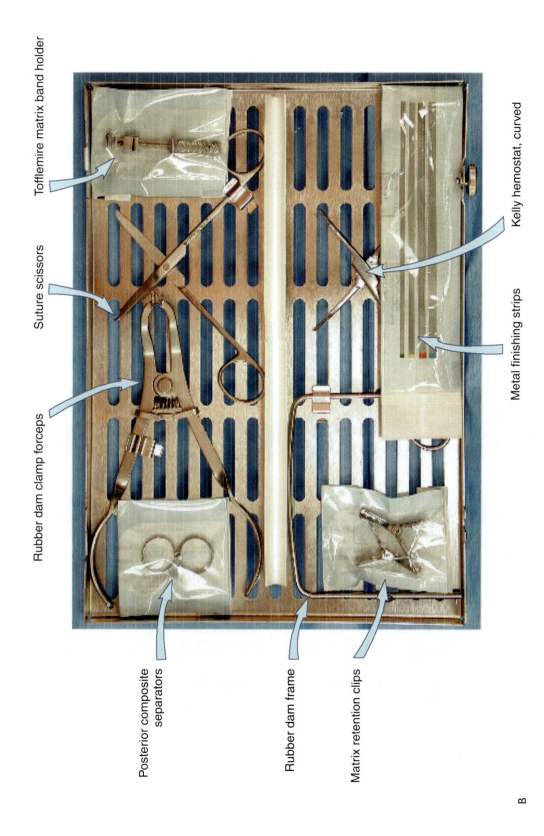

Figure B–1. *A*, Main instrument compartment of a universal restorative tray. Note that the position of the color band on each instrument indicates its proper position in the tray. Instruments are placed to work from left (examination) to right (adjustment and cementation). *B*, Cover compartment of a universal restorative tray, which includes predominantly isolation and matrix equipment.

278 Tooth-Colored Restoratives

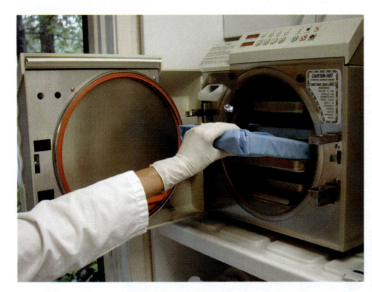

Figure B–2. Placement of wrapped tray into autoclave for final step in sterilization.

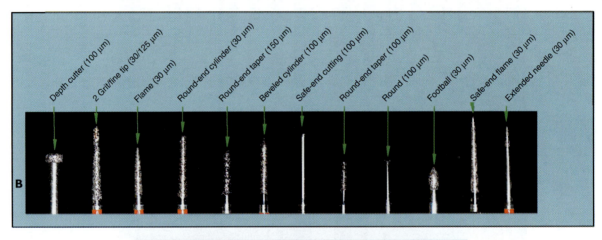

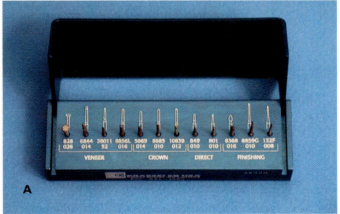

Figure B–3. *A*, Block of diamond cutting instruments. *B*, Close-up of diamond cutting instruments.

Appendix B: Universal Restorative Tray 279

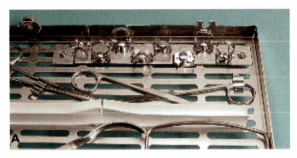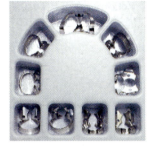

Figure B–4. *A*, Rubber dam clamps, forceps, and frame in a rubber dam clamp organizing board. *B*, Recommended array of rubber dam clamps.

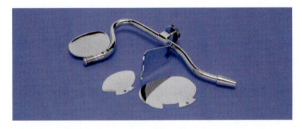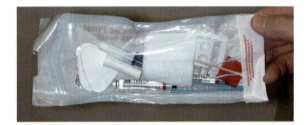

Figure B–5. A svedopter (optical saliva ejector) is used when a rubber dam is not appropriate.

Figure B–6. A universal set of consumables packed in a sterilization bag.

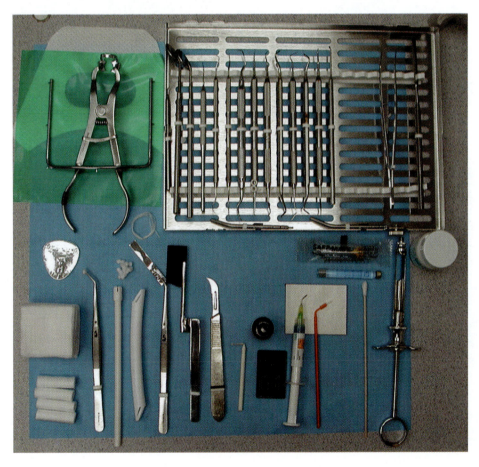

Figure B–7. A typical operatory setup. Note rubber dam instrumentation in the upper left corner, universal restorative tray in the upper right corner, consumables in the lower left corner, and specific bonding materials in the lower right corner.

Table B-1. Recommended Restorative Tray Instruments

Instrument	Company*	Model
Main Compartment		
Mouth mirror	Patterson	088-6853 Delux Handle
		88-6804 No. 5 Front Surface
	Brasseler	260 BR6082 30
		260 BR6082101
Perioprobe	Patterson	316-9935 American Eagle
	Brasseler	250N33
Explorer, pig-tail	Suter	DE Classic 2
	Brasseler	250EXPL-2XL
	Hartzell	Double End No. 2
Explorer, shepard's hook	Suter	DE Classic 5
	Brasseler	250EXPL-23-6
	Hartzell	Double End No. 5
Excavator, medium	Suter	Tru-Bal 225-4
	Brasseler	250EXC-6
	Hartzell	Disc type No. 38 39
Excavator, special	Suter	DP 7/8-4
	Brasseler	250EXC-1S
	Hartzell	Disc type No. 5
Excavator, medium with curves	Suter	Tru-Bal 245-4
	Brasseler	250EXC-8
	Hartzell	Disc type No. 13
Condenser	Suter	Hollenbeck 1–4
	Brasseler	250MOR1
	Hartzell	True UOP 1–2
Interproximal carver	Suter	IPC5-4
	Brasseler	250TINIPC, plain or serrated tips
	Hartzell	UC 1–2
Excavator, large	Suter	Tru-Bal 222-4
	Brasseler	250EXC-15
	Hartzell	Excavator No. 3L
Enamel hatchet, angled	Suter	Tru-Bal 45S-4
	Brasseler	250MT17-18
Enamel hatchet, straight	Suter	Ferrier Selection F 17/18-4
		Tru-Bal TB 204-4
	Patterson	Black's cutting instrument
		Premier 51/52-575-5137

Table B-1. *Continued*

Instrument	Company*	Model
Gracey curette	Suter	3/4–5
	Brasseler	250GR3–4
	Hartzell	UC3–4
Discoid carbide carver	Suter	Study Club Set
		Ferrier 31-4
	Brasseler	105–1700 (USA)
	Hartzell	No. 3–6
Cotton pliers, locking	Patterson	372-1859, Hu-Friedy
	Brasseler	250200
Anesthetic syringe	Patterson	222-4772
	Sullivan-Schein	100-9808
Articulating forceps	Patterson	083-8789
	Brasseler	250ART
Spatula	Patterson	089-5706 No. 24
	Brasseler	25024
Cavity liner placement instrument	Patterson	084-3359
(ball-tip applicator)	Brasseler	250CHP5
Air/water syringe tips	Patterson	103-5591 (5/pk, Adec)
	Sullivan-Schein	737-6038
Bottom Compartment		
Rubber dam clamp forceps	Patterson	373-1595
	Sullivan-Schein	100-8841
Suture scissors	Your preference	
Tofflemire matrix band holder	Patterson	088-6515, Tofflemire
(Universal)	Sullivan-Schein	100-9547
Kelly hemostat, curved	Patterson	086-3423
	Brasseler	260V97-38
Metal finishing strips	GC	000259, 600 mesh/70 m
		000255, 300 mesh/90 m
	Patterson	326-3308, 600 mesh, green 2.6 mm
		326-3225, 300 mesh, blue, 2.6 mm
Matrix retention clip, 45-degrees	Patterson	089-7116
	Sullivan-Schein	100-0025
Rubber dam frame	Patterson	769-5939, Young's style
	Sullivan-Schein	707-7305
Posterior composite separators	Patterson	Contact Matrix Kit
		Danville, 236-3646
	Sullivan-Schein	Sectional Matrix System
		Danville, 170-7747

Table B-1. Continued

Instrument	Company*	Model
Tray Cassettes		
(Hu-Friedy Instrument Management System [IMS], Signature Series)		
Large cassette (8" x 11" x 1.25")	Hu-Friedy	IM4162
Rubber dam clamp organizing board	Hu-Friedy	RDCOB
Autoclave wrap (24" x 24")	Hu-Friedy	IMS121
Air/water clip	Hu-Friedy	IM1005
Hinged instrument clip	Hu-Friedy	IM1000
(holds instruments on lid)		

Brasseler USA, One Brasseler Blvd., Savannah, GA 31419
  Tel: 800 841-4522
Danville Materials, 2021 Omega Road, San Ramon, CA 94583
  Tel: 800 822-9294 or 925 838-2793
GC America Inc., 3737 W. 127th Street, Alsip, IL 60803
  Tel: 800 323-7063 or 708 597-0900
G. Hartzell & Son, 2372 Stanwell Circle, Concord, CA 94520
  Tel: 800 950-2206 or 925 798-2206
Hu-Friedy, 3232 N. Rockwell Street, Chicago, IL 60618
  Tel: 800 483-7433
Patterson Dental Supply, Inc., 1031 Mendota Heights Road, St. Paul, MN 55120
  Tel: 800 328-5536 or 651 686-1600
Sullivan-Schein Dental, 135 Duryea Road, Melville, NY 11747
  Tel: 800 372-4346
Suter Dental Manufacturing Co., P.O. Box 1329, 632 Cedar Street, Chico, CA 95927
  Tel: 800 368-8376 or 530 893-8376

APPENDIX C

MAGNIFICATION

Magnification significantly enhances a dentist's ability to detect pathology and perform restorative dentistry. Improved vision not only increases productivity but also enhances work quality. Two-times magnification is helpful in avoiding eyestrain; 3.5 times is ideal for routine operative work. Higher magnifications have the drawback of a limited depth of field under normal operatory lighting.

Another significant benefit of magnification is reduction in eye fatigue and postural fatigue. Magnification increases the working distance between the eye and the object, allowing extra-ocular muscles to remain more relaxed (Figure C–1). The increased working distance also allows a dentist to maintain normal posture.

Adjuncts to traditional magnification loupes include intraoral cameras with magnification abilities. These are now considered essential equipment for recording preoperative and postoperative changes in a patient's mouth. Intraoral video devices that can magnify and show images on monitors and produce color prints are also becoming popular for sharing information with patients and other interested parties.

TYPES OF MAGNIFICATION

Two basic types of magnification systems are commonly used in dentistry: single-lens magnifiers (eg, clip-on, flip-up, jeweler's glasses) and multilens magnifiers (ie, loupes) (Figure C–2).

Single-lens magnifiers

Single-lens magnifiers produce what is known as diopter magnification, which is really just another way to describe the lens' focal length. Diopter magnifiers simply adjust the working distance to a set length. As the diopter increases, the working distance decreases.

Advantages of single-lens magnification are that they are

- inexpensive,
- made in a vast number of styles and shapes to attach to eyeglasses or headbands (Figure C–3), and
- usable without customized adjustments.

Disadvantages of single-lens magnification include

- a set working distance, requiring a set working posture,
- poor image quality, and
- lack of adjustable convergence angles of two oculars.

Multilens magnifiers

Three brands of multilens loupes are very popular: Surgical Loops (Designs for Vision, Inc., Ronkonkoma, New York), Dimension Three (Orascoptic Research Inc., Madison, Wisconsin) and SurgiTel (General Scientific Corp., Ann Arbor, Michigan).

Most manufacturers offer three types of multilens magnification: Keplerian, Greenough, and Galilean. Keplerian loupes are double lens and offer magnification of about 2 to 2.5 times, which is sufficient for dentists with good normal vision (Figure C–4). They are the least expensive and the lightest of the multilens options. Greenough loupes incorporate four to six lenses and offer magnification up to 3.5 times (Figure C–5). These loupes are longer and heavier than Keplerian loupes and have a narrower field of vision. Galilean loupes have five or more lenses and two or more prisms (Figure C–6). They offer magni-

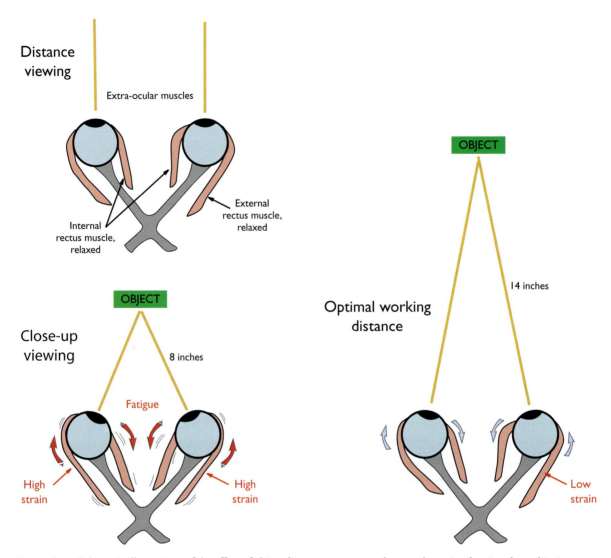

Figure C–1. Schematic illustrations of the effect of object distance on extra-ocular muscle strain, showing that achieving magnification that allows a working distance of at least 14 inches is optimal for prevention of eye fatigue.

fication of up to 6 times, and a wide field of vision. Because they are more compact and lighter than Greenough loupes, they are preferred when a magnification of greater than 3 times is needed. Most dentists operate at magnifications between 2 and 3.5 on these scales; there is no need for loupes with a magnifying power of more than 5 times (Figure C–7). Dental microscopes offer magnification of at least 10 times, which is useful for endodontics, periodontics, and some restorative procedures. They are expensive and more awkward than loupes, and are unnecessary for the majority of dental procedures.

The average dentist works comfortably at a distance of 10 to 16 inches. Most optical loupe manufacturers provide various models that can be set at the specific distance most comfortable for the wearer.

Advantages of multilens magnification include

- variable working distance,
- improved optical performance,
- adjustable convergence angle, and
- improved working range (depth of field).

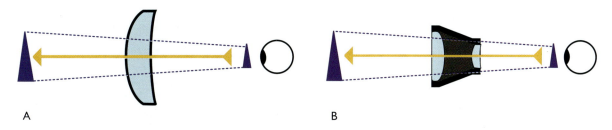

Figure C–2. Schematic of, *A*, single-lens and, *B*, multilens magnifiers, showing that multilens loupes provide greater magnification over a given working distance.

Disadvantages of multilens magnification are their

- expense and
- need to be custom-made for each operator.

CONSIDERATIONS IN MAGNIFICATION SELECTION

When selecting loupes, a dentist should choose a model that is of comfortable fit, size, and weight; compromising on these characteristics can lead to poor posture and attendant physical problems. A dentist should try many brands before choosing a magnification system.

Depth of field

With any brand of loupe, the depth of field decreases as the magnification increases. One option to minimize this effect is to increase the light source, which closes down the iris of the eye and improves the depth of field. Headlamps are available for attachment to glasses or a headband to increase lighting in the field of vision. Additional light is necessary as magnification increases.

Working distance

It is imperative that each dentist accurately measure the distance from his or her eye to the working area while in a comfortable working position. This measurement should then be used in selecting a magnification power and model. The average distance is 14 inches.

Field of view

The field of view varies depending on the design of the optics, the working distance model, and the magnification power. As with depth of field, when magnification increases, the field of view decreases.

Viewing angle

The viewing angle is key to operator comfort and should be customized to the individual. A dentist's working posture is likely to change over time, and the loupe system must be adjustable to these changes.

The ocular structure of the Designs for Vision loupe is small and lightweight and is physically secured to the lens of the glasses (see Figure C–6, *C*). The viewing angle is customized for each operator and then locked into position by building the magnifier into the lens. The ocular structures of Dimension Three and SurgiTel loupes are front-frame-mounted. These systems offer pivotal angle adjustments that can easily be altered and locked into position based on the wearer's comfortable working posture.

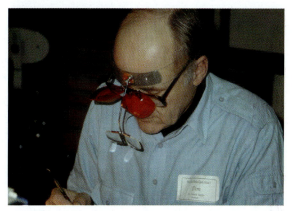

Figure C–3. Headband-mounted single-lens loupes. Single-lens loupes offer magnification of about 2 times and a narrow working field. To increase magnification requires moving the lens further from the eyes, which necessitates a headband for stabilization.

286 Tooth-Colored Restoratives

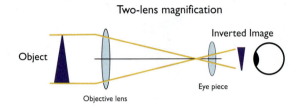

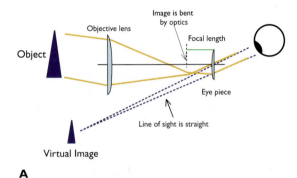

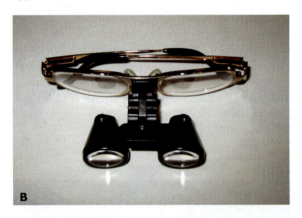

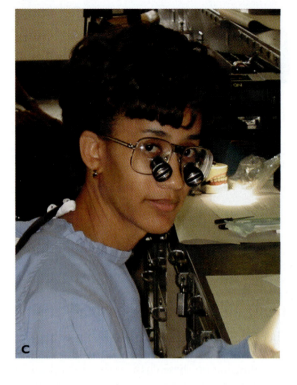

Figure C–4. *A*, Schematic of Keplerian optics compared to double-lens optics. Note that Keplerian optics result in transmission to the eye of an upright object; the object in two-lens optics is upside-down. *B*, Flip-up version of Keplerian-lens loupes. *C*, Keplerian lens mounted on glasses.

Convergence angle

The convergence angle also differs by loupe brand. Each ocular must be properly aligned with its mate and to a specific distance, or headaches and dizziness are likely for the dentist. Both SurgiTel and Designs for Vision preset this feature at the factory; Dimension Three allows the wearer to make adjustments. Many dentists feel a preset convergence angle as well as preset interpupillary distance is more user friendly, since they should not be changed once correctly positioned. An advantage of an adjustable interpupillary distance is that it allows the loupes to be used by more than one person.

Peripheral vision

The ability to maintain eye contact with patients, to watch for materials and instruments being passed into the procedure area, or to read radiographs and charts all depend on a loupe's design and allowance for peripheral vision. Front-frame-mounted loupes retain up to 90% of potential peripheral vision, and they can easily be flipped

Appendix C: Magnification 287

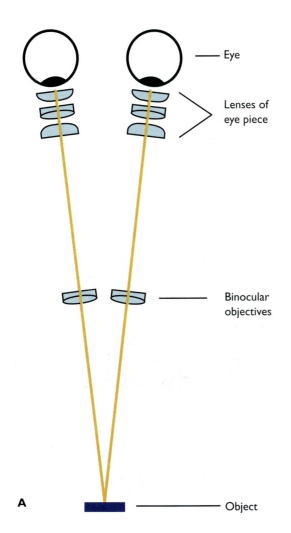

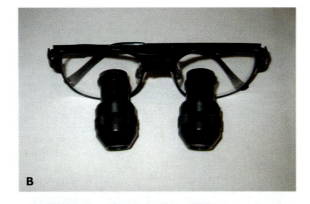

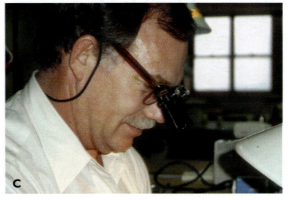

Figure C–5. *A*, Schematic of Greenough optics. *B*, Glasses-mounted Greenough lenses with adjustable magnification. *C*, Glasses-mounted Greenough lenses with fixed working distance and fixed magnification.

up, above the frame, allowing for a full facial view. This feature is useful for patient discussions and consultations. The drawback to this design is that it is slightly heavier.

Corrected vision

All currently available loupes are designed to accommodate ocular prescriptions. For a dentist to work without eyeglasses or contacts, the prescription must be added to the loupes. Prescriptions for front-frame-mounted loupes are easily installed by any optician. Inter-lens loupes are manufactured with the prescription built into the optics. When a change in ocular prescription is required, an inter-lens loupe must be returned to the manufacturer for reconfiguration.

Headband models

An alternative to frame-mounted loupes is the headband-mounted models offered by many manufacturers (see Figure C–3). Headband-mounted loupes are comfortable and allow the wearer to use his or her own prescription glasses while working. Peripheral vision is also well maintained with these loupes, and some offer a "flip-up" feature as well.

Disinfection

As with all other dental materials and equipment, cross-contamination is of concern to both patients and dentist. Unfortunately, it is difficult to disinfect most magnification systems. Refer to the manufacturer's instructions for a proper disinfection procedure.

288 Tooth-Colored Restoratives

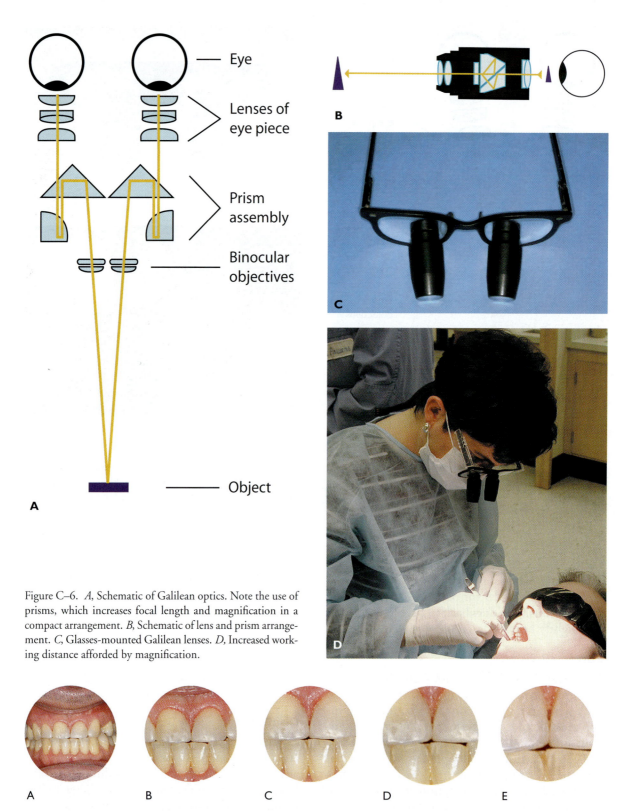

Figure C–6. *A,* Schematic of Galilean optics. Note the use of prisms, which increases focal length and magnification in a compact arrangement. *B,* Schematic of lens and prism arrangement. *C,* Glasses-mounted Galilean lenses. *D,* Increased working distance afforded by magnification.

Figure C–7. Illustration of the impact of increasing magnification: *A,* 1 time magnification (ie, normal vision); *B,* 2 times magnification; *C,* 3 times magnification; *D,* 4 times magnification; *E,* 6 times magnification.

APPENDIX D

AIR ABRASION

Air abrasion improves both speed and accuracy in treating incipient pit and fissure caries in virgin molars. Air abrasion devices are high-energy sandblasting and tooth cutting systems. The high-energy particles emitted cut faster and more precisely than traditional sandblasters. The cutting path of these devices is 100 to 1000 times smaller than that of their sandblaster counterparts. The cutting beam diameter averages about 300 µm, but they can be made as small as 100 µm.

HISTORY

Air abrasion, also referred to as advanced particle beam technology, or microabrasive technology, was invented by Dr. Robert Black in 1943.[1,2] The principles, uses, and limitations of air abrasion devices, defined in the 1950s, still provide the basis for the units currently being produced.

The first air abrasion system, which was offered as an alternative to a slow-speed, belt-driven handpiece, was the Airdent air abrasion unit (manufactured and sold by SS White Co., Piscataway, New Jersey, in 1951).[3] Its placement in over 20 dental schools around the country initiated postgraduate courses in air abrasion technology. By 1955, the Airdent had been adopted by over 2000 dentists in the United States alone.

The Airdent was heavy, weighing well over 100 pounds, and massive (over 4 feet high, over 2 feet deep, and about 18 inches wide). Its pressure tank contained carbon dioxide (or a number of other gases) to provide a high-viscosity gaseous propellant. In spite of its awkward size, the unit had a small, 0.018-inch (460-µm) tip and delivered a 30-µm beam of aluminum oxide particles; these particles left the tip traveling at over 1000 feet per second, which is in the realm of supersonics. All this was done with a divergent angle of only 3.5 degrees. The Airdent and other air abrasion devices became popular quickly in the 1950s, because they produced less heat and vibration than a belt-driven handpiece. At their introduction in 1950, Dr. Black stated that air abrasion systems were an adjunct and not a replacement for the dental handpiece.[2] This is still true.

In the late 1950s, the use of air abrasion devices declined after the introduction of the Borden Air Rotor, the first air turbine handpiece, even though both had valuable uses. The rapid cutting burs used in the Air Rotor and the almost universal acceptance of G.V. Black's extension-for-prevention preparations diverted dentists' interest in air abrasion devices. The technology went into a slumber for the next 50 years.

In December 1982, the Food and Drug Administration (FDA) approved the sale of a redesigned air abrasion device, giving rise to a reemergence of this technology in the dental profession (KV-1, Kreative Inc., Albany, Oregon; KCP series, American Dental Technologies, Corpus Christi, Texas; MicroPrep, Sunrise Technologies, Fremont, California). Currently available air abrasion devices are considerably more sophisticated and precise than the earlier units. New metering systems have been developed to control the flow of abrasive particles. Many units have cutting beams as narrow as 500 µm. By increasing the beam working distance, this beam can be increased to over 1 mm. The revamped technology offers a clinician considerable control of the particle beam as well as a pulsing feature that can double the efficiency of the device.

PHYSICAL PROPERTIES

The physics for air abrasion technology was made apparent in 1829 by Gaspard Coriolis with the discovery of the formula $E = 1/2 MV^2$. The particles from these devices are emitted as a well-defined, sharply focused beam.

A number of variables interact in the use of an air abrasion device, including the following:

- Particle energy, which is related to air pressure and other factors
- Beam intensity, which is related to the particle flow-rate, particle type, particle size, nozzle diameter, and nozzle design
- Beam working distance, which is determined by the operator
- Beam incident angle, which is determined by the operator
- Dwell time, or the time the device is held in one spot, which is determined by the operator

The controls on the devices usually include on/off, abrasion flow, air pressure, and choice of nozzle (usually 0.011 or 0.018 inches in diameter). The air sources are either an accessory compressor or compressed nitrogen. The aluminum oxide particles emitted are typically 25 to 29 μm in size (average, 27.5 μm). Some systems offer a wider range in particle size, spreading 20 μm or more. Air pressure is typically 40 to 100 psi (average, 70 psi). The average flow rate is 2 to 3 g per minute, and dwell time is typically 20 to 45 seconds per tooth.

CLINICAL USES

Air abrasion devices cut tooth structure, especially enamel, with a precise, rapid, and quiet beam of energy. They produce less heat, pressure, and vibration than conventional cutting tools, and result in less crazing on enamel. Patients treated with air abrasion require less anesthesia. In one survey, 90% of patients reported little or no discomfort after having teeth restored with this procedure.[4]

Disadvantages of air abrasion include (1) the dentist's loss of tactile sense, (2) large size of the unit, (3) high cost, (4) possible gingival tissue hemorrhage, and (5) noisy suction system for clearing the air of particles.

Debris removal

This technology can be used to remove debris and repair leaking margins of composite restorations. Likewise, it can be used to remove sealants to examine beneath them for suspected decay.

Diagnosis of pits and fissures

Air abrasion devices are useful in detecting pit and fissure caries.[5-7] When a darkened area is detected, one or more short bursts of particles removes the stain or organic plug, while removing only a few microns of healthy tooth structure. If the tooth is caries-free, a sealant can be placed as a preventive measure. When underlying decay is discovered, it can be removed by air abrasion. Since the dentist controls the duration (the dwell time) and range (the beam working distance) of these bursts, by holding the handpiece about an inch above the tooth, he or she can remove material in tiny increments and preserve the maximum amount of healthy tooth structure.

Treatment of pits and fissures

Air abrasion devices allow a trained dentist to cut conservative preparations in pits and fissures for placing preventive resin restorations (Figure D–1). It is possible to conservatively open pits and fissures in teeth where caries is suspected, and deepen pits and fissures with negligible widening between the walls.

Cleaning

Air abrasion can also be used to clean a tooth prior to etching if oil contamination from the handpiece is suspected (eg, from sterilization procedures).

Cementation of a crown

Internal (metal) surfaces of crowns and the tooth itself can be sandblasted immediately before cementation or re-cementation to improve adhesion.

Effect on bonding

Some laboratory studies show that the use of these devices improves bond strengths to enamel and dentin.[8] This may have no clinical significance, however, because almost all bonding agents have bond strengths higher than the cohesive strength of enamel and dentin.

CLINICAL SAFETY

Air abrasion devices cut hard tooth structure faster than soft tooth structure. That is, they cut enamel (and old composite) the fastest, then healthy dentin,

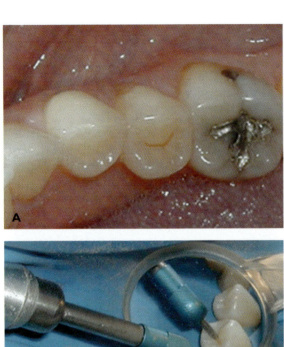
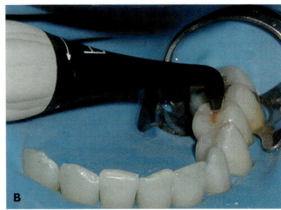
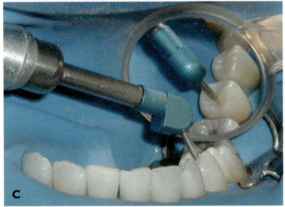
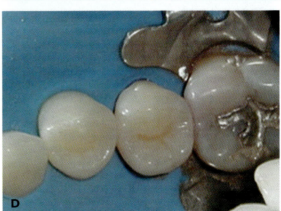
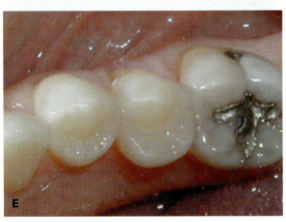

Figure D–1. *A*, Preoperative view of carious pit and fissure. *B*, Diagnosis confirmed with laser optics. *C*, Preparation cut with air abrasion. *D*, Finished preparation. *E*, Postoperative view. (Photographs courtesy of K. Kutch.)

affected dentin, infected dentin, and lastly soft tissue. In the hands of improperly trained or inexperienced dentists, air abrasion devices can be dangerous and cause significant iatrogenic destruction of tooth structure. Adequate training is important. Air abrasion devices also easily cut such hard restorative substances as porcelain, but they are less effective than burs and diamonds in removing gold or amalgam.

When an air abrasion device is used, the tip (the nozzle) should not contact the tooth. Its movement over the tooth is completely directed by what the operator sees. There is no tactile guidance. The use of magnification is a necessity, since cutting must be done with direct vision and the preparations are small. Use of a mirror while cutting is problematic because scattered particles bounce off it, turning the surface frosty and useless. Disposable mirrors have to be discarded after each use.

The clinician and assistant should wear protective eyewear (with magnification) and a face shield. It is best to isolate the working field with a rubber dam, although in some cases this is not possible (eg, for crown cementation, partially erupted teeth, etc.). The dental assistant should use high-volume evacuation to remove excess particles.

REFERENCES

1. Black RB. Airbrasive: some fundamentals. J Am Dent Assoc 1950;41:701–10.

2. Black RB. Application and reevaluation of air abrasive technique. J Am Dent Assoc 1955;50:408–14.

3. Morrison AH, Berman L. Evaluation of the Airdent unit: preliminary report. J Am Dent Assoc 1953;46:298–303.

4. Goldberg MA. Airbrasive: patient reactions. J Dent Res 1952;31:504–5.

5. Brockmann SL, Scott RL, Eick JD. The effect of an air-polishing device on tensile bond strengths of a dental sealant. Quintessence Int 1989;20:211–7.

6. Laurell K, Lord W, Beck M. Kinetic cavity preparation effects on bonding to enamel or dentin [abstract]. J Dent Res 1993;72(Spec Issue):273.

7. Burbach G. Micro-invasive cavity preparation with an air abrasive unit. GP Insider 1993;2:55–8.

8. Goldstein RE, Parkins FM. Air-abrasive technology: its new role in restorative dentistry. J Am Dent Assoc 1994;125:551–7

Index

A
A-fibers, 33
Abfraction, 34, 35f, 163f
Abrasion, 10, 10f, 35f, 178–179
Accelerators, 47–48
Acid-base reactions
  in dental materials, 1
  ionic bond formation, 14f
Acid etching. See Enamel, acid etching
Adaptic (composite resin), 111, 111f
Addent (composite resin), 111, 111f
Adherence, 13, 13f
Adhesion
  effect of wetting on, 14f
  of glass-ionomer cement, 74
Adhesive(s)
  in composites, 85
  dentin, 143
  wear, 10
Air abrasion
  clinical safety, 290–292
  clinical uses, 290
  history, 289
  as method of particle fabrication, 84
  physical properties, 289–290
Air entrapment, 73
Airdent (air abrasion unit), 289
Airosil (fumed silica), 113, 114f
Aluminosilicate polyacrylate-1, 44
Aluminum oxide, 175
Amalgam, v–vi
  in tunnel preparations, 219
  wear rate, 53f
Anorexia nervosa, 36–37
Anterior restorations. See Restorations
ASPA-1 (cement), 44
Auto Matrix, 222

B
Balance, and esthetics, 238–239, 243f
Bard Parker blades (hand instruments), 173, 175f
Barium glass, 84, 111, 112
BHT, 83
Bis-GMA, 81–82, 82f, 127–128
BiTine Ring (matrix), 222
Boeing test, 13, 13f
Bond strength, 5, 6f
Bonding
  agents
    compatibility with resins, 134
    storage, 148
    wet and dry, 145
  composite resin primers, 152
  dentin (See Dentin, bonding)
  dentin-resin, 139–142, 140f–142f
  resin-resin
    delayed, 149–152, 150f
    etching, 151, 152f
    immediate, 149, 149f, 150f
    sandblasting, 151
Bonds, 13–14, 14f, 15f
Borden Air Rotor (air abrasion unit), 289
Bowen's resin. See Bis-GMA
Brinell hardness, 9
Bruxism, 241
Bulimia, 37–38, 37f
Burs
  compared to diamonds, 170f
  use in finishing, 166–167, 166f, 167f, 169f, 176, 177f

C
C-factor, 272, 273f
C-fibers, 33
Cadurit (composite resin), 111
Camphoroquinine
  free radical formation, 88f
  role in lightening of composite resin(s), 158, 158f
Caries. See also Restorations
  detection of
    digital radiographs in, 24–25

dyes in, 28–30, 29f
electronic devices in, 30
laser fluorescence in, 30, 31f
radiographs in, 24–25
transillumination in, 25–27, 26f–27f
under existing composite, 24, 25, 27f
    incidence, 20
    occlusal, 20
    physiology, 19–20
    pit and fissure, 20
detection, 21f, 22f, 23, 290
sealing (See Sealants, pit and fissure)
treatment, 290, 291f
    proximal, 20, 24, 77f
detection, 23, 25, 26f–27f
early, 24
ranking system, 24f
role of fluoride in patterns, 22–23, 22f, 23f
root, 20
treatment, 77f
    smooth-surface, detection, 21
stages, 19f
Cementation
air entrapment prior to, 73
technique for, 73f, 75
Cement(s)
acid-base, 69, 69t
components, 44t
eugenol, 74
glass-ionomer, 43–44, 51f, 61
    clinical concerns with, 74
    hydrous, 70–71
    powder-to-liquid ratios in, 74
    schematic representation, 58f
    semihydrous, 71
    setting, 73f
    technique for using, 75
    teeth sensitivity to, 73
    wear rate, 53f

glass powder, 69
liquids, 69–70
noneugenol, 74
polyacid, 43
properties, 71, 71t
selection, 71–73
temporary, 73t, 74
zinc oxide, 69
zinc phosphate, 43
Ceramic-metal glass ionomers. See Ionomer(s), cermet
Cermets. See Ionomer(s), cermet
Cervical lesions
causes, 35f
causes of, 34–36
stress-induced, 34
Charisma (submicron hybrid composite), 119
Chemical erosion, 35–36
Chipping
composites, 116f, 180, 180f
veneers, 265–266, 268f
Chlorhexidine, 34
Class I, II, III, IV, V restorations. See Restorations
Coatings, surface, 176–178
Cohesive forces, 13
Cohesive fracture, 180, 180f
Colloidal silica, 113
Color modifiers
in composites, 119
in veneers (See Veneers, color modifiers)
Color shifts
of composites, 158, 158f
in detection of caries, 21
Color stability
of glass ionomers, 65
of initiator compounds in res in systems, 88
Command Ultrafine (micron hybrid composite), 119
Compo-strips (finishing strips), 173

Compoglass (compomer), 60
Compomers, 59–60
Composite fillers. See Filler(s), composite
Composite resin(s). See also Veneers
abrasion, 178–179
autocured, 3f
blended, 117
caries beneath existing, 24, 25, 27f
chipping, 180, 180f
classification, 111–119
cohesive fracture, 180, 180f
color modifiers, 119
color shifts, 158, 158f, 181
compared to glass ionomers, 63f
contouring, 161–162
contraction gaps, 177–178, 179f
curing techniques for, 89–93, 90f
effect of filler loading on, 85, 85f
erosion, 179
factors affecting light curing, 95–99
filler types in, 111–112, 112t
finishing, 162–163, 163f
    burs, 167, 176
    cups and wheels, 169–170, 173f, 176
    diamonds, 167, 170f, 176
    discs, 168–169, 168t, 171f, 172f, 176
    hand instruments, 173, 175f, 176
    instrumentation, 166–167
    rotational abrasive techniques, 166
    stones, 167
    strips, 170–174, 174f
    surface coatings, 176–178
flowable, 123–124
fluoride-containing, 60–61

handling, 124
heavy filled hybrid, 118–119, 119f
hybrid, 117–118, 118f
ionomer-modified, 60–61, 63f
layering, 162
light-cured, 4f, 95–96, 95f, 97f, 98f, 162
light curing systems for, 89, 99–100
longevity, 119–120
macrofilled, 112–113, 113f, 114f
maintenance, 178–181
matrices for, 159–161, 160f
microfilled, 114f
   condensed, 116
   failure, 116f, 117f
   polishing, 116f
   problems with, 114–115
   steps in manufacture, 115f
micron hybrid, 118
minifilled hybrid, 118, 118f
mixing, 159
opaquers, 119
packable, 123
pits, 180
placement instruments, 161, 161f
polishing, 113f
   cups and wheels, 169–170, 173f
   methods, 165–167, 175
   pastes, 175
   polymerization lightening, 158, 158f
   relation of filler and resin, 111t, 115t
   relation of filler size to filler loading, 112t
   relation of filler size to surface smoothness, 165f
   restorations using (See Restorations)
selection, 120–123
shade selection, 157, 159f
small-particle hybrid, 118, 176
submicron hybrid, 118
surface smoothness, 162–165, 165f
syringes, 159
wear, 178–179
   patterns, 164f
   rate, 53f
white line margins, 90f, 179–180, 179f
Conditioners, dentin. See Dentin, conditioners
Configuration factor (C-factor), 272, 273f
Contact angle, 13, 14f
Contouring, prepolymerization, 161–162
Conversion rate, in polymerization, 87
Conversions, units of measure, 15–16
Copolymer(s)
   cross-linking, 3f
   in glass-ionomer liquids, 47, 48f
   linear, 2f
Coupling agents, 85
Coupling phase, 111
Covalent bonds, 13, 15f
Cross-linking, 3f
Crown forms, 161
Curing. See also Light curing
   of composite resin(s), 89–93, 90f
   energy measurement in, 93–94
   high-energy pulse, 91f, 92
   pulse-delay, 93, 93f
   ramp, 91f, 92
   step, 91, 91f
   uniform continuous, 91, 91f
Curing lights, ocular hazards, 106–108
Curing systems, 89
Curing tips, 104
Curing units, 99–100
Cyclic fatigue, 8, 8f
Cyclic loading, 7, 7f

D

Dental esthetics. See Esthetics
Dental insurance, vi
   for veneer placement, 244
Dentin
   A-fibers, 33
   adhesives, 143, 144–145
   bonding
      effect of blood, 148
      effect on pulp, 138
      failure, 147–148
      one-component systems, 143, 146, 147f
      stability, 139
      steps, 145–146
      two-component systems, 146
      wet and dry, 145
   C-fibers, 33
   caries, 19–20
   composition, 135
   conditioners, 75, 140f, 142–143, 144, 144f
   etchants, 142–143
   histology, 32, 135–138, 136f, 138f
   effect of age, 137–138
   hypersensitivity, 32f, 33–34
   primers, 143, 144
   smear layer, 137, 137f
   thickness, 74
Dentin-resin bonding. See Bonding, dentin-resin
Dessication
   and glass ionomers, 51
   as pain stimulus of dentin, 33
DIAGNOdent (device), 30–31, 31f
Diamond Strips (finishing strips), 173, 174f

Diamond(s)
    instruments, 280f
    use in finishing, 167, 168f, 170f, 176
    compared to burs, 170f
Diastema closure
    proximal restorations, 255–256, 255f–257f
    restorative technique, 257–260, 258f, 259f
DIFOTI (device), 26–27, 27f
Digital radiographs, 24–25
Dimension Three (magnifiers), 283
Discoloration
    in resin systems, 88
    tooth (See Tooth discoloration)
Discs, finishing, 168–169, 168t, 172f, 178f
Dispersed phase, 111
Durelon (cement), 43
Dyes, in detection of caries, 27–30, 29f
Dytract (compomer), 60

E
EAS. See Energy application sequence
ED. See Energy density
EDMA, 83
Elastic modulus. See Stiffness
Electronic caries monitor (ECM), 30, 30f
Embrasure form, 239f
    and esthetics, 237, 238f
Enamel
    acid etching
        acid strength, 128
        in Class III restorations, 185
        in Class IV restorations, 189–190
        clinical procedure, 134–135
        contamination, 130–131
        drying, 130, 135f
        histologic effects, 128–129, 128f, 129f
        history, 127–128
        leakage following, 128f
        materials, 131
        in placement of veneers, 250
        in preventive resin restorations, 212, 214f
        remineralization following, 131–132
        times, 129
        washing times, 130
    bonding resins, intermediate, 133–134
    caries in, 19
    coarse finishing, 133
    composition, 135
    discing, 132
    histology, 127, 128f
    margin design, 132–133, 132f
    preparation angles, 132–133
    resin penetration, 130f
Energy application sequence (EAS), 90f, 95–96, 272
Energy density (ED), 95, 271
Energy density for optimal polymerization (EOP), 95, 272
Enhance (polishing cups and points), 170, 176
EOP. See Energy density for optimal polymerization
Erosion, 10, 10f, 35f
    as method of particle fabrication, 85
Esthetics
    and balance, 238–239, 243f
    and embrasure form, 237, 238f, 239f
    and front to back progression, 238
    and light reflection, 238
    optical principles, 237–239
    and tooth form, 238, 240f–242f
Ethyleneglycol dimethacrylate. See EDMA

Eugenol, 69
Eye protection, 108

F
Fatigue, 6
    cyclic, 8, 8f
    fracture, 115
    wear, 10
Filler(s)
    composite
        methods of particle fabrication, 84
        properties, 83–84
        relative sizes, 165f
        use of glass in, 112, 112f
        wear process in, 113f
            loading, 85, 85f
            resin
                interface with matrix, 114–115
            prepolymerized, 114
            volume, 123
Fini Finishing and Polishing Discs, 171f
Finishing
    composite
        instrumentation, 166–167, 173, 175f, 176
        materials, 167–175
        surface coatings, 176–178
        techniques, 176, 177f, 178f, 186–188, 193–194, 202, 224–230
    glass ionomers, 66
Fissure caries. See Caries, pit and fissure
Flexidiscs (finishing discs), 168–169, 171f
Flexistrips (finishing strips), 173
Flowable composites. See under Composite resin(s)
Fluoride
    affect on caries patterns, 22–23, 22f, 23f
    movement cycle, in glass-ionomer cements, 54f
    release, 11–12, 62–63

in treatment of dentin hyper sensitivity, 33
Force, units of, 16
Fracture(s)
Class IV, 190f
glass ionomer restoration, 75f
in macrofilled composites, 120
with posterior composite restorations, 204, 204f
toughness, 8–9, 9f
of heavy filled hybrid composites, 119
Free radicals, in initiation of polymerization, 86, 86f, 87t, 88f
Front to back progression, 238
Fuji Duet (resin-modified glass ionomer), 5
Fuji II LC (resin-modified glass ionomer), 62
fluoride release from, 65
Fuji Lining LC (resin-modified glass ionomer), 62
Full width at half maximum (FWHM), 271
Fumed silica, 113
FWHM. See Full width at half maximum

G

Galilean loupes (magnifiers), 283–284, 288f
GC International Metal Strips (finishing strips), 173, 174f
GIC. See Cement(s), glass-ionomer
Gingiva, and veneers, 264–265, 267f
Glass, heavy-metal, 84
Glass ionomer(s). See also Resin-modified glass ionomer(s)
accelerators in, 47–48
bases, 46
cements (See Cement(s), glass-ionomer)
ceramic-metal (See Ionomer(s), cermet)
classification, 46
compared to composite resins, 62–63, 63f, 64–66
dehydration and rehydration, 163, 163f
finishing, 66
fluoride released from, 53, 62
fracture, 75f, 77f–79f, 183–184, 213
liners, 46
liquid, 47, 47f
phases in setting, 49–50, 52f
powder, 48, 50f
properties, 51–53, 51f
recharging, 53
restorations using, 75–80
Glass powder cement, 69. See also Cement(s)
Glazes, surface, 178
Glutaraldehyde, 34
Greenough loupes (magnifiers), 283, 287f
Guides, light, 102–103, 103f, 104

H

Hand oscillation techniques, 166
Handpiece-driven oscillation techniques, 166, 166f
Hardness, surface, 9, 10f
Heat curing, of resins, 88, 99
HEMA. See Hydroxyethyl methacrylate
Herculite (submicron hybrid composite), 118
High-energy pulse cure, 91f, 92. See also Curing
Hydroxyethyl methacrylate (HEMA)
in dentin primer, 139
in resin-modified glass ionomers, 46, 61–62
Hytac (compomer), 60

I

Instruments
for restorations, 276t–278t, 279f–281f
sterilization, 280f
Ionic bonds, 13, 14f
Ionomer-modified composite resins. See Composite resin(s)
Ionomer(s)
cermet, 45, 46
wear rate, 53f
glass (See Glass ionomer(s); Resin-modified glass ionomer(s))
glass-metal, 44
resin (See Resin(s), ionomer(s))

K

Keplerian loupes (magnifiers), 283, 286f
Ketac-fil (cement), 44
Ketac-Silver (cermet), 45
Knoop hardness, 9

L

Lamps
curing, 101–103
laser, 101
light-emitting diode (LED), 101–102
spectral overlap, 94f
Laser fluorescence, in detection of caries, 30, 32f
Length, units of, 16
Lesions, cervical, 34–36, 35f
Light
intensity
as cause of color shifts in composites, 158
in light curing of composites, 96, 96f–98f
reflection, 238, 250f
Light-activated systems

ultraviolet, 89
visible, 89
Light curing. See also Curing
  factors affecting, 95–99
  guides for, 102–103, 102f, 103f, 104
  units
    heat generation by, 102
    selection and maintenance, 103–104
Luting cements, 46

M

Magnification, 283, 284f, 288f
Magnifiers
  multilens, 283–285, 285f
  selection, 285–287
  single-lens, 283, 285f
Mandrels, 168
Master shade guide systems, 157
Matrices, for composite restorations, 159–161, 160f, 222, 222f
Matrix, resin, 81, 111
Mercury, v–vi
Metallic bonds, 13, 15f
Metals, stress-strain curves, 9f
Methacrylates, 2
Micro-Fill Composite Finishing Discs, 168
Micron hybrids, 118
Mill grinding, 84
Minifilled hybrid composites, 118
Mitra (company), 45
Modulus of elasticity. See Stiffness
Monomers, 2
Moore discs (finishing discs), 171f
Moore's mandrels, 168
Moyco Metal Strips (finishing strips), 173
Moyco Plastic Strips (finishing strips), 173
Multifill (blended composite), 116

N

National Institute of Dental Research, 20
Nuva-System (light-activated system), 89, 128

O

Occlusal caries, 20. See also Caries
Occlusal wear, 53f
Oil
  effect on acid etching, 131
  effect on dentin bonding, 147
Opaquers, 119
OptiBond System, 143
Optical principles, 237, 237f, 238f
  applied to esthetics, 237–239
Oscillation techniques, 166, 166f
Oxygen
  effect on acid etching, 131
  effect on light curing of resin, 98
  role in resin polymerization, 88

P

Packable composites. See Composite resin(s)
Particle fabrication, 84–85
Particulate reinforcement, 117
Patient management, 242–243
PD. See Power density
PE. See Pulse energy
Peel
  energy, 13, 13f
  strength, 12, 12f
  vs. tensile, 12f
Phosphoric acid, 70
Photac-Fil (resin-modified glass ionomer), 65
Photoinitiator, 99
Pit caries. See Caries, pit and fissure
Pits, composite resins, 180

Plasma arc lamp, for light curing of composite resins, 101
Point 4 (submicron hybrid composite), 119
Polish, acquired vs. inherent, 162–165
Polishing methods. See under Composite resin(s)
Polyacid cements, 43
Polyacid-modified resin composites. See Compomers
Polyacrylic acid, 70
Polycarboxylate cement, 43
Polymerization
  dental terms for, 94–95
  initiation systems for, 87–88
  initiators, 86–87, 111
  lightening during, 158, 158f
  rate, 87–88
  reactions, 1–2
  resin, 83
  of resin-modified glass ionomer(s), 57–58
  shrinkage
    of Class V composite restorations, 200f, 201f
    of microfilled composites, 115
  patterns, 2–3, 3f, 4f
    of posterior composites, 204f
Polymer(s)
  branched, 81
  cross-linked, 3f, 81
  definition, 2
  dental, history, 81
  linear, 2f, 81
Pop-on mandrels, 168
Porcelains, stress-strain curves, 9f
Posterior restorations. See Restorations
Potassium nitrate, 33
Potassium oxalate, 33
Powder-to-liquid ratios, 74

Power density (PD)
  definition, 94–95, 95–96, 271
  in light curing of composite resins, 95, 96f, 97f
Power range (PR), 271
PR. See Power range
Practice building, 244
Precipitation reactions, 2–3, 4f
Primary bonds, 13, 14f, 15f
Primers
  dentin (See Dentin, primers)
  in treatment of dentin hypersensitivity, 34
Profin (handpiece attachment device), 166f
Proximal caries. See Caries, proximal; Restorations, proximal
Pulse-delay cure, 93, 93f. See also Curing
Pulse energy (PE), 273

Q
Quartz
  in micron hybrid composites, 118
  use as composite filler, 84
  use in macrofilled composites, 111

R
Radiographs, 24–25
Radiometers, 105
Radiopacity
  elements used to increase, 84
  in selection of composite, 122
Ramp cure, 91f, 92. See also Curing
Remineralization, 131–132, 131f
Resin-modified glass ionomer(s). See also Glass ionomer(s); Resin(s), ionomer(s)
  chemistry, 62
  compared to glass ionomers, 62–63, 63f, 64–66
  definition, 61
  dual-cured, 58
  finishing, 66
  history, 61–62
  photocured, 58
  polymerization, 57–58
  schematic representation, 58f, 59f
  setting reaction sequence, 59f
  types, 45–46
  wear rate, 53f
Resin-resin bonding. See Bonding, resin-resin
Resin(s)
  bonding, 133–134
  Bowen's, 82f (See also Bis-GMA)
  chemical composition, 81–82
  color stability, 88
  compatibility with bonding agents, 134
  composite (See Composite resin(s))
  control of viscosity, 83
  heat curing, 88
  ionomer(s) (See also Glass ionomer(s); Resin-modified glass ionomer(s))
    clinical uses, 64–66
    coefficient of thermal expansion, 65
    color stability, 65
    fluoride release, 63–64, 65
    properties, 64–66
    restorations using, 75–80, 76f, 77f
    shear bond strength, 64
    volume stability, 65
  matrix, composition, 81
  penetration, 130f
  polyacid-modified (See Compomers)
  polymerization (See Polymerization, resin)
  polymerizing, 81
  stress-strain curves, 9f
  in treatment of dentin hypersensitivity, 34
Restorations
  anterior, 121–122, 183
  Class I, 209–212, 211f, 212f
    adhesive enamel exit, 213f
    preparation, 212f, 213f
    procedure, 212–213
  Class II, 219
    composite placement, 222–224, 229f
    equipment, 219–220, 221f, 222f
    finishing, 224–230
    preparation, 220–222, 223f–230f
    sequence, 224–228f, 231–232f
    wedging, 233f
  Class III
    completed, 188f, 189f
    composite placement, 185–186, 187f, 188f
    finishing and polishing, 186–188
    preparation
      angle of approach, 185
      dentin-enamel, 186f
      dentin-involved, 184–185, 185f, 187f
      enamel-only, 184
      intra-enamel, 184f
    selection of material for, 121
    use of glass ionomer, 183–184
    use of proximal strip, 188f
  Class IV
    composite placement, 190–192
    finishing, 193–194
    following earlier restorations, 196–197f
    fractures, 190f
    margins, 190f, 191f
    preparation, 189–190
    beveled, 190f, 193f, 194f
    Chamfer, 190f–192f

dentin involved, 195f
selection of material for, 122, 188–189
Class V
  composite placement, 200–202, 200f
  contraction gap, 200f, 201f
  finishing and polishing, 202
  preparation
  dentin involved, 197–199, 199f, 201f
  enamel only, 197, 198f
  selection of material for, 121–123, 194, 197
    glass ionomer, 75–80, 77f–79f
    indirect resin, 152–153
    posterior
      advantages, 203
      disadvantages, 203–204
      longevity, 205
      polymerization shrinkage, 204, 204f
      proximal, 77f
      recommended instruments, 276t–278t, 279f–281f
      resin ionomer, 75–80, 76f, 77f
      sealants (See Sealants, pit and fissure)
      selection of material for, 122–123
      sensitivity following, 204–205
  slot, 213, 215f, 217f
  tunnel
    amalgam in, 216–219
    closed-bite filling technique, 219
    equipment, 215–216
    indications, 215–216
    preparation, 213–215, 218f
    procedure, 216–219, 216f
    use of periodontal probe in, 216, 218f, 219f
    universal tray setup, 275–281
Restoratives, glass ionomer, 46
Rockwell hardness, 9
Root caries. See Caries
Rotary instruments, 166–167
Roughness, 10–11, 11f

S

Saliva
  effect on acid etching, 130, 131f
  effect on dentin bonding, 148
SE. See Spectral emission; Spectral emission (SE) for photopolymerization
Sealants
  glass-ionomer, 46
  pit and fissure, 22, 22f
    caries under, 206
    long-term effectiveness, 205
    loosening, 207f
    materials, 207–208
    preparation and placement, 206
    procedure, 206f, 208–209, 209–211f
    repairs, 206–207
Secondary bonds, 13–14, 15f
Sensitivity, of teeth
  classification, 71–72
  with posterior composite restorations, 204–205
  testing, 71–72, 72f, 72t
Setting reaction sequence, 59f
Shade selection, 157, 159f
Shear bond test, 6f
Silica
  agglomerated submicron, 84
  in microfillers, 113
Silver cermets, 45. See also Ionomer(s), cermet
Silver nitrate, 33
Slot restorations. See Restorations, slot
Small-particle hybrid composites, 118
Smear layer, 137, 137f
Smoothness, 10–11
Sof-Lex Discs (finishing discs), 168, 171f
Sof-Lex Strips (finishing strips), 173, 174f
Sof-Lex XT Discs (finishing discs), 169, 171f
Spectral emission (SE) for photopolymerization, 94, 271
Spectral overlap
  lamps, 94f
  in light curing of resins, 93
Spectral requirements (SR) for photopolymerization, 94, 271
SR. See Spectral requirements; Spectral requirements (SR) for photopolymerization
Steady loading, 7
Step cure, 91, 91f. See also Curing
Stiffness, 5–6, 6f
  of microfilled composites, 115
  relation to filler loading, 85f
Stones, in composite finishing, 167
Strain, 6, 6f
Strength
  bond, 5, 6f, 136f
  compressive, 3–4, 4f
  diametrical tensile, 4
  peel, 12, 12f
  shear, 4–5, 5f
    of resin ionomers, 63
  tensile, 4, 5f
  of composites, 115, 136f
  of crown buildup materials, 53f
Stress, 6, 6f
  corrosion, treatment, 34
  units of, 16
Stress-strain curves, 9f
Strips, finishing, 170–174, 174f
Strontium, 112
Strontium chloride, 33
STT. See Surface transition time

Super-Snap Discs (finishing discs), 169, 171f
Surface
 coatings, 176–178
 glazes, 178
 hardness, 9, 10f
Surface transition time, 164–165
Surgical Loops (magnifiers), 283
Surgitel (magnifiers), 283
Synergy (submicron hybrid composite), 119
Syringe, composite, 159

T
Tartaric acid, 48, 48f
TEDMA. See TEGDMA
TEGDMA
 chemical structure, 83, 83f
 mixed with Bis-GMA, 82
 use in viscosity control, 82
TEGMA. See TEGDMA
Teledyne Proflex Scaler (finishing strips), 173
Temperature
 in light curing of composite resins, 97
 as pain stimulus of dentin, 33
 units of, 16
Tensile
 strength, 4, 5f
 vs. peel, 12f
Thermal expansion
 coefficient of, 11, 11f
 resin ionomers, 63
 of microfilled composites, 115
Tooth discoloration, and use of veneers, 240–241, 247–248, 251f, 252–255, 252f
Tooth form, and esthetics, 238, 240f–242f
Tooth-form templates, for veneers, 245

Tooth position, and veneers, 261–264, 261f–267f
Tooth sensitivity, classification, 71–72, 72f, 72t
Transillumination
 in detection of caries, 25–27, 26–27f
 devices, 25
 digital, 26
Trial buildups, 245–246, 246f
Triethylene glycol dimethacrylate. See TEGDMA
Tungsten carbide carvers (hand instruments), 173, 175f
Tungsten-halogen lamp, for light curing of composite resins, 101
Tunnel restorations. See Restorations, tunnel
Turbo (light guide), 103, 103f

U
UDM (urethane dimethacrylate)
 advantages and disadvantages, 82, 82f
 use in viscosity control, 82, 82f
Ultrasonic interaction, 84–85
Uniform continuous cure, 91, 91f. See also Curing
Units of measure, 15–16
Universal tray setup, 275–281
Urethane dimethacrylate. See UDM

V
Valux (blended composite), 117
Veneers
 chipping, 265–266, 268f
 color modifiers, 247, 248f, 253, 254f
 in correction of malposed teeth, 261–264, 261f–267f
 dental-enamel preparation, 252–255, 252f
 and dental insurance, 244

 diagnostic considerations, 239–241
 diagnostic models, 244–245
 diastema closure, 255–260, 255f–259f
 direct, 239
 and discolored teeth, 240–241, 247–248, 251f, 252–255, 252f
 equipment and materials, 248–249
 esthetic contouring, 247
 extra-enamel preparation, 243f
 failure, 264–267
 fee structure, 243–244
 finishing and polishing, 252
 indirect, 239
 intra-enamel preparation, 244f, 249–250, 249f
 layer separation, 267, 269f
 maintenance and repairs, 267–268, 269f
 marginal breakdown, 265–267, 267f, 269f
 patient management, 242–243
 periodontal involvement, 264–265, 267f
 pitting, 266, 268f
 placement, 246–247, 250–252, 254–255, 254f
 and practice building, 244
 shade records, 241–242
 tooth-form templates, 245
 treatment planning, 244
 trial buildups, 245–246, 246f
Vickers hardness, 9
Viscosity, 83
Vita Lumin system (master shade guide), 157
Vitalescence (submicron hybrid composite), 119
Vitapan system (master shade guide), 157

Vitrebond Liner/Base (resin-modified glass ionomer), 61
Vitrebond (resin-modified glass ionomer), 45, 62
Vitremer (resin-modified glass ionomer), 65
Vivadent polishing cups and wheels, 170
Vivadent Polishing Discs (finishing discs), 169
Vivadent Strips (finishing strips), 173

W

Water sorption, 11, 12f
　of microfilled composites, 115
Wear, 10, 10f
　occlusal, 53f
　patterns, 164f
　prevention, 34
　rates, 53f
Wedge test, 13, 13f
Wedging, in posterior composite restorations, 230, 233f
Wetting, effect on adhesion, 14f
White line margins, composites, 90f, 179–180, 179f

Y

Young's modulus. See Stiffness

Z

Zinc oxide cement, 69. See also Cement(s)
Zinc phosphate cement, 43. See also Cement(s)
Zirconium fillers, 84
ZOE. See Zinc oxide cement